Equine Sports Medicine

Editor

JOSÉ M. GARCÍA-LÓPEZ

VETERINARY CLINICS OF NORTH AMERICA: EQUINE PRACTICE

www.vetequine.theclinics.com

Consulting Editor
THOMAS J. DIVERS

August 2018 • Volume 34 • Number 2

ELSEVIER

1600 John F. Kennedy Boulevard ● Suite 1800 ● Philadelphia, Pennsylvania, 19103-2899

http://www.vetequine.theclinics.com

VETERINARY CLINICS OF NORTH AMERICA: EQUINE PRACTICE Volume 34, Number 2
August 2018 ISSN 0749-0739, ISBN-13: 978-0-323-61355-2

Editor: Colleen Dietzler
Developmental Editor: Donald Mumford

Veterinary Clinics of North America: Equine Practice (ISSN 0749-0739) is published in April, August, and December by Elsevier Inc., 360 Park Avenue South, New York, NY 10010-1710. Business and Editorial Offices: 1600 John F. Kennedy Blvd., Suite 1800, Philadelphia, PA 19103-2899. Subscription prices are $281.00 per year (domestic individuals), $536.00 per year (domestic institutions), $100.00 per year (domestic students/residents), $328.00 per year (Canadian individuals), $675.00 per year (Canadian institutions), $365.00 per year (international individuals), $675.00 per year (international institutions), and $180.00 per year (international and Canadian students/residents). To receive student/resident rate, orders must be accompanied by name of affiliated institution, date of term, and the signature of program/residency coordinator on institution letterhead. Orders will be billed at individual rate until proof of status is received. Foreign air speed delivery is included in all *Clinics* subscription prices. All prices are subject to change without notice. **POSTMASTER:** Send address changes to *Veterinary Clinics of North America: Equine Practice*, 3251 Riverport Lane, Maryland Heights, MO 63043. Customer Service (orders, claims, online, change of address): Elsevier Health Sciences Division, Subscription **Customer Service, 3251 Riverport Lane, Maryland Heights, MO 63043. Tel: 1-800-654-2452 (U.S. and Canada); 314-447-8871 (outside U.S. and Canada). Fax: 314-447-8029. E-mail: journalscustomerservice-usa@elsevier.com (for print support);** E-mail: **journalsonlinesupport-usa@elsevier.com (for online support).**

Reprints. For copies of 100 or more of articles in this publication, please contact the Commercial Reprints Department, Elsevier Inc., 360 Park Avenue South, New York, NY 10010-1710. Tel.: 212-633-3874; Fax: 212-633-3820; E-mail: reprints@elsevier.com.

Veterinary Clinics of North America: Equine Practice is covered in *MEDLINE/PubMed (Index Medicus), Excerpta Medica, Current Contents/Agriculture, Biology and Environmental Sciences, and ISI.*

Contributors

CONSULTING EDITOR

THOMAS J. DIVERS, DVM
Diplomate, American College of Veterinary Internal Medicine; Diplomate, American College of Veterinary Emergency and Critical Care; Steffen Professor of Veterinary Medicine, Section of Large Animal Medicine, College of Veterinary Medicine, Cornell University, Ithaca, New York

EDITOR

JOSÉ M. GARCÍA-LÓPEZ, VMD
Diplomate, American College of Veterinary Surgeons; Diplomate, American College of Veterinary Sports Medicine and Rehabilitation; Director of Equine Sports Medicine, Associate Professor of Large Animal Surgery, Department of Clinical Sciences, Cummings School of Veterinary Medicine at Tufts University, North Grafton, Massachusetts

AUTHORS

STACIE AARSVOLD, DVM
Diplomate, American College of Veterinary Radiology; Puchalski Equine Diagnostic Imaging, Petaluma, California

DANIELA BEDENICE, DrMedVet
Diplomate, American College of Veterinary Internal Medicine (Large Animal); Diplomate, American College of Veterinary Emergency and Critical Care (Equine); Associate Professor, Department of Clinical Sciences, Cummings School of Veterinary Medicine at Tufts University, North Grafton, Massachusetts

RAUL J. BRAS, DVM, CJF, APF
Podiatry Department, Rood and Riddle Equine Hospital, Lexington, Kentucky

KIRSTIN A. BUBECK, DrMedVet
Diplomate, American College of Veterinary Surgeons-Large Animal; Diplomate, American College of Veterinary Sports Medicine and Rehabilitation (Equine); Clinical Assistant Professor for Equine Sports Medicine and Surgery, Department of Clinical Sciences, Cummings School of Veterinary Medicine at Tufts University, North Grafton, Massachusetts

KATHERINE B. CHOPE, VMD
Diplomate, American College of Veterinary Sports Medicine and Rehabilitation; Clinical Assistant Professor, Department of Clinical Sciences, Cummings School of Veterinary Medicine at Tufts University, North Grafton, Massachusetts

ERIN K. CONTINO, MS, DVM
Diplomate, American College of Veterinary Sports Medicine and Rehabilitation; Assistant Professor, Equine Sports Medicine and Rehabilitation, Department of Clinical Sciences, Equine Orthopaedic Research Center, Colorado State University, Fort Collins, Colorado

ELIZABETH J. DAVIDSON, DVM
Diplomate, American College of Veterinary Surgeons; Diplomate, American College of Veterinary Sports Medicine and Rehabilitation; Associate Professor in Sports Medicine, New Bolton Center, University of Pennsylvania, Kennett Square, Pennsylvania

NICHOLAS FRANK, DVM, PhD
Diplomate, American College of Veterinary Internal Medicine; Associate Dean for Academic Affairs and Professor, Department of Clinical Sciences, Cummings School of Veterinary Medicine at Tufts University, North Grafton, Massachusetts

JOSÉ M. GARCÍA-LÓPEZ, VMD
Diplomate, American College of Veterinary Surgeons; Diplomate, American College of Veterinary Sports Medicine and Rehabilitation; Director of Equine Sports Medicine, Associate Professor of Large Animal Surgery, Department of Clinical Sciences, Cummings School of Veterinary Medicine at Tufts University, North Grafton, Massachusetts

KEVIN K. HAUSSLER, DVM, DC, PhD
Diplomate, American College of Veterinary Sports Medicine and Rehabilitation; Associate Professor, Department of Clinical Sciences, Equine Orthopaedic Research Center, College of Veterinary Medicine and Biomedical Sciences, Colorado State University, Fort Collins, Colorado

AMY L. JOHNSON, BA, DVM
Diplomate, American College of Veterinary Internal Medicine (Large Animal and Neurology); Assistant Professor, Department of Clinical Studies, University of Pennsylvania, School of Veterinary Medicine, New Bolton Center, Kennett Square, Pennsylvania

MELISSA R. MAZAN, DVM
Diplomate, American College of Veterinary Internal Medicine; Professor, Department of Clinical Sciences, Cummings School of Veterinary Medicine at Tufts University, North Grafton, Massachusetts

KYLA F. ORTVED, DVM, PhD
Diplomate, American College of Veterinary Surgeons; Diplomate, American College of Veterinary Sports Medicine and Rehabilitation; Assistant Professor of Large Animal Surgery, Department of Clinical Studies, New Bolton Center, University of Pennsylvania, Kennett Square, Pennsylvania

ERIC J. PARENTE, DVM
Diplomate, American College of Veterinary Surgeons; Professor of Surgery, Department of Clinical Studies, New Bolton Center, University of Pennsylvania, Kennett Square, Pennsylvania

RIC REDDEN, DVM
Independent practitioner, Versailles, Kentucky

ERIC LOCKWOOD SWINEBROAD, DVM
Diplomate, American College of Veterinary Internal Medicine; Newmarket-Indialantic Equine, Newmarket, New Hampshire

STEPHANIE J. VALBERG, DVM, PhD
Diplomate, American College of Veterinary Internal Medicine; Diplomate, American College of Veterinary Sports Medicine and Rehabilitation; Department of Large Animal Clinical Sciences, Michigan State University, McPhail Equine Performance Center, East Lansing, Michigan

KATHRYN B. WULSTER, VMD
Diplomate, American College of Veterinary Radiology; Clinical Assistant Professor, Diagnostic Imaging, Department of Clinical Studies, New Bolton Center, School of Veterinary Medicine, University of Pennsylvania, Kennett Square, Pennsylvania

Contents

Lameness examination is commonly performed in the athletic horse. A skilled lameness diagnostician must have keen clinical and observational skills. Evaluation starts with a detailed history and thorough physical examination. Next, gait evaluation in the moving horse is performed. Lame horses have asymmetric body movement due to unconscious shift of body weight. Recognition of the resultant head nod and pelvic hike is the basis for lameness diagnosis. Detection of lameness is enhanced by circling, limb flexions, and riding. Most lame horses do not exhibit pathognomonic gait characteristics, and therefore, diagnostic analgesia is the best way to authenticate underlying sites of pain.

This article discusses the basis of image formation of radiography, scintigraphy, PET, computed tomography (fan beam and cone beam), and magnetic resonance as it relates to imaging of musculoskeletal injury in the sport horse. The benefits and drawbacks of each modality are discussed with particular emphasis on sensitivity, specificity, and accuracy of identification of subchondral bone injury. Examples of straightforward as well as confounding lesions are provided, emphasizing the need for appropriate clinical workup and diagnostic analgesia, where appropriate.

For successful diagnosis of soft tissue injuries in the sport horse, localizing the area of injury during clinical and lameness evaluation will be followed in most cases by an ultrasonographic examination. With MRI more available in equine veterinary clinics, this modality can allow for a complete evaluation of soft tissue and osseous structures and is especially useful for the evaluation of structures within the hoot capsule. This article discusses special ultrasonographic techniques, an overview of MRI image generation, and the use of contrast computed tomography for the diagnosis of soft tissue injuries.

Pain localized to the neck, back, and/or pelvis can result in a profound effect on the horse's performance. These conditions can present with a varied and nonspecific set of clinical signs. A careful and thorough examination of these areas by means of physical examination, lameness evaluation both in hand and under saddle, diagnostic anesthesia, and the use of multiple imaging modalities in combination is often necessary to have an accurate prognosis. Medical and surgical management where appropriate of the conditions highlighted in this article are discussed as well as their individual prognosis.

Optimal function of skeletal muscle is essential for successful athletic performance. Even minor derangements in locomotor muscle function will affect power output, coordination, stamina, and desire to work during exercise. In this article, the presenting clinical signs, differential diagnoses, approach to diagnostic testing and treatment of muscle atrophy and weakness, focal muscle strain, and exertional myopathies are discussed. Exertional myopathies include polysaccharide storage myopathies, recurrent exertional rhabdomyolysis, malignant hyperthermia, and myofibrillar myopathy.

EPM, CVSM, and EDM are currently recognized as the 3 most common neurologic diseases in US horses, with the latter 2 conditions being most prevalent in young animals. Moreover, horses competing at shows and performance events are at greater risk for exposure to highly contagious, neurologic EHV-1 outbreaks. A clinical diagnosis of any neurologic disease should be based on a careful history, complete neurologic examination, and appropriate diagnostic testing and interpretation. However, mild or early neurologic signs can often mimic or be mistaken for an orthopedic condition when horses present for performance-related concerns.

Equine athletes are affected by 2 major endocrine/metabolic disorders, insulin dysregulation (ID) and pituitary pars intermedia dysfunction. ID is a risk factor for laminitis in horses, which poses the greatest threat to performance because of the damage that it causes to hoof structures. This article includes an in-depth discussion of ID and other risk factors for laminitis that are grouped together as equine metabolic syndrome. As horses age, the risk of pituitary pars intermedia dysfunction increases, and this endocrine disorder may exacerbate preexisting ID and further increase the risk of laminitis.

Given the variable clinical signs attributed to *Borrelia burgdorferi*, including infectious arthritis, neurologic disease, and behavioral changes, *B burgdorferi* is an important differential for decreased performance in sport horses. The primary vectors (*Ixodes* tick species) are expanding their

range, and thus *Borrelia* species are located in a wider area, making exposure more likely. Owing to regionally high seroprevalence and vague clinical signs, diagnosis of Lyme disease in the horse is believed
overestimated. Antibiotics are first-line treatment of confirmed Lyme disease. A single positive serologic test, by itself, is not conformation of
Lyme disease but is evidence of current or past infection.

the 2 highly respected professions each contributing to the task at hand but neither formally educated and trained as collaborative team members with a common thread of podiatry principles.

Katherine B. Chope

Cardiac murmurs are not uncommonly detected in the equine athlete. Although most are benign in nature, differentiation and quantification of murmurs due to valvular regurgitation are important for prognosis and recommendations. Arrhythmias can be associated with structural disease or occur independently and may range in severity from minimal clinical effect to poor performance to presenting a safety risk to rider and horse. This article discusses commonly encountered cardiac conditions in the sport horse. Physical examination, diagnostic approach, valvular disease, and arrhythmias with an impact on performance or ridden safety are discussed.

Eric J. Parente

Many abnormalities of the upper airway that can inhibit performance are determined on a critical resting endoscopic evaluation. Some dynamic abnormalities can be seen only during an exercising endoscopic evaluation, which should be performed whenever the history of abnormal noise or performance limitations is not completely consistent with the resting endoscopic findings. Head and neck position may play a critical role in the evaluation process, and the exact position during performance should be reproduced during the clinical examination to definitively define the abnormality. Treatments and prognoses are presented.

Melissa R. Mazan

The airways are the first part of the pathway in the oxygen transport chain that is critical to excellent athletic performance, and the lower airways are considered the final gatekeeper before oxygen enters the blood and carbon dioxide exits. Horses are blessed with large airways and lungs that allow them to be superb athletes, but the down side of this largesse on the part of evolution is that unless they are truly elite athletes they may withstand noninfectious disease of the lower respiratory tract for months to years before the owner or trainer notices. The two conditions of the lower respiratory tract that affect the athletic horse during exercise are exercise-induced pulmonary hemorrhage and inflammatory airway disease. The former may be considered, at least at the onset, as a problem of physiology rather than a disease, and the latter is a disease primarily of domestication: both are widespread among the athletic horse population and account for an impressive number of horses that fail to perform to their potential. Because of the high demands for oxygen in the athletic horse, even minor insults to the oxygen-carrying capacity of the body can affect performance, so it is of critical importance to keep the lungs as healthy as possible.

VETERINARY CLINICS OF NORTH AMERICA: EQUINE PRACTICE

THE CLINICS ARE NOW AVAILABLE ONLINE!
Access your subscription at:
www.theclinics.com

Equine Sport Medicine

VETERINARY CLINICS OF
NORTH AMERICA: EQUINE PRACTICE

FORTHCOMING ISSUES

December 2018
Wound Management
Earl M. Gaughan, Editor

April 2019
Clinical Cardiology
Colin Schwarzwald and
Katharyn J. Mitchell, Editors

August 2019
**Controversies in Equine Medicine
and Surgery**
Robert J. MacKay, Editor

RECENT ISSUES

April 2018
**Recent Advances in the Diagnosis and
Management of Equine Gastrointestinal
Diseases**
Henry Stämpfli and Angelika Schoster,
Editors

December 2017
Equine Ophthalmology
Mary Lassaline, Editor

August 2017
Orthopedic Disorders of the Foal
Ashlee E. Watts, Editor

ISSUE OF RELATED INTEREST

Veterinary Clinics of North America: Equine Practice
April 2016 (Vol. 32, Issue 1)
Rehabilitation of the Equine Athlete
Melissa R. King and Elizabeth J. Davidson, Editors

THE CLINICS ARE NOW AVAILABLE ONLINE!
Access your subscription at:
www.theclinics.com

Preface

Equine Sports Medicine: Our Daily Challenge

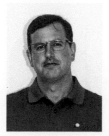

José M. García-López, VMD
Editor

The equine athlete is a display of finesse, endurance, grace, power, ability, and fragility. The field of equine sports medicine has seen a dramatic and desperately needed influx of new information and research, which continues to expand our knowledge and abilities when evaluating, diagnosing, managing, and rehabilitating these amazing athletes. Those of us who have the fortune to work daily with sport horses are all too aware of the challenges that we encounter when evaluating and treating these athletes. It is fitting with all the emphasis that we as clinicians have toward the equine athlete and all the new information available that *Veterinary Clinics of North America: Equine Practice* is dedicating an entire issue to equine sports medicine.

I am forever grateful to all the authors involved in this issue for their contributions and expertise. They made this issue not only enjoyable to put together but also enlightening. I am confident that you, the reader, will find the information included in this new issue beneficial to your everyday practice. I would like to thank Dr Thomas Divers for giving me the opportunity to make this issue, a first of its kind for *Veterinary Clinics of North America: Equine Practice*, and Donald Mumford for his guidance and patience along the way.

Vet Clin Equine 34 (2018) xiii–xiv
https://doi.org/10.1016/j.cveq.2018.05.001
0749-0739/18/© 2018 Published by Elsevier Inc.

Last, I would like to dedicate this issue to the memory of Dr Benson (Ben) Martin, VMD, DACVS (1946-2015), who to many was one of the pioneers in the specialty of equine sports medicine.

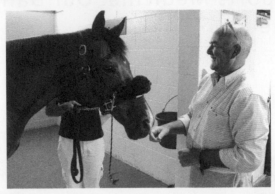

Those of us who had the fortune to be taught by or to work with Ben during his 34-year career at New Bolton Center are forever indebted to him not only for teaching and training us in how to be better clinicians and diagnosticians but also for showing us how to effectively manage the personalities of the people surrounding each case. Although he is sorely missed, his legacy and teachings will continue to have an impact for a lot of us.

José M. García-López, VMD
Large Animal Surgery
Department of Clinical Sciences
Cummings School of Veterinary Medicine at Tufts University
200 Westboro Road
North Grafton, MA 01536, USA

E-mail address:
jose.garcia-lopez@tufts.edu

Lameness Evaluation of the Athletic Horse

Check for updates

Elizabeth J. Davidson, DVM

KEYWORDS

- Lameness examination • Gait evaluation • Equine • Limb flexion tests
- Ridden gait evaluation • Diagnostic analgesia

KEY POINTS

- Lameness evaluation required keen clinical and observational skills.
- Examination starts with a thorough physical examination including visual assessment at rest, conformation, and systemic palpation.
- Gait evaluation is performed in a consistent manner over flat firm surfaces. Lunging, riding, and limb flexion tests may enhance detection of lameness.
- Most lame horses do not exhibit pathognomonic gait characteristic gait abnormalities; therefore, accurate diagnosis requires comprehensive evaluation including diagnostic analgesia.

INTRODUCTION

For years, veterinarians have been performing lameness evaluations on athletic horses. Information on the subject is plentiful dating back 100 or more years and is highlighted by today's renowned textbooks, Adams and Stashak's *Lameness in Horses*[1] and Ross and Dyson's *Diagnosis and Management of Lameness in the Horse*.[2] Throughout time, the basic concept of lameness evaluation persists: keen clinical assessment and observation (the art of lameness) combined with diagnostics (the science of lameness).

Lameness is defined as abnormal stance or gait caused by structural or functional abnormality of the locomotor system. Normal horses should move with balanced and symmetric motion; lame horses have unbalanced and/or asymmetric gaits. Lameness is a clinical sign, not a disease per se. It is a manifestation of pain, mechanical dysfunction, or neuromuscular deficit causing alteration of gait, that is, the horse limps. In certain conditions, characteristic gait abnormalities are pathognomonic, and

Disclosure Statement: The author does not have any relationship with a commercial company that has a direct financial interest in subject matter or materials discussed in article or with a company making a competing product.
Department of Clinical Studies, New Bolton Center, School of Veterinary Medicine, University of Pennsylvania, 382 West Street Road, Kennett Square, PA 19348, USA
E-mail address: ejdavid@vet.upenn.edu

therefore, recognition and location of the problem are straightforward. For example, a horse standing with its hind limb locked in extension and fetlock caudally placed and flexed is the distinctive stance of upward fixation of the patella ("locked stifle"). Unfortunately, most causes of lameness do not exhibit characteristic gait abnormalities, making diagnosis a real challenge. The lameness diagnostician then becomes the lameness detective.

Being a skilled lameness detective is critical because best treatment practices are based on accurate diagnosis of underlying cause or causes of lameness. The lameness evaluation should therefore be performed in an orderly, systemic, and thoughtful fashion except in horses with severe lameness and/or if fracture is suspected. This type of approach can be time consuming, especially when the underlying cause is not obvious. Because pain is the most common cause of lameness in the horse, an essential component of the lameness evaluation is diagnostic analgesia (nerve and joint blocks). Diagnostic analgesia authenticates the site or sites of lameness. It also establishes the clinical relevance (or not) of physical examination and/or previous imaging findings. Although valuable, diagnostic imaging is not a substitute for a detailed lameness evaluation because it is the horse that runs and jumps, not the radiograph. Once the site or sites of pain are localized, targeted therapy is initiated with the goals of returning the horse to its athletic activity.

HISTORY AND PHYSICAL EXAMINATION

A thorough and logical lameness evaluation starts with obtaining the affected horse's signalment. Age, sex, breed, and athletic use are basic vital facts that influence the predisposition of certain underlying lameness causes. For example, racehorses are prone to stress fractures and bucked shins due to the high-intensity training, whereas older seasoned show horses are prone to osteoarthritis and other degenerative musculoskeletal conditions. The horse's comprehensive medical history and past performance record are also important. Helpful information includes onset and duration of lameness, management changes, and whether lameness severity improves with rest or exercise. The shoeing interval and type should also be noted. Response to medications and/or exercise modifications, and previous lameness are also important historical data. Additional information from questions tailored to the specific horse is also useful; for example, "the horse won't pick up the left lead canter" or "the horse lunges when pulling the steer."

The next step is performing a comprehensive physical examination starting with visual inspection and conformation evaluation. The horse's demeanor, stance, and body symmetry are assessed. Obvious conformational abnormalities are commonly linked to performance-limiting lameness; however, minor abnormalities may offer little insight to the current and future sites of lameness. Abnormal posture such as "dropped elbow" stance is distinctive for upper forelimb fractures and should be investigated radiographically before observing the horse in motion. Static muscle fascinations should also be noted because they may be due to pain and/or underlying myopathic conditions. Pelvic asymmetry should be noted; however, direct correlation between pelvic abnormalities and underlying pelvic pain should be linked with caution. Muscle atrophy of the gluteal region is a common finding in horses with hind limb lameness regardless of underlying cause (lower limb, hock, stifle, or pelvis). There is no association between asymmetrical tuber sacrale ("hunter's bump") and the presence of sacroiliac pain.[3] The back and neck are also thoroughly examined. Flexibility, extensibility, and overall muscle development along the topline should also be noted.

To some degree, body and limb conformation determines the way the horse moves and therefore influences its athletic ability and soundness. Conformation assessment pervades performance horse practice and is a cornerstone of presales evaluation. However, determining what is considered ideal is complicated because desirable conformational traits vary between different breeds and athletic use. For example, long sloping shoulders are advantageous in elite show jumpers and dressage horses[4] but associated with decreased performance in National Hunt racehorses.[5] Conformation abnormalities are considered undesirable because of resultant changes in gait patterns, unbalanced limb stress, and associated lameness. Horses with base-wide, toed-in front limb conformation tend to wing out or "paddle" when walking, which overloads the medial aspect of the limb, often resulting in lameness.[6] Sickle hock conformation concentrates load to the dorsal aspect of the hock, which may predispose affected horses to curb (plantar desmitis) and distal hock pain.[7] Horses with straight hock conformation are at risk for suspensory desmitis.[8] Although not all conformation faults are detrimental in the athletic horse, most standardbreds and warmbloods have a "toe out behind" conformation,[6] suggesting this conformational fault is a normal breed characteristic with no impact on performance. Other conformational defects may even be protective for musculoskeletal injury. In racing thoroughbreds, carpal valgus decreases the incidence of carpal fracture.[9] Although an important part of the physical assessment, abnormal conformation is not synonymous with lameness.

Closer inspection during the physical examination includes systematic palpation of limbs. The hoof size and shape, shoe type, shoe wear pattern, presence of mismatched feet, low heel, upright heel (club foot), and broken pastern-foot angle should all be appreciated. Digital pulses should be assessed and increased pulse quality ascertained. Time-honored hoof tester application maintains value in modern lameness evaluation because foot pain is the most common site of lameness in the front limb. Focal areas of sole sensitivity should be investigated thoroughly. However, only 45% of horses with navicular pain will have a positive response to hoof testers[10]; false positive and false negative hoof testers responses do exist. Next, each joint and its associated joint pouches should be palpated; subtle medial femorotibial joint effusion is easily missed without careful palpation. Metacarpal/metatarsal tendon and ligaments should be palpated in the weight-bearing and non-weight-bearing position. Each structure should be isolated during palpation and assessed for focal areas of heat, sensitivity, and enlargement. Deep focal pressure along the proximal suspensory ligament is also beneficial; however, false positive and negative responses are common in horses with authentic injury in this region.[8] In the upper forelimb and pelvis regions, joint effusion is difficult to appreciate even when present because of their deep locations and overlying muscles. In addition to overall musculoskeletal palpation, it is also important to perform targeted palpation to areas of pain common to the use of the horse. For example, palpation of the dorsal aspect of each carpal bone in non-weight-bearing position is very important in the racehorse because this is a common site of injury for this breed and use.

Static manipulative tests, such as standing flexion and extension of joints, can also yield valuable information. Decreased range of motion in a young athletic horse is uncommon, and if noted, is frequently associated with underlying pain and injury. As with any type of limb manipulation, it is difficult to stress one joint in isolation, and therefore, specificity of lameness to a particular joint is almost impossible. Of all the joint flexion tests, reduced carpal flexion and/or pain during carpal flexion appears to be the most likely to be directly correlated to carpal pain. As with other physical examination findings, palpation and manipulative findings can facilitate localization of pain. However, many factors, such as individual horse responses to focal pressure and interpretation of pain, can be confounding.

GAIT EVALUATION

Next, and perhaps the most important step, evaluation of gait is performed while the horse is moving, allowing the clinician the opportunity to characterize the nature and severity of the gait abnormality. If fracture is suspected in the acute, severely lame horse, exercise should not be performed or catastrophic breakdown may result. Appropriate imaging is recommended. Key basic questions when performing gait evaluation include the following:

1. Is the horse lame?
2. What leg is lame?
3. What is the severity (grade) of lameness?
4. Is the lameness complicated, that is, observed in more than 1 limb or only under certain circumstances?

These basic inquiries are easy to answer when the horse is severely and consistently lame. However, the answers are not straightforward in the horse with an inconsistent and/or subtle lameness. Fast moving, fit athletic horses frequently exhibit quick changes of pace, speed, and direction, which compounds the clinician's accurate assessment of normal and abnormal gait patterns, especially with complicated lamenesses. Therefore, to enhance recognition of stride abnormalities, it is very important to establish consistency in the lameness examination. The horse should be handled by a skilled horseperson using a loose lead shank so the head and neck position can be evaluated, but not too loosely such that the horse's movement is not contained with a straight line. Ideal surfaces should be flat, firm, and nonslippery. Hard surfaces allow the examiner to listen as well as observe disparity in footfall patterns; the lame limb contacts the ground with less force and therefore less noise. Frequently lameness is more pronounced when exercising in a circle, and most of time, severity is increased when affected limb is on the inside of the circle. Lunging on soft surface may also be necessary, especially when faster but controlled gaits, such as canter, are evaluated. Slowing the speed, small circles, and ridden evaluations are particularly helpful for subtle lameness. In some horses, observation of gaits specific to the horse's athletic use, such as passage in the dressage horse or tölt in Icelandic horse, is also valuable. For consistency, handler, surface, speed, distance, size of circle, and gaits should remain constant and repeatable throughout the entire lameness evaluation.

The methodology to determine, the question number one: "Is the horse is lame?," is clinician preference. The examiner must rely on one's keen observation skills as they formulate the subjective assessment of the horse's gait. First, the diagnostician gets an overall impression of the horse's movement. The horse is observed as it walks away (evaluating from behind) and then as it walks toward (evaluating from the front). The sound horse should bear weight equally on each individual limb as it ambulates. Foot flight pattern is best observed from the front, and most horses will have a slight lateral-to-medial foot flight pattern.[11] The horse's limb movement should also be observed while considering the effects of conformation on limb flight patterns. Perfectly straight limbs travel even in all planes, whereas conformational abnormalities result in uneven limb flight patterns. Front limbs that are toed in or toed out may wing in or wing out when exercising. Foot placement relative to midline should also be assessed. Does one limb or foot consistently land closer to or farther away (placed laterally) of midline? Does the horse drift? If the horse drifts, does it drift with the front end or the hind end and to which direction? For the expert lameness diagnostician, these observations are performed quickly and instinctively as the horse walks down and back. For the inexperienced clinician, the horse may be walked several times down and back to target their visual acuity on specific regions of the moving parts (eg, the feet, front feet, back end).

Next, the horse is evaluated at the trot, the most useful gait for lameness evaluation. The horse is trotted away and then toward the clinician. The trotting horse should also be evaluated from the side. Again, gait characteristics should be noted. Sound horses move with a symmetric trotting gait, each limb bearing equal weight with a uniform limb flight pattern, and the horse travels freely forward without hesitation. Lame horses have asymmetrical gait patterns, which is commonly classified as weight-bearing or non-weight-bearing (swinging leg) lameness. Weight-bearing lameness is used to describe when the horse reduces the amount of time (decreases the force) applied to the weight-bearing phase of stride. Swinging leg lameness is described as lameness that affects the way the horse carries the painful limb. However, most horses with painful lameness conditions will alter *both* the weight-bearing and non-weight-bearing phases of stride with distinction between the 2 all but impossible to the human eye. Lame horses consistently shorten the cranial phase of stride, a reliable gait characteristic that is best observed from the side. Other gait alternations include the degree of fetlock drop or full extension during weight-bearing. Bear in mind that all limb movement is somewhat dependent on conformation, anatomy, and function. In limbs with abnormal function, for instance, suspensory desmitis with associated loss of functional support to the fetlock, the affected horse may have increased full extension (increased fetlock drop) because of underlying pathologic condition and therefore the opposite occurs (more fetlock drop with lameness). The lame horse will exhibit some or all abnormal (asymmetrical) gait characteristics, which highlights the importance of comprehensive, consistent, and repeatable lameness examination.

After determining the presence of lameness, the examiner moves onto the second question, "In which leg is the lameness?" Recognition of asymmetric body motion patterns is the first and basic way to allocate lameness to a specific limb. The lame horse shifts their center of body mass away from the painful limb. Forelimb lameness is usually easier to recognize as a head nod. The lame horse's head and neck nod consists of elevation during the weight-bearing stance of the lame leg; the head goes up and back (caudally directed). In addition, the horse's head and neck nods downward when the sound leg hits the ground, down and cranially directed. Hence, the phase "down on the sound" is commonly used. Being very mobile, head and neck nod is a consistent gait asymmetry noted. This head and neck nod is best observed from the side but can also be observed from the front/behind evaluation position. Hind limb lameness is more difficult to identify. Affected horses will exhibit an alteration in movement of the pelvis. During the weight-bearing stance of the lame hind limb, the affected side moves upward, a "hip hike" or preferably "pelvic hike." Alternatively, "pelvic drop" can be observed during the non-weight-bearing phase of the lame leg. Another tendency for hind limb lameness is drifting away from the lameness. The horse with left hind limb lameness often travels with haunches to the right. These head nods and pelvic movements are unconscious, occurring when the horse unloads the lame leg and loads the sound leg. Identification of these shifts in body mass is the basis for determining if the lameness is in a front or hind limb, right or left.

The severity of the lameness is determined next; question number 3. Ideally, a lameness grading system should be consistent, applicable to all types of lameness, and universally accepted; no such scale exists. In North America, the most common lameness scoring system is the 0 to 5 American Association of Equine Practitioners lameness scale[12] (**Table 1**). Although useful, this system has limitations because it grades lameness at *both* the walk and trot and does not account for the horse that is lame at the walk and sound at the trot, or vice versa. In addition, horses that are only lame when trotting in a circle are commonly scored grade 1 lameness when by definition, should be grade 2 lameness. An alternative scoring system has been described by Dr Mike Ross[13] (**Table 2**) based on observations of the horse when trotting. The system can be used for lameness in the front and hind limbs. However, this system also has limitations, and differentiation between grades 2 and 3 is not straightforward. In the United Kingdom, a subjective scoring system from 0 to 10 is regularly used,[14] where 0 indicates the horse is sound and 10 indicates complete inability to use the limb. This grading system is reasonably reliable among clinicians, but less consistent with inexperienced examiners.[15] Dr Sue Dyson describes a 0 to 8 grading system,[16] which is independently applied to the walk and trot and under different circumstances, such as straight lines, circles, and while ridden. Whichever scoring system the clinician uses, it is important for the examiner to be as consistent as possible when grading lameness.

If the answer to the fourth question, "Is the lameness complicated?," is yes, accurate lameness is even more challenging. Horses that are lame in more than 1 limb, lame only under certain circumstances, and/or have bilateral lameness are difficult to evaluate. As previously discussed, the horse shifts its weight away from the lame limb, in a side-to-side and front-to-back fashion. As a result, horses with a pelvic hike may also exhibit a head nod, and vice versa. In these horses, distinction between primary and compensatory "false" lameness is not easy. The "law of sides"[17] would suggest that horses with ipsilateral concurrent front and hind limb lameness are predominantly lame in the hind end. Explanation for this phenomenon includes the following. A horse with right hind limb lameness transfers load to the left hind limb but also cranially to the contralateral left front limb resulting in a horse that appears to have ipsilateral right hind *and* right front limb lameness. Compensatory body movement is not restricted to a caudal to cranial direction, and some horses with front limb lameness also have concurrent pelvic movement that mimics contralateral hind limb lameness. Other conditions that complicate the lameness evaluation are horses with bilateral lameness, horses appearing symmetric (sound) in a straight line, and horses with subtle lameness observed only under certain conditions. Observation of gait while circling may be helpful in these horses, and in most instances, mild low-grade lameness is accentuated when circling. However, lunging can induce

Table 1	
The American Association of Equine Practitioners lameness grading system	
Grade 0	Lameness is not perceptible under any circumstances
Grade 1	Lameness is difficult to observe and is not consistently apparent, regardless of circumstances (eg, under saddle, circling, inclines, hard surfaces)
Grade 2	Lameness is difficult to observe at a walk or when trotting in a straight line but consistently apparent under certain circumstances (eg, weight-carrying, circling, inclines, hard surfaces)
Grade 3	Lameness is consistently observable at a trot under all circumstances
Grade 4	Lameness is obvious at the walk
Grade 5	Lameness produces minimal weight-bearing in motion and/or at rest or complete inability to move

From Anonymous. Guide to veterinary services for horse shows. 7th edition. Lexington (KY): American Association of Equine Practitioners; 1999; with permission.

Table 2 Alternative lameness scoring system	
Grade 0	Sound
Grade 1	Mild lameness observed while the horse is trotted in a straight line. When the lame forelimb strikes, a subtle head nod is observed; when the lame hind limb strikes, a subtle pelvic hike occurs. The head nod and pelvis hike may be inconsistent at times.
Grade 2	Obvious lameness is observed. The head nod and pelvic hike are seen consistently, and excursion is several centimeters.
Grade 3	Pronounced head nod and pelvic hike of several centimeters are noted. If the horse has unilateral singular hind limb lameness, a head and neck nod is seen when the diagonal forelimb strikes the ground (mimicking ipsilateral forelimb lameness).
Grade 4	Severe lameness with extreme head nod and pelvic hike is present. The horse can still be trotted, however.
Grade 5	The horse does not bear weight on the limb. If trotted, the horse carries the limb. Horses that are non-weight-bearing at the walk or while standing should not be trotted.

Lameness grades based on trotting in a straight line, in hand, on a firm surface.
From Ross MW. Movement. In: Ross MW, Dyson SJ, editors. Diagnosis and management of lameness in the horse. 2nd edition. St Louis (MO): Elsevier; 2011. p. 64–80; with permission.

movement asymmetries in sound horses[18]; mild inside hip hike and outside head nod-down occurs. These "normal" body movement adaptations on the lunge may therefore result in lameness to be more or less visible depending on circle direction and location of pain. Because correct identification of the lame limb is prerequisite, both circle-dependent and compensatory front/hind limb movement mechanisms must be taken into account when evaluating lame horses.

LAMENESS EXAMINATION IN THE RIDDEN HORSE

For some horses, lameness is only apparent when ridden, whereby certain movements, sport-specific gaits, changes of pace such as canter-to-trot transitions, can be reliably reproduced. In the lame riding horse, abnormal gait characteristics are highly variable, such as overt limping, reluctance to go forward, resistance in the bridle, bucking, and rearing.[19] The addition of a rider's weight causes increased limb loading[20] affecting both sound and lame horses. Posting trot causes uneven loading of the left and right limbs with peak forces on the sitting trot diagonal higher than the rising trot diagonal.[21] On the left diagonal, the rider sits when the left front and right hind limbs are bearing weight. This uneven weight distribution during rising trot may enhance detection of lameness; hind limb lameness is often worse when the rider sits on the diagonal of the lame leg.[19] In addition to changes in limb forces, sitting trot also exerts greater stress on the horse's spine resulting in increased back extension.[22] Like limb-loading patterns, rising trot creates uneven stresses on the back. Maximal back flexion occurs during unloaded rising trot stride and maximal extension during loaded sitting trot stride. However, changes in back movement are not strictly limited to rider positions. Lame horses adapt their gaits by stiffening the thoracolumbar-sacral region.[23] The resultant trunk stiffness is often perceived as back pain by the rider even when the underlying pain and decreased back flexibility are due to limb lameness. Although the mere presence of a rider can influence the incidence of lameness, rider effects in individual horse cannot be predicted.[24] Some horses will be lame in hand and sound with a rider, and vice versa, and the prevalence of may be related to the rider's skill level.[24] Professional riders may mask underlying gait abnormalities, whereas unbalanced beginners may exaggerate asymmetrical gait conditions. For all riders, accurate identification of lameness and localization of the lame limb are often difficult, and a high proportion of "owner-sound" is lame when assessed comprehensively by a skilled lameness diagnostician.[25] Although ridden evaluation is not a substitute for in-hand lameness assessment, it can enhance the clinician's ability to detect and localize lameness. Keen observations in the horse moving with or without a rider are paramount for the lameness diagnostician.

FLEXION TESTS

Flexion tests have been an integral part of the gait assessment and are routinely used in the lameness examination. This longstanding clinical tool often highlights the presence of lameness. Although common practice, subjective flexion testing is not standardized, and evidence-based support for its specificity in lameness localization is lacking. In fact, only 1 of 57 horses had both a positive flexion test and lameness in the same limb.[25] Numerous factors, such as variations in technique, degree of flexion, and amount of force applied to the flexed limb, prevail among clinicians and influence posttesting response. Duration of limb flexion period before trotting off varies from 15 to 90 seconds and may account for variable results. In one study,[26] a 60-second proximal hind limb flexion test was more likely than a 5-second flexion test to produce a positive response. With all these variables, the reproducibility of testing between examiners is unreliable, although individual repeatability is reportedly good.[27] Most sound[28,29] and lame horses[25] will be positive to limb flexion, which emphasizes the lack of sensitivity with limb flexion tests to detect authentic sites of pain. Reasons flexion testing is not a precision diagnostic tool may be due to the inability to stress a single joint without also exerted force to other joints and nearby tissues. The terms lower limb flexion test and upper limb flexion test are more appropriate than fetlock and hock flexion tests, respectively, because they more accurately describe flexion mechanics. Subjectivity of hind limb flexions is further hindered by the reciprocal apparatus, which ensures unison movement of upper hind limb joints. Two different research teams investigated which structures may be responsible for a positive distal limb flexion test, and both concluded that the metacarpophalangeal joint pain is the primary cause of a positive response.[30,31] Although these findings are interesting, debate continues regarding limb flexion testing and its inherent value in the lameness examination.

DIAGNOSTIC ANALGESIA

With careful and comprehensive gait assessment, a skilled clinician may be able to formulate a reasonable list of potential pain sources during the lameness examination. However, in most horses, diagnostic analgesia will be required to truly authenticate and localize the lameness site. With few exceptions, gait abnormalities are not specific to injury type, and examination findings can be misleading. A horse with foot pain may be lame when trotting in a straight line and/or while lunging and/or when ridden, exhibiting lameness gait characteristics in any or all of these conditions. Severity of front limb lameness may be exacerbated when circling to the right or the left or both. Lame horses also may have pain in more than one site and/or more than one limb, further complicating identification of pain by observation alone. Therefore, diagnostic analgesia is essential, perhaps the most essential, diagnostic tool for the lameness detective.

Perineural and joint blocks should be performed in a systematic and thoughtful manner. Diagnostic analgesia is time consuming but extremely rewarding because "best guesses" frequently result in improper treatment, return to training before adequate healing, and chronicity of injury in the lame horse. Albeit extremely important, interpretation of lameness severity changes after diagnostic analgesia is not always straightforward. When the same clinician performs the lameness examination and the diagnostic analgesia, there may be interpretation bias; the attending clinician expects improvement in lameness severity after blocking. Arkell and colleagues[15] demonstrated that unblinded observers allocated larger changes in lameness grades, increased effect of a nerve block, compared with blinded observers. It is also important to recognize that the intended region to desensitize may differ from what structures are actually desensitized. This sequel may be due to inadvertent penetration of a synovial structure during perineural injections and/or incorrect placement of anesthetic solution. Adequate patient restraint and a solid working knowledge of neuroanatomy can minimize but not completely abolish these complications. Even with good technique, anesthesia of adjacent structures occurs after intra-articular analgesia due to diffusion of anesthetic solution across anatomic borders and/or blockade of peripheral nerves that course through or near joint outpouchings. For example, intra-articular anesthesia of the distal interphalangeal joint improves pain not only in the joint but also in the navicular bursa, the navicular bone and associated soft tissue structures, and the toe region of the sole.[32] Diffusion also occurs after perineural injections with significant proximal dissemination occurring within 10 minutes of the procedure.[33] This rapid proximal distribution may also contribute to desensitization of unintentional structures. Small volumes of anesthetic solution and time-sensitive lameness reevaluation may diminish these untoward complications. Diagnostic analgesia is not an exact science, and high specificity within anatomic regions may not be possible. Despite these pitfalls, nerve and joint blocks combined with thorough gait assessment remain the best approach to localize pain and lameness.

REFERENCES

1. Baxter GM. Adams and Stashak's Lameness in Horses. 6th edition. Chichester, West Sussex, UK: Balckwell Publishing, Ltd; 2011.
2. Rss MW, Dyson SJ. Diagnosis and Management of Lameness in the Horse. 2nd edition. St Louis, MO: Elsevier; 2011.
3. Dyson S, Murray R. Pain associated with the sacroiliac region: a clinical study of 74 horses. Equine Vet J 2003;35:240–5.
4. Holmstrom M, Magnusson LE, Philipsson J. Variation in conformation of Swedish Warmblood horses and conformational characteristics of elite sport horses. Equine Vet J 1990;22:186–93.
5. Weller R, Pfau T, Verheyen K, et al. The effect of conformation on orthopaedic health and performance in a cohort of National Hunt racehorses: preliminary results. Equine Vet J 2006;38:622–7.
6. Ross MW, McIlwraith CW. Conformation and lameness. In: Ross MW, Dyson SJ, editors. Diagnosis and management of lameness in the horse. 2nd edition. St Louis (MO): Elsevier; 2011. p. 15–32.
7. Gnagey L, Clayton MH, Lanovaz JL. Effect of standing tarsal angle on joint kinematics and kinetics. Equine Vet J 2006;38:628–34.
8. Dyson S. Diagnosis and management of common suspensory lesions in the forelimb and hindlimbs of sport horses. Clinic Techniques in Equine Pract 2007;6: 179–88.

9. Anderson TM, McIlwraith CW, Douay P. The role of conformation in musculoskeletal problems in the racing Thoroughbred. Equine Vet J 2004;36:571–5.

10. Turner TA. Predictive value of diagnostic tests for navicular pain. Proc Am Assoc Equine Pract 1996;42:201–4.

11. Heel MCV, Barneveld A, van Weeren PR, et al. Dynamic pressure measurements for detailed study of hoof balance: the effect of trimming. Equine Vet J 2004;36: 778–82.

12. Anonymous. Guide to veterinary services for horse shows. 7th edition. Lexington (KY): American Association of Equine Practitioners; 1999.

13. Ross MW. Movement. In: Ross MW, Dyson SJ, editors. Diagnosis and management of lameness in the horse. 2nd edition. St Louis (MO): Elsevier; 2011. p. 64–80.

14. Jones W. Equine lameness. Oxford (United Kingdom): Blackwell Scientific Publications; 1988. p. 5.

15. Arkell M, Archer RM, Guitian FJ, et al. Evidence of bias affecting interpretation of the results of local anaesthetic nerve blocks when assessing lameness in horses. Vet Rec 2006;159:346–9.

16. Dyson S. Can lameness be graded reliably? Equine Vet J 2011;43:379–82.

17. Keegan KG. Evidence-based lameness detection and quantification. Vet Clin Equine 2007;23:403–23.

18. Starke SD, Willems E, May SA, et al. Vertical head and truck movement adaptations of sound horses in a circle on a hard surface. Vet J 2012;193:73–80.

19. Dyson S. Equine performance and equitation science: clinical issues. Appl Anim Behav Sci 2017;190:5–17.

20. Clayton HM, Lanovaz JL, Schamhardt HC, et al. The effects of a rider's mass on ground reaction forces and fetlock kinematics at the trot. Equine Vet J Suppl 1999;30:218–21.

21. Roepstorff L, Egenvall A, Rhodin M, et al. Kinetics and kinematics of the horse comparing left and right rising trot. Equine Vet J 2009;41:292–6.

22. De Cocq P, Prinsen H, Springer NCN, et al. The effect of rising and sitting trot on back movements and head-neck position in the horse. Equine Vet J 2009;41: 423–7.

23. Gomez-Alvarez CB, Bobbert MF, Lamers L, et al. The effect of induced hindlimb lameness on thoracolumbar kinematics during treadmill locomotion. Equine Vet J 2008;40:147–52.

24. Licka T, Kapaun M, Peham C. Influence of rider on lameness in trotting horses. Equine Vet J 2004;36:734–6.

25. Dyson S, Greve L. Subjective gait assessment of 57 sports horses in normal work: a comparison of response to flexion tests, movement in hand, on the lunge, and ridden. J Equine Vet Sci 2016;38:1–7.

26. Armentrout AR, Beard WL, White BJ, et al. A comparative study of proximal hindlimb flexion in horses: 5 versus 60 seconds. Equine Vet J 2012;44:420–4.

27. Keg PR, van Weeren PR, Back W, et al. Influence of the force applied and its period of application on the outcome of the flexion test of the distal forelimb of the horse. Vet Rec 1997;141:463–6.

28. Starke SD, Willems E, Head M, et al. Proximal hindlimb flexion in the horse: effect on movement symmetry and implications for defining soundness. Equine Vet J 2012;44:657–63.

29. Busschers E, van Weeren PR. Use of the flexion test of the distal forelimb in the sound horse: repeatability and effect of age, gender, weight, height, and fetlock range of motion. J Vet Med A Physiol Pathol Clin Med 2001;48:413–27.

30. Meijer MC, Busschers E, van Weeren PR. Which joint is most important for the positive outcome of a flexion test of the distal forelimb of a sound horse? Equine Vet Educ 2001;13:319–23.
31. Kearney CM, van Weeren PR, Cornelissen BPM, et al. Which anatomical region determines a positive flexion test of the distal limb in a nonlame horse? Equine Vet J 2010;42:547–51.
32. Schumacher J, Schramme MC, Schumacher J, et al. Diagnostic analgesia of the equine digital. Equine Vet Educ 2013;25:408–21.
33. Nagy A, Bodo G, Dyson SJ, et al. Diffusion of contrast medium after perineural injection of the palmar nerves: an in vivo and in vitro study. Equine Vet J 2009; 41:379–83.

Diagnosis of Skeletal Injury in the Sport Horse

Kathryn B. Wulster, VMD

KEYWORDS

- Horse • MRI • Standing CT • Cone beam • Subchondral bone injury

KEY POINTS

- Imaging modalities have variable sensitivity and specificity to detect skeletal injury, which often occurs in a discipline-specific pattern.
- Increased knowledge from advanced imaging (computed tomography/magnetic resonance) is improving the ability to detect corresponding changes on radiographs.
- Nontraditional radiographic projections can be used in the field to improve recognition of bone injury.
- MRI remains the gold standard for whole joint organ evaluation, but notable differences are present between high- and low-field magnets for evaluation of cartilage and subchondral and trabecular bone lesions.
- Standing computed tomography is a novel technique that requires refinement, particularly for cone beam imaging, but there is increased availability in both academia and private practice.

INTRODUCTION

With the exception of acute fracture secondary to a monotonic episode of supraphysiologic loading, skeletal injury in the sport horse is typically a manifestation of stress-induced overload injury secondary to cyclical loading.[1–3] The subchondral bone is a commonly affected region with the location of injury dependent on discipline.[4–9] Osteoarthritis is a common sequela, which may become performance limiting.[10,11] Stress fractures of equine long bones (eg, tibia, humerus) occur due to an analogous process of cyclical loading similar to humans.[12–15] Both subchondral and cortical cyclical loading can lead to catastrophic failure of the affected bone, a consequence most commonly seen in the Thoroughbred racehorse.[4,15,16]

Diagnosis of bone injury relies on recognition of pathophysiologic changes to bone that occur in the limb as it responds to stress according to Wulff's law, namely modeling and remodeling. These initially adaptive responses occur at predictable

Department of Clinical Studies, New Bolton Center, School of Veterinary Medicine, University of Pennsylvania, 382 West Street Road, Kennett Square, PA 19348, USA
E-mail address: kwulster@upenn.edu

Vet Clin Equine 34 (2018) 193–213
https://doi.org/10.1016/j.cveq.2018.04.014
0749-0739/18/© 2018 Elsevier Inc. All rights reserved.
vetequine.theclinics.com

locations depending on the discipline performed by the horse and affect diarthrodial joints, various long bones, and tendon and ligament entheses.[17–21] This adaptive response is often referred to as a repetitive stress response. The point at which adaptive changes to bone become pathologic is influenced by numerous factors, intrinsic, such as genetics, age, and size, as well as extrinsic, such as discipline, footing, training schedule, and exercise intensity.[9,22,23] Repetitive stress injuries follow discipline-specific patterns that mirror the location of the repetitive stress response.[17,24–26] With some exceptions, the distinction between adaptive response and pathologic condition can be unclear and should be based on the presence of clinical lameness with corroboration of imaging findings and response to diagnostic analgesia, where appropriate, as opposed to diagnostic imaging findings alone.[14,27,28]

The appearance of bone injury on any particular diagnostic imaging modality is dependent on what the image represents and is predominantly qualitative. For instance, computed tomography (CT) reflects tissue density relative to water,[29] whereas nuclear scintigraphy of bone reflects osteoblastic activity.[10,30–33] For certain modalities, the degree of bone change can be quantified.[34–36] Some modalities represent only morphologic changes, such as radiography and CT, whereas others reflect physiologic changes (nuclear scintigraphy and PET). MRI is unique in that it provides both morphologic and physiologic information. Representing only a snapshot of a dynamic and changing pathophysiologic process, all imaging modalities have benefits and drawbacks, and they tend to complement each rather than make any imaging modality obsolete.[37] Emerging technologies and research are focusing on the early recognition of subchondral bone and cartilage injury, allowing for more specific diagnoses and targeted therapies.[38–43]

The various manifestations of skeletal injury as identified using radiography, scintigraphy/Positron emission tomography (PET), CT, and MRI are described.

Radiography

Radiography remains the mainstay for diagnosis of skeletal injury in the sport horse because of its affordability, portability, and ease of use for the sport horse practitioner. Radiography is a planar (2-dimensional [2D]) imaging modality that reflects 5 radiographic opacities determined by tissue atomic number, thickness, overlap with other tissues, angulation of the x-ray beam, and tissue homogeneity. The main limitations of radiography include superimposition, lack of direct visualization of cartilage, and the relatively large (30%–50%) degree of bone change required before lesion visualization.[31]

Diagnosis of bone injury on radiographs includes direct fracture visualization, but is otherwise inferred from secondary changes that are associated with whole organ dysfunction leading to degenerative joint disease. Such radiographic changes include thickening and increased opacity of the subchondral and surrounding trabecular bone, subchondral osteolysis, periarticular new bone formation, and joint space narrowing. Increased radiopacity is commonly referred to as sclerosis, although strictly speaking sclerosis reflects bone strength, which cannot be evaluated with any imaging modality. Loss of cartilage can be inferred from decreased joint space, but this depends on proper positioning and is typically only recognized in advanced stages of disease. Thus, radiographs are insensitive, but reasonably specific for bone injury in the sport horse.

Repetitive stress injuries routinely diagnosed with radiographs include, but are not limited to, complete and incomplete fractures of the third metacarpal/

metatarsal condyles, osteochondral fragmentation ("chip fractures"), sagittal fractures of the proximal phalanx, wing fractures of the distal phalanx, slab fractures of the carpal and tarsal bones, and proximal sesamoid bone fractures. Compared to overt fracture, subchondral osteolytic lesions are a more subtle radiographic manifestation of subchondral bone injury, but can be associated with severe lameness. The lesions are often found in sites susceptible to fracture, such as the parasagittal groove of the metacarpal/tarsal condyles of the Thoroughbred racehorse. Lesions of the dorsomedial metacarpal/tarsal condyle and proximal phalanx sagittal groove are manifestations of subchondral osteolysis in the non-racing sport horse. Damage to the navicular bone as part of a multi-injury complex involving the podotrochlear apparatus structures, including flexor cortical lysis, has also been hypothesized to be due to repetitive trauma, although there is no current consensus for the cause of this disease, and injury to the navicular bone may in fact be a common manifestation of several etiopathologies.[44] Some of these pathologic conditions can also occur as acute monotonic events and are not exclusively a sequela of repetitive trauma.

For both repetitive trauma and monotonic injuries, it is prudent to repeat a radiographic study at 10 to 14 days if initial radiographs of a suspected region of skeletal injury do not demonstrate an abnormality. Lesion visualization after this time period is attributable to early osteoclastic activity, which increases the conspicuity of radiolucent lesions (**Fig. 1**). Early periosteal reaction may also be present at this stage if an occult fracture (eg, radius, proximal phalanx) is suspected.

Because CT and MRI have become increasing accessible to sport horse practitioners, radiographic techniques have improved to highlight commonly affected areas that correspond to pathologic regions identified with advanced imaging. Nonstandard projections that can be used to interrogate specific regions of pathologic condition include, but are not limited to, the following:

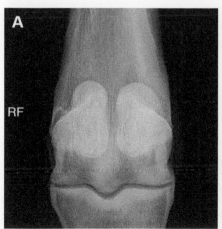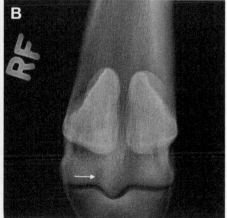

Fig. 1. Dorsopalmar (A) and flexed dorsopalmar (B) radiographs of the right metacarpophalangeal joint of a 3-year-old Thoroughbred racehorse with acute right forelimb lameness that improved following diagnostic analgesia (low 4 point) taken 14 days apart. Medial is to the right. A radiolucent, incomplete fracture plane is identified within the lateral parasagittal groove (*arrow*) on the follow-up radiographs (B), but is not identified on the initial study (A).

- Flexed dorsopalmar projection of the metacarpophalangeal/metatarsophalangeal joints to demonstrate palmar/plantar unicortical fracture
- Flexed dorsoproximal-dorsodistal oblique projection of the dorsal third metacarpal condyle (**Fig. 2**)
- Variable angle dorsoproximal-palmarodistal oblique projections to highlight proximal phalanx sagittal groove lucencies (**Fig. 3**)
- Variable angle dorsomedial-plantarolateral oblique projections of the central or third tarsal bone to demonstrate slab fractures
- Variable angle palmaroproximal-palmarodistal oblique (navicular skyline) projection to highlight the distal border of the navicular flexor cortex (**Figs. 4** and **5**)
- The cranio 5° disto10° lateral-caudoproximomedial oblique (flexed lateral oblique) is a view that isolates the medial femoral condyle

Evaluation of cartilage with radiography continues to be limited and requires contrast arthrography except in cases of advanced disease.

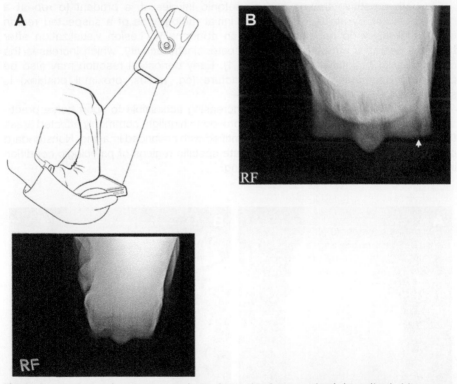

Fig. 2. Positioning and projection angle to obtain the dorsoproximal-dorsodistal oblique projection of the dorsal aspect of the third metacarpal condyle. The medial aspect of the dorsal condyle is radiopaque relative to the lateral aspect, which was considered a normal adaptive response to training in this sound middle-aged warmblood jumper (*A*). Same projection highlighting an ovoid region of radiolucency ovoid region of radiolucency (*white arrow*) and irregular margination of the dorsomedial aspect of the right third metacarpal condyle in a middle-aged warmblood with lameness localized by intra-articular analgesia of the fetlock joint (*B*). (*From* Drs Laura Faulkner, Christopher Miller, and Sarah Puchalski. Originally presented at the 2017 AAEP Convention "Diagnosis of subchondral bone injury of the fetlock joint in sport horses using field radiography"; with permission.)

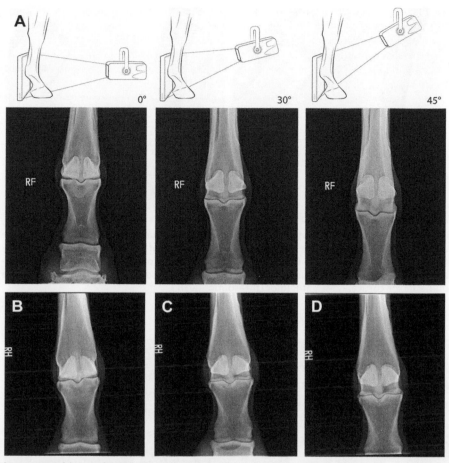

Fig. 3. Variable angle (0°–30°–45°) dorsoproximal-palmarodistal oblique projections of a normal metacarpophalangeal joint (*A*). Variable angle: 0° (*B*), 30° (*C*), 45° (*D*) dorsoproximal-palmarodistal oblique projections demonstrating variability in appearance of a horse with subchondral bone trauma/fissure fracture (parallel lesion configuration) of the sagittal groove with lameness localized by perineural analgesia (low 4 point). (*From* Drs Laura Faulkner, Christopher Miller, and Sarah Puchalski. Originally presented at the 2017 AAEP Convention "Diagnosis of subchondral bone injury of the fetlock joint in sport horses using field radiography"; with permission.)

Scintigraphy

As a highly sensitive and noninvasive modality, nuclear scintigraphy remains a useful tool in the diagnosis of musculoskeletal injury of the sport horse. Image production in scintigraphy relies on gamma-ray emission from a metastable radionuclide that is captured by a gamma camera following intravenous administration of the parent radionuclide, but is limited to planar (2D) images with inherently poor spatial resolution.[45] Lesions reflect the degree of radiopharmaceutical uptake in bone and are typically visualized as increased density of black pixels on a white background, although other displays are also used and may even improve sensitivity for lesion detection.[46] Comparison between right and left symmetry and knowledge of normal uptake patterns based on discipline is imperative for interpretation.

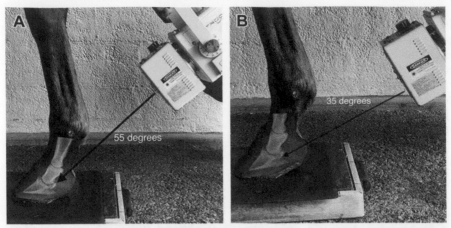

Fig. 4. Variable angle palmaroproximal-palmarodistal oblique projections (55°–35°) of the navicular bone highlighting the proximal and distal aspects of the flexor cortex, respectively (*A, B*). (*Data from* Johnson SA, Barrett MF, Frisbie DD. Effect of additional palmaropoximal-palmarodistal oblique projections on the accuracy of detection and characterization of equine flexor cortical lysis. Vet Radiol Ultrasound, 2018.)

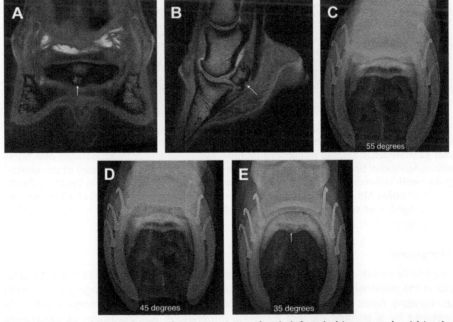

Fig. 5. Dorsal and sagittal MRIs demonstrating a focal defect (*white arrows*) within the distal aspect of the navicular flexor cortex on midline (*A, B*, respectively). Corresponding radiographic images at variable projection angles (55–45–35) highlighting the proximal, mid, and distal aspects of the navicular flexor cortex, respectively (*C–E*). An ovoid radiolucent lesion (*arrowhead*) is visualized best on the 35° projection and corresponds to the erosion identified on MRI. (*Courtesy of* Sherry A. Johnson, Myra F. Barrett, and David D. Frisbie, Fort Collins, Colorado; with permission.)

Numerous intravenously administered radioisotopes are available for nuclear imaging, but the most common isotope used for skeletal scintigraphy in the horse is technetium-99m linked to a phosphonate radiopharmaceutical (eg, methylene diphosphonate [MDP]) because of its high degree of incorporation into bone, specifically by binding to hydroxyapatite crystal in proportion to regional blood flow and osteoblastic activity.[10,47–49] As osteoblastic activity can be increased in pathologic and nonpathologic processes, increased radiopharmaceutical uptake is not synonymous with lameness-causing injury and knowledge of normal radiopharmaceutical uptake patterns is crucial for accurate diagnosis[35,50–57] (**Fig. 6**). False negative findings can also occur and are dependent on the timing of the study relative to the initial

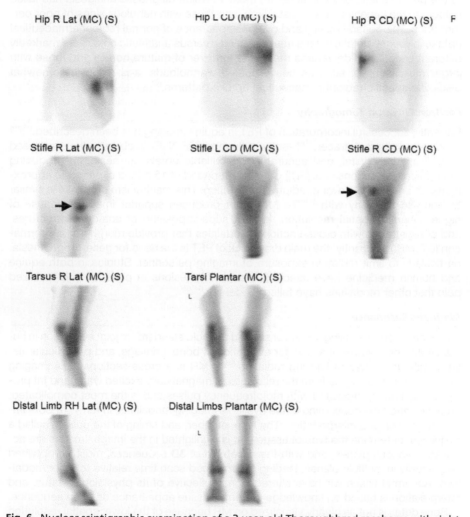

Hip R Lat (MC) (S)   Hip L CD (MC) (S)   Hip R CD (MC) (S)   F

Stifle R Lat (MC) (S)   Stifle L CD (MC) (S)   Stifle R CD (MC) (S)

Tarsus R Lat (MC) (S)   Tarsi Plantar (MC) (S)
L

Distal Limb RH Lat (MC) (S)   Distal Limbs Plantar (MC) (S)
L

Fig. 6. Nuclear scintigraphic examination of a 3-year-old Thoroughbred racehorse with right hind limb lameness localized to the distal limb via perineural diagnostic analgesia. Focal, intense, increased radiopharmaceutical uptake (*black arrow*) is present within the region of the right medial femoral condyle. Radiography confirmed a clinically silent osseous cyst-like lesion. The cause of lameness, oblique distal sesamoidean ligament desmopathy, was identified with MRI.

injury, the thickness of overlying soft tissues, and the specific region of bone affected. For instance, subchondral lysis tends to have more intense uptake compared with osteophytosis.[58] Some body parts require advanced disease before visualization, whereas others, such as osteoarthritis of the distal interphalangeal joint and carpus, can produce negative results even in the presence of severe disease.[59–61]

The high metabolic rate and bone turnover of Thoroughbred and Standardbred racehorses as well as their propensity for repetitive stress injury and fracture make this an ideal tool in these populations to avoid potentially catastrophic exacerbation of injury. For nonracing sport horses, nuclear scintigraphy is useful in horses that are behaviorally refractory to diagnostic analgesia, horses that have pain localized to the proximal limb or axial skeleton, those in which diagnostic analgesia has failed to localize the lameness to the distal limb, and those with nebulous signs of poor performance. The general quality and overall appearance of normal radiopharmaceutical uptake in young, athletic versus mature, athletic versus unathletic horses are markedly different because of decreased metabolic turnover of mature horses and those with larger muscle mass, such as heavy-bodied warmbloods, and result in somewhat discipline-specific radiopharmaceutical uptake patterns.[62]

Positron Emission Tomography

Recently, successful incorporation of PET in equine imaging has been described.[63,64] A bone-specific radiotracer, ^{18}F-sodium fluoride (^{18}F-NaF), is absorbed into exposed hydroxyapatite crystal, and accurately quantifiable uptake is measured producing tomographic (3-dimensional [3D]) data over a period of 15 minutes (per area) approximately 45 minutes following radiotracer injection. This mechanism of uptake is similar to bone scintigraphy with ^{99m}Tc MDP, but produces superior images because of higher inherent spatial resolution, lack of superimposition of anatomic structures, and coregistration with cross-sectional modalities that provide morphologic information (CT, MRI). Currently, the main drawback of PET is the need for general anesthesia, particularly to limit radiation exposure of imaging personnel. Studies in both equine and human medicine have used PET to identify lesions in patients with localized pain that other modalities have failed to identify.[64,65]

Magnetic Resonance

Whole organ scoring using MR is considered the gold standard for joint evaluation in human medicine because it allows for evaluation of bone, cartilage, and periarticular tissues without the use of ionizing radiation.[66,67] MR is a cross-sectional (3D) imaging modality that maps signal from the relaxation of magnetically excited water and fat protons, which are manipulated with radiofrequency pulses and is the most complicated, nuanced, and time consuming of the available imaging modalities, in terms of both image acquisition and interpretation. The type, number, and timing of the pulses, called a sequence, determine the type of tissue that is highlighted in the image. Images are acquired in various planes, and with the exception of 3D sequences, must be obtained sequentially in multiple planes, leading to prolonged scan time relative to other modalities. Abnormal tissue will have altered signal reflective of its physiologic status, and interpretation is based on knowledge of normal tissue appearance on each sequence.

Bone detail is not as clearly visualized on MR because of the lower spatial resolution relative to CT, but MR provides superior contrast resolution and physiologic information that CT does not. The sequences used in equine musculoskeletal imaging are similar to those used in human medicine (eg, short tau inversion recover [STIR], fat-saturated T2-weighted fast spin echo), with emphasis on detection of high fluid signal within the subchondral and regional trabecular bone by marrow fat-suppression techniques because this high signal is associated with lameness, cartilage damage, and osseous cystlike lesion formation.[21,68–74] Historically, the terms "bone edema," "bone bruise," and "bone contusion" have been used to describe bone marrow with abnormally high fluid signal. However, numerous studies have demonstrated that the histologic composition of such lesions is variable and associated with different pathologic processes. Osteonecrosis, fat necrosis, fibrosis, edema, and hemorrhage can all result in high fluid signal, and thus, the more generic term "high fluid signal" is recommended.[75] Similar to other modalities, bone lesions on MR imaging often exhibit discipline-specific patterns.[9,26,68]

In human medicine, high intraosseous fluid signal can persist despite resolution of clinical signs.[76–78] Persistent high intraosseous fluid signal has also been demonstrated by Holowinski and colleagues,[79] in equine cases, but this may be site dependent and has not been thoroughly investigated in the horse. Some studies have demonstrated that the resolution of high fluid signal on MR is correlated with resolution of lameness.[70,79] Inconveniently, high intraosseous fluid signal can also be identified in sound horses, which may represent physiologic stress remodeling. The distal aspect of the middle phalanx tends to be overrepresented in this respect[80,81] (**Fig. 7**). Depending on the timing of imaging relative to the onset of lameness, initial MR examination may not reveal a cause of lameness, in which case recheck MRI may demonstrate high fluid signal several months after initial injury (**Fig. 8**).

Low-field magnets (<0.3 T) provide a highly accessible and relatively affordable means to evaluate distal limb musculoskeletal injury without the need for general anesthesia, which is particularly beneficial for the competitive sport horse. However, bone lesion identification is superior with high-field (>1.0 T) magnets because of the higher spatial resolution, signal-to-noise ratio, diagnostic confidence, and decreased motion artifact. Although false positives and negatives can occur at either field strengths, both are more common at lower-field strengths.[82–84]

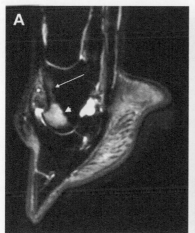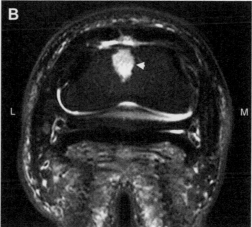

Fig. 7. Sagittal (*A*) and transverse (*B*) STIR images of the distal right forefoot of an 8-year-old warmblood equitation horse. The patient was presented for unilateral left forelimb lameness localized with palmar digital perineural analgesia that did not result in subsequent right forelimb lameness. Marked distal (*arrowhead*) and moderate proximal (*arrow*) high fluid signals are identified within the dorsal aspect of the right fore middle phalanx, which was attributed to physiologic stress remodeling. Distal interphalangeal joint effusion and synovial proliferation were also identified.

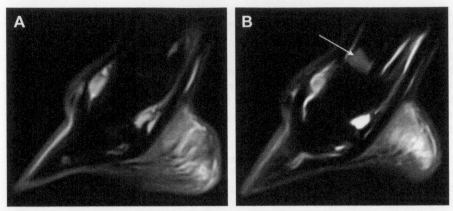

Fig. 8. (*A*) Sagittal STIR image of the left forefoot of a 10-year-old warmblood show jumper obtained 2 months after the onset of acute left forelimb lameness localized to the proximal interphalangeal joint. A cause for lameness referable to the proximal interphalangeal joint was not identified. Moderate distal interphalangeal joint effusion is present. (*B*) Recheck MR at 4 months due to persistent lameness localized to the proximal interphalangeal joint. Marked intraosseous fluid signal (*arrow*) is now identified within the dorsal, distal aspect of the proximal phalanx. The distal interphalangeal effusion has progressed.

Cartilage Imaging

Because subchondral bone and cartilage injury are intimately associated, a discussion of skeletal injury would be incomplete without at least a brief discussion of cartilage imaging. Injury to or degeneration of subchondral bone is commonly associated with regional cartilage abnormalities and vice versa (**Fig. 9**). Injury to either tissue can lead

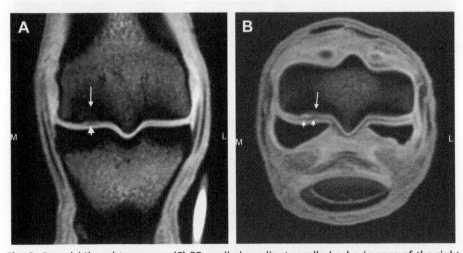

Fig. 9. Dorsal (*A*) and transverse (*B*) 3D spoiled gradient recalled echo images of the right metacarpophalangeal joint. Medial is to the left. Focal irregularity and altered signal intensity of the cartilage signal of the medial metacarpal condyle are identified (*arrowheads*). The adjacent subchondral bone exhibits heterogeneous hyperintense signal surrounded by hypointense trabecular bone (*arrow*). Subchondral bone thickening and trabecular hypointensity are also present within the proximomedial aspect of the proximal phalanx in (*A*).

to injury of the other, with subsequent development or progression of osteoarthritis. However, identification of cartilage damage remains a diagnostic challenge with no consensus on an ideal sequence for consistent and early identification, although spoiled gradient recalled echo sequences are commonly noted in both the human and the equine literature.[38,85] In human medicine, higher magnet field strength is associated with higher sensitivity, accuracy, and confidence scores for detecting cartilage injury.[39,40,86] Low-field magnets may identify articular cartilage damage in joints with relatively thick cartilage, such as the distal interphalangeal joint, but the diagnosis of articular cartilage damage on low-field MR is typically reliant on inference from adjacent subchondral bone damage.[87] Semiquantitative and quantitative measures to evaluate cartilage are also available, but are beyond the scope of this article.[41,42]

Computed Tomography

Computed tomography (CT) is a cross-sectional (3D) imaging modality that uses ionizing radiation to display morphologic information based on tissue radiodensity.[29,88] Data are acquired by measuring the degree of x-ray attenuation as an x-ray beam passes through tissues at different angles. Pixel grayscale values called CT numbers are then assigned based on the attenuation and are based on the average radiodensity of a small volume of tissue. In order to standardize CT numbers between various machines, the attenuation values are compared with the radiodensity of distilled water and referred to as Hounsfield units. Because the tissue data are acquired as a volume, images can be reconstructed in multiple planes following a single scan of the region of interest.

Similar to radiographs, evaluation of skeletal injury on CT consists of identification of secondary changes to bone, as evidenced by increased subchondral and trabecular attenuation (density), decreased attenuation of subchondral bone (eg, subchondral lysis, osseous cystlike lesions) that may or may not communicate with the articular surface or be surrounded by hyperattenuating bone, irregular subchondral margination, loss of normal trabecular pattern, free osseous fragments, periarticular new bone formation, and increased size and number of vascular channels. Evaluation of bone injury on CT has several advantages compared with radiographs, including lack of superimposition of anatomic structures and increased sensitivity to changes in bone density due to higher contrast resolution.[89–92] CT is considered the gold standard for evaluation of skeletal injury/trauma in humans, particularly in regions of complex anatomy, such as the skull, with numerous human and veterinary studies demonstrating benefits of improved diagnostic confidence and surgical planning due to its higher spatial resolution relative to MR.[92–95] Evaluation of bone density or attenuation can be evaluated both qualitatively and quantitatively using $K_2HPO_4^-$ (mg/mL) calibrated Hounsfield units and peripheral CT.[3,96–98] The main drawbacks of CT include a lack of information about bone physiology and relatively poor soft tissue contrast resolution, although the latter can be mitigated with intra-arterial contrast techniques.[99,100] Cartilage cannot be directly visualized with CT, but inferred using arthrography. Normal cartilage will create a smooth band of hypoattenuation with relatively uniform thickness between the hyperattenuating subchondral bone and contrast medium. Subtle changes in margination and shape of the contrast as well as loss of separation between subchondral bone and contrast material indicate cartilage thinning, fibrillation, and/or partial thickness defects.[101–103] Until recently, the need for general anesthesia and fixed annular scanner geometry was the major limiting factor in the routine use of CT the diagnosis of skeletal injury in sport horses.

Given the large amount of radiation typically used in conventional CT imaging, approximately 50 times the dose of a radiographic study, as well as the preponderance of scatter in all CT imaging, monitoring exposure of imaging personnel restraining horses for standing CT is of vital importance. Radiation safety measures should be implemented based on the principle of ALARA ("as low as reasonably achievable") with the stationing of horse handlers as far as possible from the radiation source.

Conventional (Fan Beam) Computed Tomography

Conventional CT uses a fan-shaped x-ray beam that rotates around a patient. A multi-element detector directly opposite and synced to the x-ray source records how the x-ray energy is attenuated as it passes through various portions of the patient. The detector provides superior contrast resolution because of the narrow beam geometry and absorption of scatter between the detector elements via thin lead septa. This information is then compiled to create volumetric data about the imaged tissue and is reconstructed as a set of contiguous 2D slices, typically in a transverse/axial plane. Both anisotropic and isotropic volume data can be acquired, although the latter typically requires a higher patient dose. The subject is advanced through the CT scanner while the tube and detector rapidly rotate. This helical acquisition allows for rapid data acquisition of large sections of the body in a relatively short period of time (eg, a 16-slice CT scanner can image a 40-cm area of interest in <30 seconds). The rapid scan time limits motion artifact. If present, motion is typically limited to a small portion of the study if the motion is transient. Fan beam CT is considered the gold standard for CT imaging.

Modifications to a conventional CT scanner has allowed for imaging of the standing equine head and cranial cervical spine.[98] A separate unit developed from a modified quantitative CT scanner was used to successfully image the distal limb, but was labor intensive and limited to tractable animals because of safety concerns.[99] More recently, a fan beam system with a relatively large gantry based on an airport security scanner (Asto CT, LLC, Madison, WI, USA) has been proposed to simultaneously image the distal forelimbs or distal hind limbs, although clinical case results and radiation safety data from this system are not yet available.

Cone Beam Computed Tomography

Introduced in human medicine in the early 2000s with worldwide availability beginning in the 2010s, cone beam CT is most commonly used in dental, breast, and extremity imaging.[104,105] Isotropic volume data are acquired from a high number of 2D x-ray projections that are acquired in a circular orbit around a region of interest. The images can be constructed in any plane, although the sagittal and dorsal planes tend to be of the highest diagnostic quality. Unlike conventional CT, cone beam CT is not limited by a fixed annulus geometry.

Image quality of cone beam CT is heavily influenced by scatter and motion. Many cone beam systems claim lower radiation doses relative to fan beam CT, but in order to image thick body parts and obtain image quality similar to that of fan beam systems, the patient dose is similar or sometimes greater with the cone beam system.[106,107] In addition, the issue of motion correction in cone beam CT is not a trivial one, because motion during any point in the scan will affect the image quality of the entire study. The issue of motion applies to macroscopic motion as well as imperceptible motion from breathing.

The use of cone beam CT for equine musculoskeletal imaging is in its infancy, but 2 systems are used routinely at several university and private practice hospitals to perform standing imaging in the horse. Both systems use proprietary reconstruction algorithms that use a combination of filtered back projection and iterative reconstruction.

One system (Pegaso CT; Epica, San Clemente, CA, USA) has a fixed annular geometry with a large gantry (120 cm), capable of imaging from the skull to the caudal cervical spine. Image acquisition takes 45 to 90 seconds. Imaging of the distal limb requires the horse to be placed in lateral recumbency under general anesthesia.

A second system (4DDI Equine; Equimagine, Holbrook, NY, USA) uses a high-output x-ray tube and large (43 cm × 43 cm) indirect flat panel detector mounted to synced car-manufacturing robotic arms (ABB Group, Zurich, Switzerland). This system is capable of imaging from the skull to the cervicothoracic junction as well as from the foot to the mid-radius and distal tibia in the standing horse rotating a minimum of 190° (180° + beam angle) around the region of interest. The system requires an elaborate motion correction system based on tracking of reflective markers affixed to the region of interest (Vicon, Oxford, UK) (**Fig. 10**). The lack of fixed geometry for this system gives more flexibility in the image acquisition, but path geometry is still limited by the combination of the shape of the equine body and robotic arms.

Standing cone beam CT has several significant limitations that are inherent to the technology, including a high degree of scatter, which leads to decreased contrast. Even with using high-contrast techniques (eg, low kilovolt peak), the images do not have the contrast resolution of conventional fan beam images. In addition to scatter, cone beam images are plagued with artifacts. Artifacts refer to structures visualized in the reconstructed data that are not truly present in the patient. Although the artifacts can be due to a variety of causes, most cone beam artifacts manifest as a streaklike appearance oriented along projection lines.[108] When acquired in the standing horse, even visually imperceptible motion renders the studies unreadable without motion correction (**Fig. 11**). Some investigators report that the spatial resolution of cone beam images is superior to fan beam. Although diagnostic value decreases with increasing slice thickness, the absolute slice thickness for ideal image interpretation and the clinical utility of achieving a slice thickness less than 0.625 mm is currently unknown.[106] Finally, the accuracy of measuring Hounsfield units for cone beam systems is variable and is best performed by direct measurement with a hydroxyapatite (or bone density equivalent) phantom compared with pixel grayscale values, as Hounsfield unit calculations based on effective energy calculations are inaccurate. For some systems, even the use of a known bone density phantom will produce inaccurate Hounsfield units because of system-dependent inherent nonuniformity of the reconstruction algorithm or nonuniformity due to artifacts.

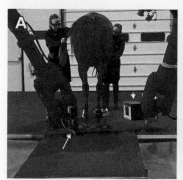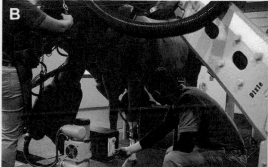

Fig. 10. Standing cone beam CT linked to robotic arms (*A*). The detector (*arrow*) is fixed to the robot on the left. The x-ray tube (*arrowhead*) is fixed to the robot on the right. A plastic cuff with reflective markers is present on the lateral aspect of the right metatarsophalangeal joint. In the upper right corner (*asterisk*), the motion correction cameras are visible. Close-up image (*B*) of the detector, motion correction cuff and markers, and the detector. (*Courtesy of* the New Bolton Center/University of Pennsylvania, Philadelphia, PA; with permission.)

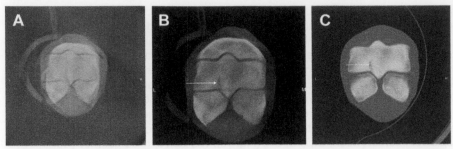

Fig. 11. Transverse standing cone beam CT of the metacarpophalangeal joint of a 3-year-old Thoroughbred racehorse with lameness localized to the fetlock region. No appreciable patient motion was noted during the scan. Lateral is to the left. The study was reconstructed without motion correction (*A*) and considered nondiagnostic; numerous streak artifacts are identified. Following reconstruction with motion correction, an incomplete unicortical fracture/fissure of the lateral parasagittal groove is identified with surrounding sclerosis (*arrow*) (*B*). Recumbent fan beam CT image (*C*) of the metacarpophalangeal joint reformatted at approximately the same level as in (*B*). Although the image quality is superior in (*C*), the lesion location, morphology, and size are similar between the 2 modalities. This lesion was not identified on survey radiographs, including the flexed dorsopalmar oblique projection.

Despite these limitations and the fact that cone beam images have lower contrast resolution compared with conventional CT, early data suggest that clinically significant lesions are detected on cone beam CT that are not apparent on radiographs. Clinically significant lesions have been demonstrated in both racehorses (see **Fig. 11**) and sport horses (**Fig. 12**), although the former are more frequently evaluated.

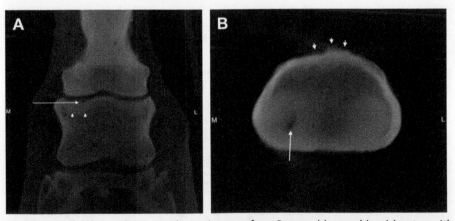

Fig. 12. Dorsal (*A*) standing cone beam image of an 8-year-old warmblood hunter with lameness localized to the proximal interphalangeal joint. Medial is to the right. Radiographs revealed only mild dorsal osteophytosis of the proximal interphalangeal joint. Standing CT demonstrated a proximomedial subchondral lesion (*arrow*) with hyperattenuating surrounding subchondral and trabecular bone (*arrowheads*). The corresponding transverse image (*B*) demonstrates the linear shape of the subchondral defect (*arrow*) and dorsal periarticular new bone formation (*arrowheads*). Medial is to the right; dorsal is to the top of the image.

SUMMARY

Knowledge of the pathophysiology of skeletal injury and imaging in the sport horse is rapidly advancing. Each imaging modality provides useful clinical information provided judicious patient selection. Although advanced imaging early in the course of lameness may be indicated in some cases, it should not be a replacement for more cost-effective and straightforward modalities, such as radiography. Interpretation of musculoskeletal injury for all imaging modalities requires consideration of the patient's presenting complaint, lameness grade, results of diagnostic analgesia, and correlation with other imaging modalities.

REFERENCES

1. Burr DB, Radin EL. Microfractures and microcracks in subchondral bone: are they relevant to osteoarthrosis? Rheum Dis Clin North Am 2003;29(4):675–85.
2. Radin EL, Parker HG, Pugh JW, et al. Response of joints to impact loading - III. Relationship between trabecular microfractures and cartilage degeneration. J Biomech 1973;6(1):51–7.
3. Loughridge AB, Hess AM, Parkin TD, et al. Qualitative assessment of bone density at the distal articulating surface of the third metacarpal in Thoroughbred racehorses with and without condylar fracture. Equine Vet J 2017;49(2):172–7.
4. Janes JG, Kennedy LA, Garrett KS, et al. Common lesions of the distal end of the third metacarpal/metatarsal bone in racehorse catastrophic breakdown injuries. J Vet Diagn Invest 2017;29(4):431–6.
5. Murray RC, Branch MV, Dyson SJ, et al. How does exercise intensity and type affect equine distal tarsal subchondral bone thickness? J Appl Physiol 2007; 102(6):2194–200.
6. Dyson S. Lameness and poor performance in the sport horse: dressage, show jumping and horse trials. J Equine Vet Sci 2002;22(4):145–50.
7. Singer ER, Barnes J, Saxby F, et al. Injuries in the event horse: training versus competition. Vet J 2008;175(1):76–81.
8. Murray RC, Dyson S, Tranquille C, et al. Association of type of sport and performance level with anatomical site of orthopaedic disease. Equine Vet J Suppl 2006;(36):411–6.
9. Olive J, Serraud N, Vila T, et al. Metacarpophalangeal joint injury patterns on magnetic resonance imaging: a comparison in racing Standardbreds and Thoroughbreds. Vet Radiol Ultrasound 2017;58(5):588–97.
10. Christensen SB. Osteoarthrosis. Changes of bone, cartilage and synovial membrane in relation to bone scintigraphy. Acta Orthop Scand Suppl 1985;214:1–43. Available at: http://www.ncbi.nlm.nih.gov/pubmed/3161266.
11. Norrdin RW, Kawcak CE, Capwell BA, et al. Subchondral bone failure in an equine model of overload arthrosis. Bone 1998;22(2):133–9.
12. Milner CE, Ferber R, Pollard CD, et al. Biomechanical factors associated with tibial stress fracture in female runners. Med Sci Sports Exerc 2006;38(2):323–8.
13. Dimock AN, Hoffman KD, Puchalski SM, et al. Humeral stress remodelling locations differ in Thoroughbred racehorses training and racing on dirt compared to synthetic racetrack surfaces. Equine Vet J 2013;45(2):176–81.
14. Ramzan PHL, Newton JR, Shepherd MC, et al. The application of a scintigraphic grading system to equine tibial stress fractures: 42 cases. Equine Vet J 2003; 35(4):382–8.

15. Vallance SA, Entwistle RC, Hitchens PL, et al. Case-control study of high-speed exercise history of Thoroughbred and Quarter Horse racehorses that died related to a complete scapular fracture. Equine Vet J 2013;45(3):284–92.

16. Riggs CM. Fractures - a preventable hazard of racing Thoroughbreds? Vet J 2002;163(1):19–29.

17. Murray RC, Vedi S, Birch HL, et al. Subchondral bone thickness, hardness and remodelling are influenced by short-term exercise in a site-specific manner. J Orthop Res 2001;19(6):1035–42.

18. Boyde A, Firth EC. Musculoskeletal responses of 2-year-old Thoroughbred horses to early training. 8. Quantitative back-scattered electron scanning electron microscopy and confocal fluorescence microscopy of the epiphysis of the third metacarpal bone. N Z Vet J 2005;53(2):123–32.

19. Branch MV, Murray RC, Dyson SJ, et al. Is there a characteristic distal tarsal subchondral bone plate thickness pattern in horses with no history of hindlimb lameness? Equine Vet J 2005;37(5):450–5.

20. Holmes JM, Mirams M, Mackie EJ, et al. Thoroughbred horses in race training have lower levels of subchondral bone remodelling in highly loaded regions of the distal metacarpus compared to horses resting from training. Vet J 2014;202(3):443–7.

21. Powell SE, Ramzan PHL, Head MJ, et al. Standing magnetic resonance imaging detection of bone marrow oedema-type signal pattern associated with subcarpal pain in 8 racehorses: a prospective study. Equine Vet J 2010;42(1):10–7.

22. Kawcak CE, McIlwraith CW, Norrdin RW, et al. Clinical effects of exercise on subchondral bone of carpal and metacarpophalangeal joints in horses. Am J Vet Res 2000;61(10):1252–8.

23. Stock K, Distl O. Genetic correlations between conformation traits and radiographic findings in the limbs of German Warmblood riding horses. Genet Sel Evol 2006;38(6):657.

24. Jacklin BD, Wright IM. Frequency distributions of 174 fractures of the distal condyles of the third metacarpal and metatarsal bones in 167 Thoroughbred racehorses (1999-2009). Equine Vet J 2012;44(6):707–13.

25. Tranquille CA, Parkin TDH, Murray RC. Magnetic resonance imaging-detected adaptation and pathology in the distal condyles of the third metacarpus, associated with lateral condylar fracture in Thoroughbred racehorses. Equine Vet J 2012;44(6):699–706.

26. Gray SN, Spriet M, Garcia TC, et al. Preexisting lesions associated with complete diaphyseal fractures of the third metacarpal bone in 12 Thoroughbred racehorses. J Vet Diagn Investig 2017;29(4):437–41.

27. Ramzan PHL, Palmer L, Powell SE. Unicortical condylar fracture of the Thoroughbred fetlock: 45 cases (2006-2013). Equine Vet J 2015;47(6):680–3.

28. Tranquille CA, Murray RC, Parkin TDH. Can we use subchondral bone thickness on high-field magnetic resonance images to identify Thoroughbred racehorses at risk of catastrophic lateral condylar fracture? Equine Vet J 2017;49(2):167–71.

29. Hounsfield GN. Computerized transverse axial scanning (tomography): I. Description of system. Br J Radiol 1973;46(552):1016–22.

30. Francis MD, Ferguson DL, Tofe AJ, et al. Comparative evaluation of three diphosphonates: in vitro adsorption (C- 14 labeled) and in vivo osteogenic uptake (Tc-99m complexed). J Nucl Med 1980;21(12):1185–9. Available at: http://www.ncbi.nlm.nih.gov/pubmed/6449567.

31. Harris WH, Heaney RP. Skeletal renewal and metabolic bone disease. N Engl J Med 1969;280(4):193–202.

32. Wong KK, Piert M. Dynamic bone imaging with 99mTc-labeled diphosphonates and 18F-NaF: mechanisms and applications. J Nucl Med 2013;54(4):590–9.
33. Lamb CR, Koblik PD. Scintigraphic evaluation of skeletal disease and its application to the horse. Vet Radiol 1988;29(1):16–27.
34. Walker JE, Lewis CW, MacLeay JM, et al. Assessment of subchondral bone mineral density in equine metacarpophalangeal and stifle joints. Biomed Sci Instrum 2004;40:272–6.
35. Weekes JS, Murray RC, Dyson SJ. Scintigraphic evaluation of the proximal metacarpal and metatarsal regions in clinically sound horses. Vet Radiol Ultrasound 2006;47(4):409–16.
36. Olive J, D'Anjou MA, Alexander K, et al. Correlation of signal attenuation-based quantitative magnetic resonance imaging with quantitative computed tomographic measurements of subchondral bone mineral density in metacarpophalangeal joints of horses. Am J Vet Res 2010;71(4):412–20.
37. Nelson BB, Kawcak CE, Goodrich LR, et al. Comparison between computed tomographic arthrography, radiography, ultrasonography, and arthroscopy for the diagnosis of femorotibial joint disease in western performance horses. Vet Radiol Ultrasound 2016;57(4):387–402.
38. Olive J, D'Anjou MA, Girard C, et al. Fat-suppressed spoiled gradient-recalled imaging of equine metacarpophalangeal articular cartilage. Vet Radiol Ultrasound 2010;51(2):107–15.
39. Wong S, Steinbach L, Zhao J, et al. Comparative study of imaging at 3.0 T versus 1.5 T of the knee. Skeletal Radiol 2009;38(8):761–9.
40. Kijowski R, Blankenbaker DG, Davis KW, et al. Comparison of 1.5- and 3.0-T MR imaging for evaluating the articular cartilage of the knee joint. Radiology 2009; 250(3):839–48.
41. Carstens A, Kirberger RM, Dahlberg LE, et al. Validation of delayed gadolinium-enhanced magnetic resonance imaging of cartilage and T2 mapping for quantifying distal metacarpus/metatarsus cartilage thickness in thoroughbred racehorses. Vet Radiol Ultrasound 2013;54(2):139–48.
42. Carstens A, Kirberger RM, Velleman M, et al. Feasibility for mapping cartilage T1 relaxation times in the distal metacarpus3/metatarsus3 of thoroughbred racehorses using delayed gadolinium-enhanced magnetic resonance imaging of cartilage (DGEMRIC): normal cadaver study. Vet Radiol Ultrasound 2013; 54(4):365–72.
43. Gold GE, Chen CA, Koo S, et al. Recent advances in MRI of articular cartilage. Am J Roentgenol 2009;193(3):628–38.
44. Dyson S, Murray R, Schramme M, et al. Current concepts of navicular disease. Equine Vet Educ 2011;23(1):27–39.
45. Selberg K, Ross M. Advances in nuclear medicine. Vet Clin North Am Equine Pract 2012;28(3):527–38.
46. Eksell P, Carlsson S, Lord P, et al. Effects of different colour displays on detectability of a phantom lesion in an equine scintigram. Acta Universitatis Agriculturae Suecicae, Veterinaria 76, p. 1–19
47. Archer DC, Boswell JC, Voute LC, et al. Skeletal scintigraphy in the horse: current indications and validity as a diagnostic test. Vet J 2007;173(1):33–46.
48. Kanishi D. 99mTc-MDP accumulation mechanisms in bone. Oral Surg Oral Med Oral Pathol 1993;75(2):239–46. Available at: http://www.ncbi.nlm.nih.gov/pubmed/8381217. Accessed April 6, 2018.

49. Einhorn TA, Vigorita VJ, Aaron A. Localization of technetium-99m methylene diphosphonate in bone using microautoradiography. J Orthop Res 1986;4(2): 180–7.

50. Weekes JS, Murray RC, Dyson SJ. Scintigraphic evaluation of metacarpophalangeal and metatarsophalangeal joints in clinically sound horses. Vet Radiol Ultrasound 2004;45(1):85–90.

51. Didierlaurent D, Contremoulins V, Denoix J-M, et al. Scintigraphic pattern of uptake of 99mTechnetium by the cervical vertebrae of sound horses. Vet Rec 2009; 164(26):809–13.

52. Dyson S, Murray R, Branch M, et al. The sacroiliac joints: evaluation using nuclear scintigraphy. Part 1: the normal horse. Equine Vet J 2003;35(3):226–32. Available at: https://www.scopus.com/record/display.uri?eid=2-s2.0-0141889525&origin= inward&txGid=9a724251e79ee96d5b63f25ffc81ad51. Accessed April 6, 2018.

53. Dyson S, McNie K, Weekes J, et al. Scintigraphic evaluation of the stifle in normal horses and horses with forelimb lameness. Vet Radiol Ultrasound 2007;48(4):378–82.

54. Erichsen C, Eksell P, Roethlisberger Holm K, et al. Relationship between scintigraphic and radiographic evaluations of spinous processes in the thoracolumbar spine in riding horses without clinical signs of back problems. Equine Vet J 2004;36(6):458–65. Available at: https://www.scopus.com/record/display.uri? eid=2-s2.0-4544328801&origin=inward&txGid=38879eb195659d4d0023606708b e8330. Accessed April 6, 2018.

55. Erichsen C, Eksell P, Widstrom C, et al. Scintigraphy of the sacroiliac joint region in asymptomatic riding horses: scintigraphic appearance and evaluation of method. Vet Radiol Ultrasound 2003;44(6):699–706.

56. Erichsen C, Eksell P, Widstrom C, et al. Scintigraphic evaluation of the thoracic spine in the asymptomatic riding horse. Vet Radiol Ultrasound 2003;44(3):330–8.

57. Murray RC, Dyson SJ, Weekes JS, et al. Nuclear scintigraphic evaluation of the distal tarsal region in normal horses. Vet Radiol Ultrasound 2004;45(4):345–51.

58. Murray RC, Dyson SJ, Weekes JOS, et al. Scintigraphic evaluation of the distal tarsal region in horses with distal tarsal pain. Vet Radiol Ultrasound 2005;46(2): 171–8.

59. Graham S, Solano M, Sutherland-Smith J, et al. Diagnostic sensitivity of bone scintigraphy for equine stifle disorders. Vet Radiol Ultrasound 2015;56(1): 96–102.

60. Squire KRE, Fessler JF, Cantwell HD, et al. Enlarging bilateral femoral condylar bone cysts without scintigraphic uptake in a yearling foal. Vet Radiol Ultrasound 1992;33(2):109–13.

61. Dyson S. Musculoskeletal scintigraphy of the equine athlete. Semin Nucl Med 2014;44(1):4–14.

62. Bailey REA, Dyson SJ, Parkin TDH. Focal increased radiopharmaceutical uptake in the dorsoproximal diaphyseal region of the equine proximal phalanx. Vet Radiol Ultrasound 2007;48(5):460–6.

63. Spriet M, Espinosa P, Kyme AZ, et al. Positron emission tomography of the equine distal limb: exploratory study. Vet Radiol Ultrasound 2016;57(6):630–8.

64. Spriet M, Espinosa P, Kyme AZ, et al. 18F-sodium fluoride positron emission tomography of the equine distal limb: exploratory study in three horses. Equine Vet J 2018;50(1):125–32.

65. Draper CE, Fredericson M, Gold GE, et al. Patients with patellofemoral pain exhibit elevated bone metabolic activity at the patellofemoral joint. J Orthop Res 2012;30(2):209–13.

66. Peterfy CG, Gold G, Eckstein F, et al. MRI protocols for whole-organ assessment of the knee in osteoarthritis. Osteoarthr Cartil 2006;14(suppl 1):95–111.
67. Hunter DJ, Lo GH, Gale D, et al. The reliability of a new scoring system for knee osteoarthritis MRI and the validity of bone marrow lesion assessment: BLOKS (Boston–Leeds Osteoarthritis Knee Score). Ann Rheum Dis 2008;67(2):206–11.
68. Gold SJ, Werpy NM, Gutierrez-Nibeyro SD. Injuries of the sagittal groove of the proximal phalanx in warmblood horses detected with low-field magnetic resonance imaging: 19 cases (2007–2016). Vet Radiol Ultrasound 2017;58(3): 344–53.
69. Biggi M, Zani DD, De Zani D, et al. Magnetic resonance imaging findings of bone marrow lesions in the equine distal tarsus. Equine Vet Educ 2012;24(5): 236–41.
70. Dyson S, Nagy A, Murray R. Clinical and diagnostic imaging findings in horses with subchondral bone trauma of the sagittal groove of the proximal phalanx. Vet Radiol Ultrasound 2011;52(6):596–604.
71. Powell SE. Low-field standing magnetic resonance imaging findings of the metacarpo/metatarsophalangeal joint of racing Thoroughbreds with lameness localised to the region: a retrospective study of 131 horses. Equine Vet J 2012;44(2):169–77.
72. Małkiewicz A, Dziedzic M. Bone marrow reconversion - imaging of physiological changes in bone marrow. Pol J Radiol 2012;77(4):45–50.
73. Carrino JA, Blum J, Parellada JA, et al. MRI of bone marrow edema-like signal in the pathogenesis of subchondral cysts. Osteoarthr Cartil 2006;14(10):1081–5.
74. Vanhoenacker FM, Snoeckx A. Bone marrow edema in sports: general concepts. Eur J Radiol 2007;62(1):6–15.
75. Smith MRW, Kawcak CE, Mcilwraith CW. Science in brief: report on the Havemeyer Foundation workshop on subchondral bone problems in the equine athlete. Equine Vet J 2016;48(1):6–8.
76. Boks SS, Vroegindeweij D, Koes BW, et al. Follow-up of occult bone lesions detected at MR imaging: systematic review. Radiology 2006;238(3):853–62.
77. Dobrindt O, Hoffmeyer B, Ruf J, et al. Estimation of return-to-sports-time for athletes with stress fracture - an approach combining risk level of fracture site with severity based on imaging. BMC Musculoskelet Disord 2012;13:139.
78. Chiba M, Kumagai M, Fukui N, et al. The relationship of bone marrow edema pattern in the mandibular condyle with joint pain in patients with temporomandibular joint disorders: longitudinal study with MR imaging. Int J Oral Maxillofac Surg 2006;35(1):55–9.
79. Holowinski M, Judy C, Saveraid T, et al. Resolution of lesions on stir images is associated with improved lameness status in horses. Vet Radiol Ultrasound 2010;51(5):479–84.
80. Werpy NM. Recheck magnetic resonance imaging examinations for evaluation of musculoskeletal injury. Vet Clin North Am - Equine Pract 2012;28(3):659–80.
81. Olive J, Mair TS, Charles B. Use of standing low-field magnetic resonance imaging to diagnose middle phalanx bone marrow lesions in horses. Equine Vet Educ 2009;21(3):116–23.
82. Werpy NM, Ho CP, Pease AP, et al. The effect of sequence selection and field strength on detection of osteochondral defects in the metacarpophalangeal joint. Vet Radiol Ultrasound 2011;52(2):154–60.
83. Smith MA, Dyson SJ, Murray RC. The appearance of the equine metacarpophalangeal region on high-field vs. standing low-field magnetic resonance imaging. Vet Radiol Ultrasound 2011;52(1):61–70.

84. Murray RC, Mair TS, Sherlock CE, et al. Comparison of high-field and low-field magnetic resonance images of cadaver limbs of horses. Vet Rec 2009;165(10): 281–8.
85. Choi JA, Gold GE. MR imaging of articular cartilage physiology. Magn Reson Imaging Clin N Am 2011;19(2):249–82.
86. De Maeseneer M, Shahabpour M, Van Roy P, et al. MRI of cartilage and subchondral bone injury. A pictorial review. JBR-BTR 2008;91(1):6–13. Available at: http://www.ncbi.nlm.nih.gov/pubmed/18447123.
87. Olive J. Distal interphalangeal articular cartilage assessment using low-field magnetic resonance imaging. Vet Radiol Ultrasound 2010;51(3):259–66.
88. Ambrose J. Computerized transverse axial scanning (tomography): II. Clinical application. Br J Radiol 1973;46(552):1023–47.
89. Crijns CP, Martens A, Bergman HJ, et al. Intramodality and intermodality agreement in radiography and computed tomography of equine distal limb fractures. Equine Vet J 2014;46(1):92–6.
90. Rose PL, Seeherman H, O'Callaghan M. Computed tomographic evaluation of comminuted middle phalangeal fractures in the horse. Vet Radiol Ultrasound 1997;38(6):424–9.
91. Morgan JW, Santschi EM, Zekas LJ, et al. Comparison of radiography and computed tomography to evaluate metacarpo/metatarsophalangeal joint pathology of paired limbs of thoroughbred racehorses with severe condylar fracture. Vet Surg 2006;35(7):611–7.
92. Crijns CP, Weller R, Vlaminck L, et al. Comparison between radiography and computed tomography for diagnosis of equine skull fractures. Equine Vet Educ 2017. https://doi.org/10.1111/eve.12863.
93. Marinaro J, Crandall CS, Doezema D. Computed tomography of the head as a screening examination for facial fractures. Am J Emerg Med 2007;25(6):616–9.
94. Getman LM, Davidson EJ, Ross MW, et al. Computed tomography or magnetic resonance imaging-assisted partial hoof wall resection for keratoma removal. Vet Surg 2011;40(6):708–14.
95. Gasiorowski JC, Richardson DW. Clinical use of computed tomography and surface markers to assist internal fixation within the equine hoof. Vet Surg 2015; 44(2):214–22.
96. Olive J, D'anjou MA, Alexander K, et al. Comparison of magnetic resonance imaging, computed tomography, and radiography for assessment of noncartilaginous changes in equine metacarpophalangeal osteoarthritis. Vet Radiol Ultrasound 2010;51(3):267–79.
97. Bogers SH, Rogers CW, Bolwell C, et al. Quantitative comparison of bone mineral density characteristics of the distal epiphysis of third metacarpal bones from Thoroughbred racehorses with or without condylar fracture. Am J Vet Res 2016;77(1):32–8.
98. Bogers SH, Rogers CW, Bolwell CF, et al. Impact of race training on volumetric bone mineral density and its spatial distribution in the distal epiphysis of the third metatarsal bone of 2-year-old horses. Vet J 2014;201(3):353–8.
99. Puchalski SM, Galuppo LD, Hornof WJ, et al. Intraarterial contrast-enhanced computed tomography of the equine distal extremity. Vet Radiol Ultrasound 2007;48(1):21–9.
100. Puchalski SM. Advances in equine computed tomography and use of contrast media. Vet Clin North Am - Equine Pract 2012;28(3):563–81.
101. Valdés-Martínez A. Computed tomographic arthrography of the equine stifle joint. Vet Clin North Am - Equine Pract 2012;28(3):583–98.

102. Powell SE. Standing computed tomography (CT) of the equine head. Proc Am Coll Vet Surg 2011;57:67–8.
103. Desbrosse FG, Vandeweerd JMEF, Perrin RAR, et al. A technique for computed tomography (CT) of the foot in the standing horse. Equine Vet Educ 2008;20(2): 93–8.
104. Kiljunen T, Kaasalainen T, Suomalainen A, et al. Dental cone beam CT: a review. Phys Med 2015;31(8):844–60.
105. Berris T, Gupta R, Rehani MM. Radiation dose from cone-beam CT in neuroradiology applications. Am J Roentgenol 2013;200(4):755–61.
106. Lechuga L, Weidlich GA. Cone beam CT vs. fan beam CT: cone beam CT vs. fan beam CT: a comparison of image quality and dose delivered between two differing CT imaging modalities. Cureus 2016;8(9):e778.
107. Kan MWK, Leung LHT, Wong W, et al. Radiation dose from cone beam computed tomography for image-guided radiation therapy. Int J Radiat Oncol Biol Phys 2008;70(1):272–9.
108. Schulze R, Heil U, Groß D, et al. Artefacts in CBCT: a review. Dentomaxillofac Radiol 2011;40(5):265–73.

Diagnosis of Soft Tissue Injury in the Sport Horse

Kirstin A. Bubeck, DrMedVet[a],*, Stacie Aarsvold, DVM[b]

KEYWORDS

- Soft tissue injury • Horse • Ultrasound • MRI

KEY POINTS

- Soft tissue injuries are common in sport horses and due to the long lay-up period, it is important to have an accurate diagnosis.
- Ultrasonographic evaluation is mainly used in horses to evaluate soft tissue injuries, and special techniques can help further characterize the severity and duration of injury.
- MRI has recently become more available for diagnosis of soft tissue injury, and it is important for the equine practitioner to understand basic principles as well as in what situations MRI can provide additional valuable information.
- Contrast computed tomography may give additional information about soft tissue injuries in the equine foot and distal limb in case MRI is not available.
- MRI and computed tomography can add additional information to ultrasonography, given the ability to evaluate the internal bone structure and structures within the hoof capsule.

INTRODUCTION

Soft tissue injuries are a common cause of lameness in the sport horse. Because the recovery time from soft tissue injuries is in most cases more than 6 to 12 months, and in most cases results in a certain loss of muscle mass and conditioning, it is important that the diagnosis is accurate. The clinical examination, results of diagnostic analgesia, and diagnostic imaging must be correlated to determine the clinical significance of each lesion. With portable ultrasound machines becoming more powerful and more affordable, a wide range of examinations can be done in the field. Depending on the lesion, MRI can be used as a second imaging modality, as it has inherently high contrast resolution allowing for detection of lesions within soft tissue structures, as

Disclosure Statement: The authors have no relationship with a commercial company that has a direct financial interest in subject matter or materials discussed in article or with a company making a competing product.

[a] Department of Clinical Sciences, Cummings School of Veterinary Medicine, Tufts University, 200 Westboro Road, North Grafton, MA 01536, USA; [b] Puchalski Equine Diagnostic Imaging, 911 Mustang Court, Petaluma, CA 94954, USA
* Corresponding author.
E-mail address: kirstin.bubeck@tufts.edu

well as differentiation of adjacent soft tissue structures from one another, and the cross-sectional nature of MRI is unaffected by surrounding structures. As such, it is particularly useful for imaging the soft tissues within the hoof capsule that cannot be evaluated with ultrasound and the area of the proximal suspensory where smaller lesions can be missed on ultrasonographic examination.

CLINICAL EXAMINATION AND DIAGNOSTIC ANALGESIA

During clinical evaluation, certain information can give the clinician hints of soft tissue injury.

1. *History*: Lameness is reported to improve with rest, but worsens again with exercise. In some instances (superficial digital flexor tendon [SDFT] lesion, suspensory branch injury, or inferior check ligament injury), lameness can resolve quickly, but the underlying soft tissue injury may get worse with continued exercise.
2. *Visual examination*: Soft tissue injury may be characterized by visual swelling or asymmetry between corresponding limbs.
3. *Palpation*: Soft tissue swelling might be felt in acute cases of soft tissue injury and if the injured structure is superficial enough. Focal pain to palpation and increased heat can be noted as signs of inflammation, but their absence will not exclude soft tissue injury. Injury of the distal sesamoidean ligaments, impar ligament, proximal suspensory ligament, or collateral ligaments may not be identified with palpation.
4. *Examination during motion*: Lameness caused by soft tissue injury is often more pronounced when the horse is worked on soft ground versus on harder ground. Flexion tests on the contralateral limb might increase the lameness on the affected limb due to increased weight bearing and can be seen in horses with deep digital flexor tendon (DDFT) lesions.[1] Lower and upper limb flexion tests may both be positive if the soft tissue structure spans over a longer area, for example, suspensory ligament. In the hind limb, upper or lower limb flexion test can be falsely positive due the reciprocal apparatus.
5. *Diagnostic analgesia*: To confirm the location of injury, diagnostic analgesia is an important step during the examination process. Ligamentous injury in close proximity to the joint (eg, collateral ligaments, impar ligament, distal aspect of suspensory branches) will be desensitized by intra-articular diagnostic analgesia. This should be taken in consideration when radiographs are within normal limits. In some cases, it is beneficial to perform diagnostic analgesia after ultrasonographic evaluation to avoid air shadow (reverberation) artifacts (eg, proximal suspensory ligament). In horses with multiple injuries to soft tissue and/or bone, diagnostic analgesia also can be used to further weigh the significance of diagnostic imaging findings.

ULTRASONOGRAPHIC EXAMINATION

Ultrasonographic examination is a very effective method to diagnose soft tissue injuries in the equine patient. Although MRI is considered the gold standard for the diagnosis of soft tissue lesions, the ultrasonographic examination can provide important information of most anatomic regions where ultrasound can penetrate the tissues and in regions not amendable to MRI because of the size limitations. In addition, radiographic evaluation and nuclear scintigraphy are useful to evaluation bony involvement at the origin and insertion of soft tissue.

The combination of clinical examination, diagnostic analgesia, and ultrasonographic examination will give the equine practitioner valuable insight of soft tissue injuries. Combining baseline examination with recheck ultrasonographic examinations can be used to monitor progressive healing of soft tissue injuries and regression or reinjury in case of overuse.

Equipment and Patient Preparation

For the evaluation of soft tissue injuries in the equine patient, the necessary equipment depends on the structure size and depth. For most soft tissue structures, a linear transducer with a frequency of 10 to 13 MHz is sufficient. For deeper and larger structures, for example, the coxofemoral joint or areas of the biceps tendon, a curvilinear transducer with a frequency of 2.5 to 5.0 MHz will be necessary. Curvilinear microconvex transducers will allow the ultrasonographer to evaluate smaller structures in curved regions (eg, lower pastern region or the origin of the medial and lateral collateral ligament of the femoro-tibial joint).

Patient preparation is one key aspect during ultrasonography. The quality of ultrasonographic images is dependent on contact between the transducer and the horse's skin. The best image quality is achieved by clipping the area with a #40 blade and cleaning the skin with water and soap before applying ultrasound gel. For transcuneal ultrasound, it is best to soak the hoof for 30 minutes or longer after removing a superficial horn layer from the frog and preparing a flattened surface for even placement of the transducer. Depending on the temperament of the horse, light sedation can facilitate the examination.

How to Examine Soft Tissue Injuries

Tendon and ligament structures are best imaged in transverse and longitudinal planes. In the transverse plane, the cross-sectional area can be measured and compared with the contralateral limb (**Fig. 1**) or compared with known, normal breed-dependent sizes. During reevaluation, this measurement can be repeated at the same location and compared. If a lesion is present, the cross-sectional area of the lesion should be measured as well as a baseline value for further comparison. The longitudinal view is evaluated for fiber pattern and the lesion's length can be measured within this view. For archiving images, split screens with transverse and longitudinal views in one image can be very valuable.

To ensure comparable images during reevaluation of a soft tissue injury, the metatarsus and metacarpal region is divided in zones (each 4-cm wide), or the distance to the accessory carpal bone or to the point of the hock can be noted. This will allow reproduction of the same image during reevaluation examination and accurate comparison of images for cross-sectional area and lesion size.

A standoff pad can facilitate examination of superficial structures or structures in areas with uneven bony surfaces. The standoff pad provides good contact between skin and transducer, but can in some situations interfere with transducer handling. It is useful to produce images with and without standoff pad from the same location and interpret both images for best results.

Type of Lesions

Acute

Acute lesions are characterized by increase of ligament/tendon cross-section, reduction of echogenicity, and loss of normal striated fiber pattern, and are often poorly defined and heterogeneous. Because of similar echogenicity of intact fibers and accumulation of hemorrhage and debris, the lesion might be difficult to visualize in the early acute stage of injury.

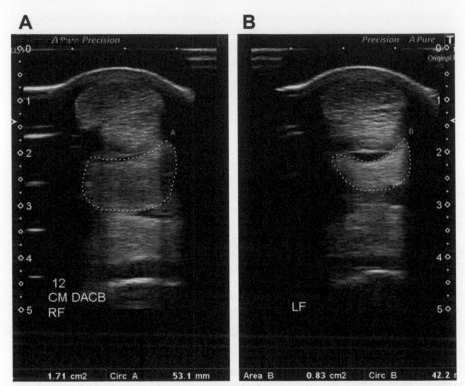

Fig. 1. Comparison of the transverse view between right (*A*) and left (*B*) front limb at 12 cm distal to the accessory carpal bone. The accessory ligament of the DDFT is increased in size and shows reduced echogenicity in image (*A*; dotted line) versus image (*B*; dotted line).

Subacute

Subacute lesions show increased hypoechogenicity and are better defined than acute lesions due to resorption of blood and ingrowing granulation tissue (**Fig. 2**).

Chronic

Chronic lesions can be of variable appearance and can be subtle. Often the cross-sectional area is diffusely enlarged, and the lesion shows mixed echogenicity (hypoechoic, normoechoic, and hyperechoic). On the longitudinal plane, the fiber pattern is missing striations and the parenchymal pattern is coarser. Mineralization within the tissue might be seen as small hyperechoic areas with an associated acoustic shadow.

Chronic active

Chronic active lesions are variable and can range from a diffuse hypoechogenic area superimposed on scar tissue or discrete hypoechoic regions in other parts of the tendon or ligament, often in close proximity to the previous injury (**Fig. 3**).

Core lesions

Core lesions are hypoechoic lesions in the core of the tendon or ligament.

Border lesions

Border lesions are hypoechoic lesions at the periphery, which often include the paratenon and may alter the shape of the tendon or ligament.

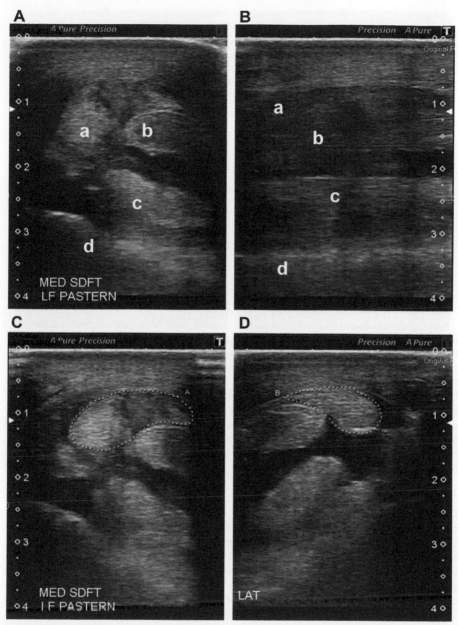

Fig. 2. Subacute injury to the medial branch of the SDFT at the level of mid first phalanx (P1B). (*A*) Transverse view, (*B*) longitudinal view (*C, D*) comparison of injured medial branch of the SDFT (*C*, dotted line) versus normal lateral branch of SDFT (*D*, dotted line) in transverse view.[a], SDFT; [b], DDFT; [c], DSSL; [d], P1.

When to Perform the Ultrasonographic Examination

Ultrasonographic examination of an acute soft tissue injury is best performed approximately 48 to 72 hours after the incident. At this time, peritendinous edema is reduced and will not obscure the ultrasonographic image. A second baseline ultrasound should

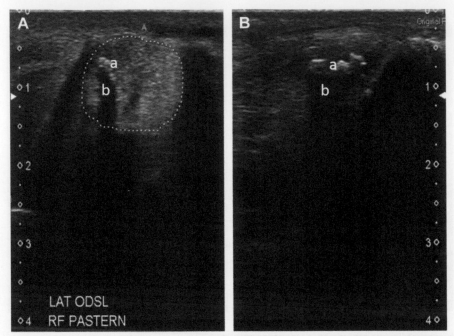

Fig. 3. Transverse (*A*) and longitudinal (*B*) views of a chronic active lesion in the lateral oblique distal sesamoidean ligament (dotted line) of the pastern. [a] Hyperechoic mineralization, [b] casting shadow due to tissue mineralization.

be performed approximately 3 weeks from injury to visualize the full extent of the injury. In the acute inflammatory phase, enzymatic processes can lead to progression of the tendon or ligament damage. This process should have resolved at 2 to 3 weeks from injury with rest and anti-inflammatory management. Hypoechoic areas at 3 weeks from injury reflect fiber bundle disruption because edema and hemorrhage should have resolved by this time.[2]

Ultrasonographic Reevaluation

During reevaluation of a soft tissue lesion, it is important to evaluate an image produced at the same location as during the previous examination. Progression of healing is seen as an increase in echogenicity, increase of parallel fiber pattern, and reduction of cross-sectional area (CSA) (**Fig. 4**). Often an increase in echogenicity is seen before improvement of fiber pattern. Therefore, reexamination of the lesion in a longitudinal view is important. During reevaluation, the tendon/ligament CSA should stay stable or decrease over time. A >10% increase of CSA at any level compared with the previous examination indicates that the current exercise level is too high. A delay in realignment of fibers should caution the clinician, and the increase of exercise level should be more conservative to give the scar tissue more time to remodel and to prevent reinjury.[2,3] Ultrasonographic reevaluation is performed at 6-week to 12-week intervals or before any increase in exercise level.

Special Ultrasonographic Techniques

Angle contrast ultrasonography

For ultrasonographic evaluation of the front and hind limb suspensory ligament, angle contrast ultrasonography has been used as an additional technique to further assess

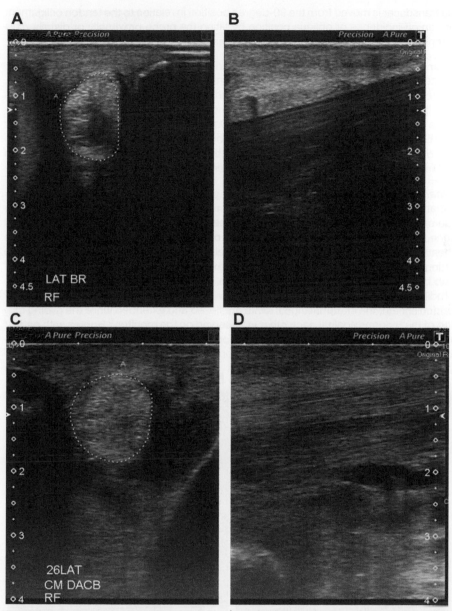

Fig. 4. Reevaluation of the lateral suspensory branch of the right front limb at 26 cm distal to the accessory carpal bone in transverse (*A, C*) and longitudinal (*B, D*) view. (*A, B*) Subacute injury of 3-week duration; (*C, D*) reevaluation after 15 months from injury.

the different tissue components of this structure. It has been shown[4–7] that angle contrast ultrasonography results in transverse images of the suspensory ligament similar to images seen on MRI examinations. This allows the examiner to differentiate between different tissues (ligamentous fibers, fat, muscle). In addition, the borders of soft tissue structures can be easier identified with this technique. This technique also can highlight poorly organized scar tissue.[2] The examination is performed in the transverse plane and the transducer is moved from the 90-degree position in relation to the tendon or ligament into an off-incidence or oblique position by tilting the probe proximally or distally. This technique can be performed on the weight-bearing or non–weight-bearing limb.

Color Doppler ultrasonography to evaluate neovascularization

For color Doppler ultrasonography, the tendons are examined in a non–weight-bearing, relaxed position to avoid any mechanical occlusion of the vessels. The transducer is kept in place for approximately 30 seconds and the tendon can be examined in a transverse and longitudinal plane. Low-flow color Doppler without standoff pad is used. No or very limited blood flow is seen in normal tendons. After injury, increased blood flow can be noted. This should subside at 3 to 6 months from injury. If increased blood flow is visible at a later date during the healing process, reinjury has likely occurred[2,8] (**Fig. 5**).

Dynamic ultrasonography

Dynamic sonography can be used to further investigate for adhesions between soft tissue structures and a bony exostosis of the second and fourth metacarpal/metatarsal bone, the SDFT, and the accessory ligament of the DDFT or structures within a tendon sheath. For this technique, the front limb is held in flexed position and stabilized on the sitting ultrasonographer's leg. For hind limb examination, an assistant flexes the distal limb by lifting the limb at the level of the tibia. With the linear probe placed in the longitudinal direction onto the area of interest, for example, flexor tendons within the distal tendon sheath, the interphalangeal joints are flexed and extended while the gliding motion of the tendons against each other is observed on the monitor.[9] Horses with palmar or plantar annular ligament desmitis were found to have restricted gliding motion between the SDFT and the annular ligament on pretenoscopic sonographic evaluation.[9]

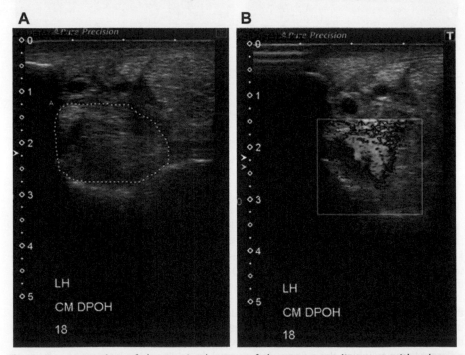

Fig. 5. Transverse view of the proximal aspect of the suspensory ligament with subacute injury (A). Color Doppler is used to evaluate for blood flow (neovascularization) within the lesion (B).

In our experience, adhesions also can be seen in cases with axial exostosis of the second or forth metacarpal/metatarsal bones, which will result in reduced gliding motion between the suspensory ligament and the bony aspect.

Although a fairly rarely seen condition in horses, dynamic sonography also is an important technique for evaluation of subluxation of the coxofemoral joint as consequence of traumatic partial tearing of the ligament of the head of the femur and accessory ligament.[10] With a low-frequency (2.5–5.0 MHz) curvilinear probe placed over the coxofemoral joint, the position of the femur relative to the acetabulum changes from the weight-bearing to non–weight-bearing position of the limb.[10]

Elastography

At this time, grayscale ultrasonography is in most cases sufficient to detect soft tissue injuries in horses by assessing morphologic changes of the fiber pattern and changes in CSAs. To date, it is still difficult in some cases to characterize the lesion as chronically active or healed scar tissue. Elastography is an ultrasonographic method to estimate tissue strain and may be an additional evaluation technique in the future providing in vivo and real-time mechanical properties of soft tissues. This technique is based on alterations of sound waves traveling through compressed tissue and results in a color image from blue via green to red depending on the stiffness of tissue (hard, soft, respectively).[11] Recently, it has been shown that this examination is feasible and results are repeatable in healthy horses.[11] In a study examining naturally occurring tendon and ligament lesions, it was noted that acute lesions appear as softer on elastography and chronic lesions as harder.[12] With more experience, this technique may add additional information about the healing status of a soft tissue lesion in the future.

Ultrasonography versus MRI

Ultrasonography is allowing the veterinarian to assess soft tissues for injury stall side, with the horse sedated or unsedated, depending on the cooperation level of the patient. There are a few areas that can be difficult to fully access via ultrasonography: soft tissue injury with In the hoof capsule (eg, the distal aspect of the collateral ligaments of the distal interphalangeal joint, the middle and distal aspect of the navicular bursa and the associated DDFT) and the proximal aspect of the suspensory ligament. In some horses, transcuneal ultrasound through the frog is obscured by inferior frog health or contracted or very long heels. It also has been shown that MRI is more sensitive than ultrasound when evaluating the proximal aspect of the suspensory ligament and can detect subtle lesions in this region that may be missed on ultrasonographic evaluation. MRI also can be used to identify bone changes in the proximal third metacarpus that may be missed with radiographs and ultrasonography alone. MRI is helpful in cases in which the lameness has been localized to a certain area, but radiography and ultrasonography did not show any abnormal or only slightly abnormal tissue.

USE OF MRI FOR DIAGNOSIS OF SOFT TISSUE INJURIES
Basic Physics

The region to be imaged is placed within a strong magnetic field that causes all of the hydrogen atoms (protons) within that structure to become aligned. A pulse of radiofrequency energy is applied to the tissue to knock the protons out of alignment. Once out of alignment, the protons want to return to their aligned state, producing a radiofrequency signal that the MRI machine detects.[13] No ionizing (x-ray) energy is used.

The degree to which the protons are bound within a tissue determines how quickly they will return to their aligned state. Protons in fluid return to alignment quickly, whereas those in organized tendinous or ligamentous tissue return slowly. When tendons/ligaments are injured, they become more edematous, inflamed, or necrotic, producing a signal that can be differentiated from normal tendon. As they heal, the tissue can be organized differently from normal tendinous tissue, which allows for visualization of chronic lesions.[13]

Equipment

Magnets currently used in equine practice range from 0.2 T to 3.0 T, with the most common magnet strengths being 0.3 T or 1.5 T. Imaging in low-field magnets (0.3 T) can be performed standing (with sedation) or under general anesthesia, whereas imaging in high-field magnets must be performed under general anesthesia.

High field (1.5 T–3.0 T)

The primary benefit of using a high field strength magnet is improved image quality. High-field magnets allow for better spatial resolution and better signal-to-noise ratio, allowing for better identification of structures and lesions. This may allow for more accurate diagnoses.

The largest drawback to using a high field strength magnet is the size of the bore (magnet tunnel). Often the bore of the magnet is relatively long (up to 1.5 m), and the region of interest is ideally placed in the center of the length of the bore. Depending on the conformation of the horse, imaging the carpus or tarsus is a challenge, and imaging anything proximal to these structures is generally not possible.

An additional drawback to using a high field strength magnet is that it may increase certain artifacts, such as susceptibility artifact (created by metal or blood) and chemical shift artifact, which is typically not a problem in equine imaging.[13]

Low field (0.3 T)

Compared with a high-field magnet, low-field magnets have decreased spatial resolution and signal-to-noise ratio, which leads to overall decreased image quality. The difference in image quality between low field and high field is discernible, although rarely affects lesion detection.

Standing The main benefit to a low-field, standing magnet is that horses do not need to be put under general anesthesia. This is particularly beneficial if repeat imaging is warranted.

The primary drawback of standing MRI is the motion artifact, which degrades image quality. This is rarely an issue in the foot or distal limb, but if more proximal regions (suspensory, carpus, tarsus) are imaged, this may significantly degrade image quality. The amount of image degradation is highly dependent on the patient, and is also dependent on the image sequence being acquired. Some imaging sequences are faster, which reduces the risk of motion during acquisition.

General anesthesia Low-field MRI under general anesthesia reduces the concern of motion artifact, which can increase image quality. Many of these magnets also have a large bore, so imaging of more proximal structures is easier.

Open-bore (U-shaped) low-field magnets also exist, which can allow for MRI of the stifle if the gantry is large enough.

Imaging Sequences

There are 5 main imaging sequences used in equine MRI. Additional sequences are sometimes added depending on the location and type of lesion suspected, but are rarely routinely used. Images generated by different sequences are typically evaluated together to determine the composition of a material (fluid vs fat vs organized tissue).

Typically, images are acquired in multiple planes through each structure or region of interest. Because of the way MRI is acquired, there is often a small gap between slices and the slices are not infinitely thin. This is important for 2 reasons. First, image information on one slice is averaged from information adjacent to the middle of a slice. This can create volume-averaging artifacts, in which a structure is a different intensity than expected because it averaged information of the actual tissue imaged and the tissue next to it. Second, imaging in multiple planes is extremely beneficial, if not necessary to facilitate lesion detection. If there is a small lesion and it is between slices, it can be missed. The use of multiple planes increases the chances of a small lesion being caught on a slice in at least one plane.

T1 weighted
In T1-weighted (T1W) images, fat is bright and fluid is dark (**Fig. 6**). This sequence typically has a high level of anatomic detail. It is also helpful in low-field imaging because thinner slices can be acquired without increasing noise. In high-field imaging, T1W sequences can be run as a 3-dimensional (3D) sequence, which allows for contiguous imaging without a gap between slices.

T1W sequences are also helpful for detecting subacute or chronic tendinous lesions that have changes in the tissue organization without significant fluid accumulation. If these lesions do not have fluid within them, they can be difficult to identify on other imaging sequences.

Slightly less important in equine imaging, T1W sequences are used to identify the uptake of contrast medium within lesions. The contrast medium used in MRI shortens T1W relaxation time (speed at which protons return to alignment), which causes tissues that take up the contrast medium (vascularized tissue) to appear bright on T1W images.

T2 weighted
In T2W images, fat and fluid are bright (**Fig. 7**). This sequence is good for identifying lesions within tendons and ligaments, especially if they are active lesions with fluid accumulation or edema.

Short tau inversion recovery
Short tau inversion recovery (STIR) sequences use a technique that suppresses the signal from fat, which causes fluid signal to be bright and fat signal to be dark, increasing lesion conspicuity (**Fig. 8**). This sequence is more useful for evaluation of intraosseous fluid accumulation, but soft tissue lesions with fluid will be bright on STIR images.[14]

Proton density weighted
Similar to T2W images, in proton density–weighted (PDW) images, fluid and fat are bright. However, PDW images allow for better anatomic delineation. In high-field

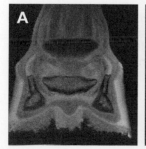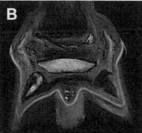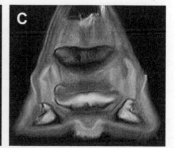

Fig. 6. Comparison of dorsal plane T1W images at the level of the navicular bone acquired at (A) 1.5 T, (B) 0.3 T under general anesthesia, and (C) 0.3 T standing.

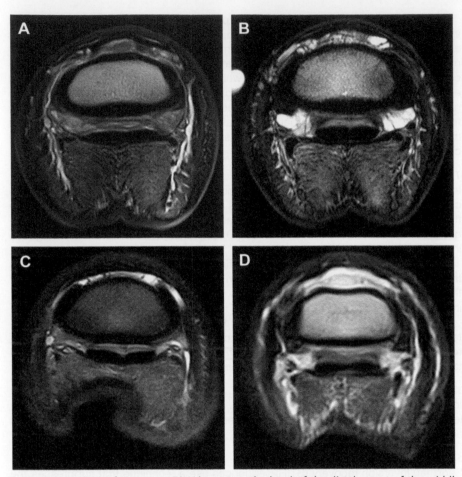

Fig. 7. Comparison of transverse T2W images at the level of the distal aspect of the middle phalanx acquired at (*A*) 3.0 T, (*B*) 1.5 T, (*C*) 0.3 T under general anesthesia, and (*D*) 0.3 T standing.

magnets, this sequence can be acquired at the same time as the T2W images and may be used in place of T1W images to decrease anesthesia time.

T2* weighted

T2*W images are gradient sequences, which means that they are sensitive to local changes within the magnetic field. These sequences are most commonly used in low-field standing magnets, as they are less sensitive at detecting fluid with STIR sequences than other MRI systems. Materials that have an inherent magnetic field (metal, blood) create a susceptibility artifact that causes a void (black region) in the image in the region of the material.

Artifacts

There are many different artifacts that occur in MRI. Similar to radiography and ultrasound, artifacts on MRI may be useful or may inhibit image interpretation. The 3 most important when evaluating equine studies are listed in the following sections.

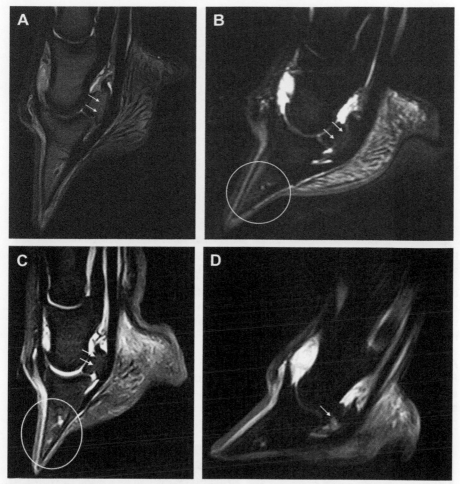

Fig. 8. Comparison of parasagittal STIR images of the distal limb acquired at (*A*) 3.0 T, (*B*) 1.5 T, (*C*) 0.3 T under general anesthesia, and (*D*) 0.3 T standing. Note that STIR hyperintensity, consistent with intraosseous fluid accumulation is present within the distal phalanx (*white oval*) and navicular bone (*white arrows*) in some images.

Magic angle
Magic angle artifact occurs when a well-organized structure (tendon, ligament) is oriented in a certain configuration with respect to the main magnetic field (**Fig. 9**). For equine patients, this artifact often occurs within the distal portion of the DDFT, as it curves around the navicular bone or within the collateral ligaments of the distal interphalangeal joint. This causes the affected structure to be artifactually hyperintense and is most pronounced on T1W and PDW sequences.[15]

Susceptibility
As discussed previously, this artifact is due to a change in the local magnetic field due to a material that has its own, smaller magnetic field.[16] The most common causes of this in equine patients is residual metallic debris associated with the hoof capsule or degrading blood, which may be traumatic or iatrogenic in origin. This artifact is often also seen after surgery and can be identified for many weeks postoperatively.[17] The

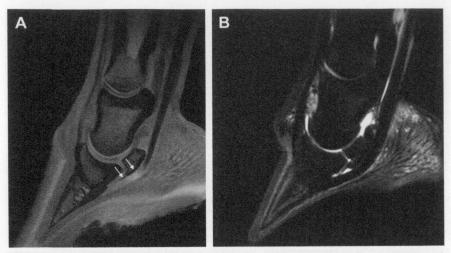

Fig. 9. Sagittal images of a distal limb acquired at 1.5 T. Magic angle artifact (*arrows*) can be seen in (*A*) T1W images but is not identified in (*B*) T2W images.

artifacts are often small, and thus unlikely to significantly hamper evaluation so long as care is taken to remove all metal fragments from the hoof. This artifact is sometimes useful to help determine if blood is present within a joint and is increased at higher magnetic field strengths.

Flow

Flow artifact or phase-encoded motion artifact is due to the motion of structures during a study.[16] In horse limbs, this is most commonly secondary to blood flow (**Fig. 10**). This artifact causes a repeating pattern of the moving structure, so for blood vessels it is a repeating pattern of hyperintense ovals on cross-sectional images. This artifact can

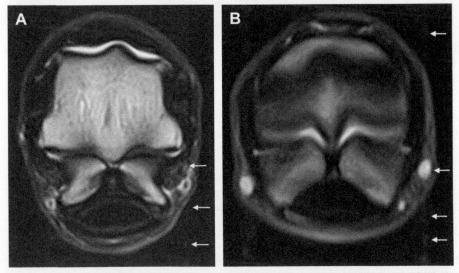

Fig. 10. Transverse T2W images acquired in a 0.3 T standing magnet at the level of (*A*) the mid aspect of the proximal sesamoid bones and (*B*) the metacarpophalangeal joint with flow artifact (*arrows*) associated with a palmar digital vessel.

mimic pathology if one of the repeating foci is transposed onto a tendinous or ligamentous structure. Although this artifact cannot be eliminated, there are techniques to change the direction of the artifact so that it is not transposed onto the areas of interest.

Types of Lesions

Substance ("core") lesions

These are probably the most common type of injury seen in equine imaging. Substance lesions are within the mid aspect of the tendon or ligament and are typically cylindrical in shape. These lesions can be seen in any tendinous or ligamentous structure, but are commonly seen in the DDFT or proximal aspect of the suspensory ligament (**Figs. 11** and **12**).

Fibrillation/longitudinal tear

Small fibrillations of the dorsal border of the DDFT are commonly seen in the region of the navicular bursa and navicular bone and are characterized by mild irregularity of the dorsal margin. More significant longitudinal tears are commonly associated with the dorsal margin of the DDFT, especially if there is concurrent change of the palmar aspect of the navicular bone. These lesions are uncommon in other tendinous or ligamentous structures, but can be seen secondary to direct trauma, such as with a penetrating foreign body.

Parasagittal or sagittal split

These lesions can be seen associated with the DDFT or the suspensory branches. When seen in the DDFT (**Fig. 13**), these lesions are often found in combination with a substance lesion. If these lesions are identified within the distal aspect of the suspensory branches, the proximal sesamoid bones should be evaluated for signs of remodeling, such as sclerosis or fluid accumulation.

Avulsion

Avulsions are typically seen secondary to hyperextension injuries and can affect any tendon or ligament at its origin or insertion. The proximal suspensory ligament is a

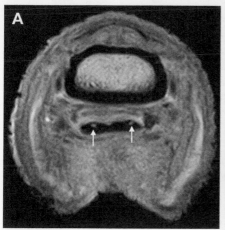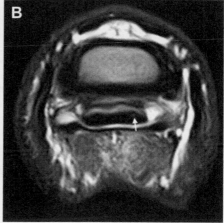

Fig. 11. Transverse images of the distal limb showing substance lesions. (*A*) T1W images at the level of the distal aspect of the middle phalanx with hyperintense foci within the dorsal aspects of both lobes of the DDFT (*arrows*). (*B*) T2W images at the level of the distal aspect of the middle phalanx with a small hyperintense focus within the dorsal aspect of one lobe of the DDFT (*arrow*).

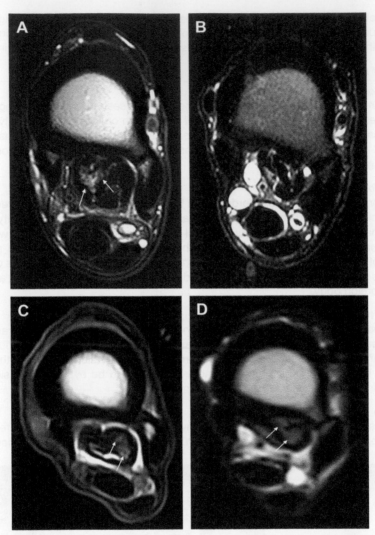

Fig. 12. Transverse T2W images of the proximal metatarsus of multiple horses acquired at (A) 3.0 T, (B) 1.5 T, (C) 0.3 T under general anesthesia, and (D) 0.3 T standing. Some horses have a substance lesion within either the medial (A) or lateral (C, D) aspect of the proximal suspensory ligament (arrows).

common site for this type of injury in equine athletes. When evaluating avulsions, the parent bone should be evaluated for signs of active remodeling, such as STIR hyperintensity.

Use of Contrast

Systemic intravenous contrast is not widely used in equine patients, partially because of the large volume (and cost) of required contrast medium. There are some reports describing the use of contrast medium to help with soft tissue injury detection.[18] More recently, contrast administered via regional limb perfusion has been studied and shown to be an effective method of delivery to the distal limb[19]

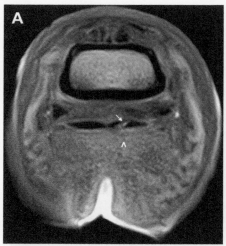
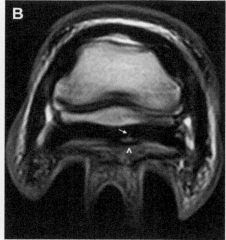

Fig. 13. Transverse (*A*) T1W and (*B*) T2W images of the distal limb at the level of the proximal aspect of the navicular bone. A complete parasagittal split of one lobe of the DDFT is identified (*arrow*). There is a small accumulation of fluid between the DDFT and the distal digital annular ligament (*caret*) that can occur if the split communicates with the navicular bursa.

(**Fig. 14**). Use of contrast material in this manner did increase conspicuity of certain lesions, but often did not add clinical data that would alter the treatment plan for the horse. The use of contrast does help to identify regions of neovascularization, which may help to further define chronicity or activity of certain lesions. Further study in this area is warranted.

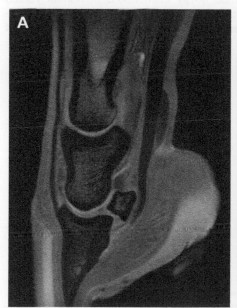
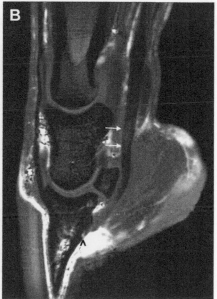

Fig. 14. Parasagittal T1W images (*A*) before and (*B*) after contrast administration of a distal limb with a penetrating foreign body trauma. The postcontrast image shows contrast enhancement of the distal phalanx (*caret*) and the DDFT at the level of the proximal aspect of the middle phalanx (*arrows*).

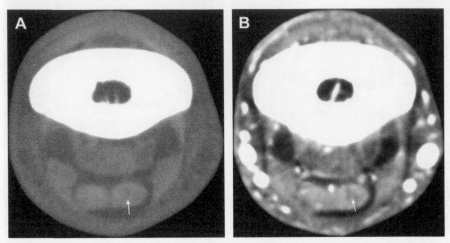

Fig. 15. Transverse CT images at the level of the distal aspect of the proximal phalanx (*A*) before and (*B*) after intra-arterial contrast administration. A substance lesion of one lobe of the DDFT can be identified before, but is better defined after contrast administration (*arrows*).

USE OF COMPUTED TOMOGRAPHY FOR DIAGNOSIS OF SOFT TISSUE INJURIES

Computed tomography (CT) is an imaging modality that uses x-rays to create a 3D image. Because CT is essentially radiography in 3D, it is not as good as MRI at differentiating soft tissue lesions because of similar x-ray attenuations of normal versus diseased tendons and ligaments. Identification of these lesions requires there to be a difference in the attenuation of normal and abnormal tissue (eg, due to an influx of

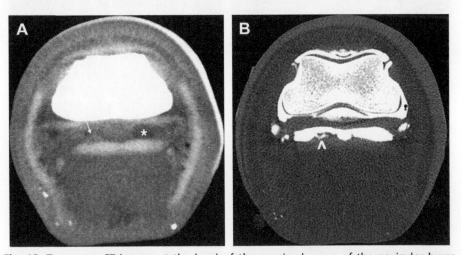

Fig. 16. Transverse CT images at the level of the proximal recess of the navicular bursa (*A*) before and (*B*) after intrasynovial contrast administration. Precontrast hyperattenuating tissue is identified within the proximal recess of the navicular bursa (*arrow*) and moderate navicular bursal effusion is present (*asterisk*). Postcontrast, a dorsal longitudinal tear of one lobe of the DDFT can be identified with contrast extending into the lesion (*caret*).

fluid and/or inflammatory cells), typically causing the abnormal tissue to be darker (hypoattenuating) compared with normal tissue. Lesion conspicuity on CT imaging can be dramatically increased with the use of contrast, either intrasynovial[20] or intra-arterial.[21] Intra-arterial contrast is helpful for identifying substance or peripheral lesions (**Fig. 15**), whereas intrasynovial contrast is helpful for identifying cartilage defects and synovitis (**Fig. 16**).

REFERENCES

1. Ross MW. Manipulation. In: Ross MW, Dyson SJ, editors. Diagnosis and management of lameness in the horse. 2nd edition. St Louis (MO): Elsevier Saunders; 2011. p. 80–8.
2. Rantanen NW, Joergensen JS, Genovese RL. Ultrasonographic evaluation of the equine limb: technique. In: Ross MW, Dyson SJ, editors. Diagnosis and management of lameness in the horse. 2nd edition. St Louis (MO): Elsevier Saunders; 2011. p. 182–205.
3. Smith RKW, Cauvin ERJ. Ultrasonography of the metacarpus and metatarsus. In: Kidd JA, Lu KG, Frazer ML, editors. Atlas of equine ultrasonography. Chichester (England): Wiley; 2014. p. 73–105.
4. Werpy NM, Denoix JM. Imaging of the equine proximal suspensory ligament. Vet Clin North Am Equine Pract 2012;28:507–25.
5. Denoix JM. Angle contrast ultrasound technique (ACUST) improves diagnosis and prognosis of tendon and ligament injuries. In: Proceedings of the Havemeyer Symposium 2012. Estes Park, Colorado, September 23–26, 2012. p. 35–6.
6. Werpy NM, Denoix JM, McIlwraith CW, et al. Comparison between standard ultrasonography, angle contrast ultrasonography, and magnetic resonance imaging characteristics of the normal equine proximal suspensory ligament. Vet Radiol Ultrasound 2013;54:536–47.
7. Denoix JM, Bertoni L. The angle contrast ultrasound technique in the flexed limb improves assessment of proximal suspensory ligament injuries in the equine pelvic limb. Equine Vet Educ 2015;27:209–17.
8. Bosch G, Moleman M, Barneveld A, et al. The effect of platelet-rich plasma on the neovascularization of surgically created equine superficial digital flexor tendon lesions. Scand J Med Sci Sports 2011;21:554–61.
9. DiGiovanni DL, Rademacher N, Riggs LM, et al. Dynamic sonography of the equine carpo(tarso)phalangeal digital flexor tendon sheath. Vet Radiol Ultrasound 2016;57:621–9.
10. Brenner S, Whitcomb MB. Ultrasonographic diagnosis of coxofemoral subluxation in horses. Vet Radiol Ultrasound 2009;50:423–8.
11. Lustgarten M, Redding WR, Labens R, et al. Elastographic characteristics of the metacarpal tendons in horses without clinical evidence of tendon injury. Vet Radiol Ultrasound 2014;55:92–101.
12. Lustgarten M, Redding WR, Labens R, et al. Elastographic evaluation of naturally occurring tendon and ligament injuries of the equine distal limb. Vet Radiol Ultrasound 2015;56:670–9.
13. Curry TS, Dowdey JE, Murry RC. Magnetic resonance imaging. In: Christensen's physics of diagnostic radiology. 4th edition. Philadelphia: Lippincott Williams & Wilkins; 1990. p. 471–504.
14. Holowinski M, Judy C, Saveraid T, et al. Resolution of lesions on STIR images is associated with improved lameness status in horses. Vet Radiol Ultrasound 2010; 51(5):479–84.

15. Busoni V, Snaps F. Effect of deep digital flexor tendon orientation on magnetic resonance imaging signal intensity in isolated equine limbs—the magic angle effect. Vet Radiol Ultrasound 2002;43:428–30.
16. Bushberg JT, Seibert JA, Leidholdt EM, et al. Magnetic resonance imaging artifacts. In: The essential physics of medical imaging. 2nd edition. Philadelphia: Lippincott Williams & Wilkins; 2002. p. 447–57.
17. Thomas AL, Schramme MC, Lepage OM, et al. Low-field magnetic resonance imaging appearance of post arthroscopic magnetic susceptibility artifacts in horses: postoperative magnetic susceptibility artifact. Vet Radiol Ultrasound 2016; 57(6):587–93.
18. Saveraid TC, Judy CE. Use of intravenous gadolinium contrast in equine magnetic resonance imaging. Vet Clin North Am Equine Pract 2012;28(3):617–36.
19. Aarsvold SA, Solano MS, Garcia-Lopez J. Magnetic resonance imaging following regional limb perfusion of gadolinium contrast medium in 26 horses. Equine Vet J 2018. https://doi.org/10.1111/evj.12818.
20. Puchalski SM. Advances in equine computed tomography and use of contrast media. Vet Clin North Am Equine Pract 2012;28(3):563–81.
21. Puchalski SM, Galuppo LD, Hornof WJ, et al. Intraarterial contrast-enhanced computed tomography of the equine distal extremity. Vet Radiol Ultrasound 2007;48:21–9.

Neck, Back, and Pelvic Pain in Sport Horses

José M. García-López, VMD

KEYWORDS

- Nuchal • Bursa • Cervical • Vertebrae • Back • DSP • Pelvis • Sacroiliac joint

KEY POINTS

- Acute cases of nuchal bursitis with little or no evidence of synovial proliferation can be managed with intrabursal therapy of anti-inflammatories; other cases benefit from nuchal bursoscopy.
- Osteoarthritis of the articular vertebral facets can be treated successfully with ultrasound-guided therapy of anti-inflammatory medications.
- Proper diagnosis of impingement or overriding of the dorsal spinous processes of the thoracolumbar spine requires the use of radiography and nuclear scintigraphy.
- Medical and surgical management of impingement or overriding of the dorsal spinous processes can be highly effective.
- Thorough evaluation of the sacroiliac region is imperative to correctly identify cases suffering from pain arising from this region.

NECK

Neck pain or stiffness in horses can limit their athletic potential and can develop secondary to a number of different conditions.[1,2] Definitive diagnosis can be difficult due to the variability in clinical signs and the common presence of concurrent lameness. In this article, we discuss disorders of the neck that can have a significant impact on the horse's performance, such as nuchal bursitis and osteoarthritis of the cervical articular facets. Neurologic conditions created by impingement of the spinal cord are discussed elsewhere in this issue.

Nuchal Bursa

The nuchal ligament is a structure that helps support the weight of the horse's head. It consists of 2 clearly defined portions or segments: funicular and laminar. The funicular (dorsal) portion is a thick cord extending between the highest spinous processes of the withers and the external occipital protuberance of the skull. The laminar portion forms

Disclosure Statement: No conflicts or commercial affiliations to disclose.
Department of Clinical Sciences, Tufts University Cummings School of Veterinary Medicine, 200 Westboro Road, North Grafton, MA 01536, USA
E-mail address: jose.garcia-lopez@tufts.edu

Vet Clin Equine 34 (2018) 235–251
https://doi.org/10.1016/j.cveq.2018.04.002
0749-0739/18/© 2018 Elsevier Inc. All rights reserved.

a fenestrated sheath that fills the space between the funicular portion and the cervical vertebrae. In horses, there are 2 bursae associated with the nuchal ligament in the cervical region. These are the atlantal or cranial nuchal bursa (*bursa subligamentosa nuchalis cranialis*), which is consistently present above the dorsal arch of the atlas (C1) and ventral to the funicular portion of the nuchal ligament, and the caudal nuchal bursa (*bursa subligamentosa nuchalis caudalis*), which is inconsistently present in horses and is located between the spinous process of the axis (C2) and the funicular portion of the nuchal ligament.[3,4] The cranial nuchal bursa, which is the bursa most commonly affected and the one that is consistently present, is bilobed with an incomplete septum separating the left and right lobes. The bursa is composed of synovium, a variable amount of fat tissue, and bundles of fibers of the laminar part of the nuchal ligament.[4]

Cranial nuchal bursitis is a relatively uncommon disease, but a differential diagnosis in horses suffering from pain associated with the neck region.[3–5] Clinical signs of nuchal bursitis include swelling and pain on palpation around the poll (**Fig. 1**), and unwillingness of the horse to flex the neck. Some horses will carry the head in a locked extended position (**Fig. 2**). Aseptic and septic nuchal bursitis has been reported in recent years, with isolates such as *Staphylococcus* spp. and *Streptococcus* spp. identified.[3] Although the use of nuclear scintigraphy and MRI have been used to diagnose this condition, definitive diagnosis is best achieved with the use of ultrasound and radiographs.[3,5] An unaffected nuchal bursa will show minimal fluid during ultrasonographic examination[4]; however, affected bursae will show a variable amount of wall thickening, synovial proliferation, and fluid distention that can range from anechoic to markedly echogenic, especially in cases with copious amounts of rice bodies within the bursa[3,5,6] (**Fig. 3**). Radiographic evaluation of the affected region often shows a variable amount of mineralization of the surrounding soft tissues or bony involvement of the atlas or axis in more chronic cases[3,5] (**Fig. 4**). Ultrasound-guided fluid aspirate for cytologic analysis and culture should be performed to assess the degree of inflammation within the bursa and to differentiate septic and nonseptic cases.[3,5]

Management of nuchal bursitis includes the use of anti-inflammatory and antimicrobial medications, both systemic and locally, as well as endoscopic debridement and lavage.[3,5] In 2017, Bergren and colleagues[5] published the largest retrospective study to date of horses suffering from cranial nuchal bursitis. In that study, 30 horses were

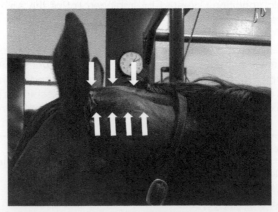

Fig. 1. Horse with swelling in the poll region (*arrows*) secondary to aseptic cranial nuchal bursitis.

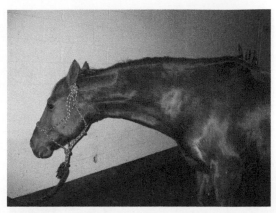

Fig. 2. Horse with aseptic cranial nuchal bursitis showing a persistent head and neck extension.

included with follow-up examinations of at least 12 months. Fourteen of the 30 horses were treated medically by means of ultrasound-guided intrabursal therapy with a combination of corticosteroids (methylprednisolone acetate or triamcinolone acetonide) and hyaluronic acid, together with systemic nonsteroidal anti-inflammatories (NSAIDs). Of these, 4 horses had recurrence of clinical signs and required surgical intervention. Of the horses treated solely medically, 33% had recurrence of clinical signs and 68% were able to return to their previous level of exercise.[5] Sixteen horses in that study were treated solely surgically by means of nuchal bursoscopy (**Fig. 5**) and underwent a thorough lavage and debridement of the affected tissue, with 29% having

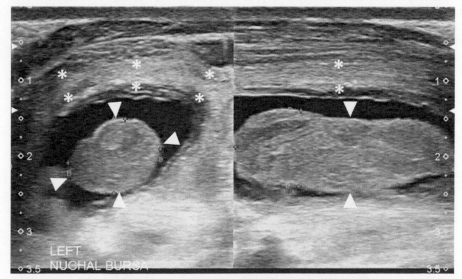

Fig. 3. Cross-sectional (*A*) and longitudinal (*B*) ultrasound image of the cranial nuchal bursa of the horse depicted in **Fig. 1** exhibiting moderate nonpeptic bursitis. Note the capsular thickness (*asterisks*) and echogenic material (*arrowheads*) within the bursa. (*Courtesy of Dr Katherine B. Chope, North Grafton, MA; with permission.*)

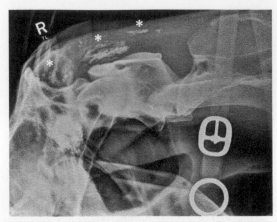

Fig. 4. Lateral radiographs of the poll region of the horse depicted in **Fig. 1**. Note the degree of mineralization (*asterisks*) dorsal and cranial to the first cervical vertebra.

a recurrence of clinical signs and 79% able to return to their previous level of exercise.[5] Only 25% of the horses treated surgically following failed medical therapy were able to return to their previous level of exercise.[5] It has been this author's experience, both in those cases published by Bergren and colleagues[5] and in those cases seen since, that the best candidates for successful medical management by means of intrabursal therapy are those with only anechoic fluid distention of the bursa with little to no capsular thickening and echogenic material. The presence of significant synovial proliferation and echogenic tissue within the bursa on ultrasound is in this author's opinion an indication to pursue surgical debridement and lavage as soon as possible, bypassing intrabursal medical therapy, as these horses do not appear to respond well to such treatment and are more likely to develop complications and return of clinical signs, thus rendering a worse prognosis for successful return to their previous level of exercise.

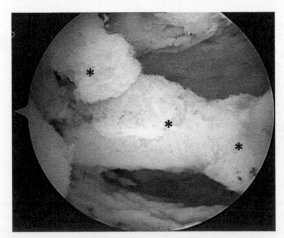

Fig. 5. Endoscopic view of the cranial nuchal bursa in horse depicted in **Fig. 1**. Note the large and copious amount of debris (*asterisks*) within the bursa.

Cervical Region

Cervical problems in the horse can be caused by an acute fall, rearing and falling over backward, or by collision with another horse or an object. Alternatively, horses may display neck stiffness, difficulties lowering or raising the head, or abnormal posture of the neck without known trauma. Other symptoms that can lead to problems in the cervical region can be unwillingness to work on the bit, unsteady head carriage, abnormal head position during exercise, and a forelimb lameness that cannot be localized to the forelimb. Stumbling hind limb gait can be caused by a compressive cervical lesion.[2]

Examination of the horse's neck should include a thorough visual examination for conformation of the neck, body conditioning score of the horse, neck carriage, and asymmetries. Some horses may show intermittent focal sweating because of peripheral nerve damage. Palpation should include muscular tissue, cervical vertebra, region of the cranial nuchal bursa, and the nuchal ligament. Focal areas of heat, discomfort, or swelling might be noted. Active range of motion can be tested to either side of the body, as well as toward the fetlock joints, and to an upper horizontal line by bribing the horse with food. The horse should then be examined in motion by trotting in hand, and exercising on the lunge line and under the rider. Any limb lameness should be excluded, and the neck position should be observed during different speeds and different stages of bending. In addition, horses with neck pain may show forelimb lameness or a reduced cranial phase of the stride, so other causes of forelimb lameness should be excluded. Neurologic evaluation should be included in the examination. Further diagnostics of the cervical region include radiographic evaluation of the vertebra and synovial joints (facet and intervertebral joints), as well as ultrasonographic evaluation of any swelling, painful areas of the nuchal ligament, the nuchal bursa, and intervertebral facet joints.[4,7,8] In addition, nuclear scintigraphy can help evaluate for acute inflammation of intervertebral facet joints, vertebral fractures, and insertional desmopathy of the nuchal ligament.

Intervertebral facet joint osteoarthritis can lead to unwillingness to bend the neck, refusing jumps, difficulties with collection, or even neurologic signs primarily in the hind end.[1,2] Neurologic deficits can occur when intervertebral facet joints show severe remodeling and compress the spinal cord. Severe findings are most often in the caudal cervical spine.[1,2] Diagnosis of osteoarthritis of the intervertebral facet joints can be made via radiographic, ultrasonographic, and nuclear scintigraphic examination. Lateral and right-45° proximal to left distal and left-45° proximal to right distal views allow visualization of the facet joint space (**Fig. 6**). For complete radiographic evaluation of the cervical spine, 4 to 5 views are typically necessary. Ultrasonographic evaluation of the intervertebral facet joint can be performed using a linear or convex 5.0 to 7.5-MHz transducer and using a depth of 4 to 8 cm, depending on the muscle thickness.[7] The transducer is placed first parallel to the long axis of the neck, approximately 8 to 10 cm higher than the palpated transverse process. By sliding downward on the neck, the most dorsal aspect of the vertebra is located and the transducer is then oriented cranio-dorsally in a 45-degree angle to open up the joint space between cranial and caudal facet.[7] The joint should be evaluated and the probe moved farther up and down the neck to evaluate the next intervertebral facet joint. The cervical facets typically present a relatively smooth hyperechoic bony contour with a small but appreciable anechoic discontinuity representative of the joint space (**Fig. 7**). The capsule can be visualized closely overlying the joint, but normally no joint fluid or synovium can be seen. Normal variations in anatomy can occur and should be interpreted with caution. The significance of small osteophytes should be weighed with caution.

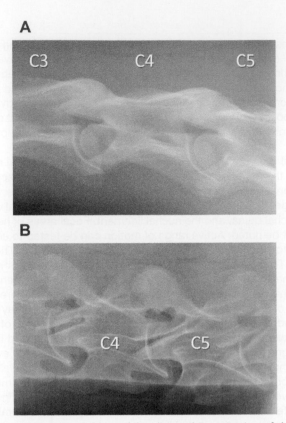

Fig. 6. Lateral (*A*) and 45-degree oblique (*B*) radiographic projection of the mid-cervical region. (*Courtesy of* Dr Gabriel Manso- Díaz, Madrid, Spain; with permission.)

Features of abnormal facet joints include significant bony irregularity or proliferation, lipping or osteophytes at the joint margin, detection of joint fluid or synovial thickening, and widening of the visible margins of the joint space.[8]

Treatment options for cervical facet joint osteoarthritis include oral NSAIDs and ultrasonographic-guided intra-articular injection with corticosteroids and hyaluronic

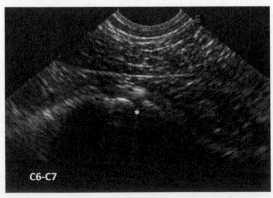

Fig. 7. Ultrasound examination of the articular facet of C6-C7. The articular space appears as a small anechoic discontinuity (*asterisk*) from the bony surface. E, dorsal.

acid.[1,7,9] In our hospital we typically use a 3.5-inch-long, 20-gauge or 18-gauge spinal needle and inject a total volume of 2.5 mL using 40 mg of methylprednisolone acetate in combination with a hyaluronic acid product. As for all intra-articular injections, aseptic technique is imperative and adequate sedation is necessary for this procedure. In a retrospective study by Birmingham and colleagues,[10] 124 symptomatic performance horses were treated via ultrasonographic-guided injection of cervical facet joints. Radiographic findings were of 4 grades (0 = normal, 1 = mild changes, 2 = moderate, 3 = severe). In that study, 59 horses could be followed, and of those 32% returned to normal function, 39% improved in performance, and 25% did not show any change after treatment. Duration of improvement ranged between 1 month and 5 years. No correlation between radiographic findings and treatment response was found.[10]

BACK

Back problems in horses can be of either primary or secondary (in combination with limb lameness) nature. Because of the thick muscular layer covering the thoracolumbar spine, diagnosis of vertebral lesions is difficult, and therefore treatment of back problems in the equine patient can be challenging. Clinical symptoms of back problems include behavioral changes, such as bucking, unwillingness moving forward or to jump, as well as pain on palpation and reduced back motion seen during exercise on a lunge line. Evaluation for back problems should include a thorough clinical examination with inspection, palpation, and mobilization of the back, as well as evaluation during motion.[11-15] Further diagnostics can be performed with radiographic, ultrasonographic, and nuclear scintigraphic examination. Diagnostic analgesia by infiltrating the identified lesion with local anesthetic can be helpful in cases with questionable or multiple lesions. The horse should be ridden before and 15 to 20 minutes after infiltration, and improvement should be noted by the rider as well as the clinician on the ground.

Impinging or Overriding Dorsal Spinous Processes

Dorsal spinous process (DSP) impingement or overriding (ORDSP), often referred to as "kissing spines" has been reported as the most common cause of back pain in the horse. Impingement of the DSPs is found mostly at the level of T13-T18, but it also can affect the lumbar DSPs.[11,13] Factors historically associated to this condition include poor conformation, poor conditioning, rider-horse mismatch, and chronic use of an ill-fitted saddle. Clinical signs may include a vague history of poor performance, change in head/neck carriage, unwillingness to move in a certain direction, concurrent hindlimb lameness, unwillingness to bend, and pain of varying degrees of intensity on firm palpation of the affected region.[13]

Diagnosis of active ORDSP can be challenging at times because radiography alone does not tell the clinician the amount of current inflammation present, and the presence of bony remodelling, impingement, and/or overriding does not mean that the horse is suffering from this condition, as radiographic signs of ORDSP have been reported in clinically normal horses.[12] Townsend and colleagues[12] reported of the presence of ORDSP during postmortem examination in 83% of 23 horses with functionally normal thoracolumbar spines. There are several radiographic grading scales used by clinicians to classify the degree of ORDSP. The 2 probably most commonly used are those described by Pettersson and colleagues[14] and by Denoix and Dyson,[13] using a 1 to 3 and 1 to 4 grading scale, respectively (**Fig. 8**). Although not in sport horses, Cousty and colleagues[16] reported their findings when evaluating the thoracolumbar spine of 106 French trotters with signs of back pain. When looking at those horses with

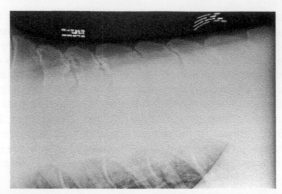

Fig. 8. Lateral radiographic projection of the caudal thoracic DSPs exhibiting severe osteolysis, remodeling, and overriding. These changes can be considered Grade 3 (Pettersson) or Grade 4 (Dyson and Denoix).

impingement of the DSP, they found no difference in the number of affected horses between the control and clinical group, but the number of lesions and severity grade were significantly higher in the clinical group.[16]

To better correlate any radiographic findings with its potential role clinically, as well to provide certain degree of "objectivity," the use of nuclear scintigraphy of this region, together with the physical examination findings and lameness workup, can be a critical imaging tool[17,18] **(Fig. 9)**. However, it is very important to remember that the presence of increased radiopharmaceutical uptake at the level of the DSPs alone does not automatically mean that the horse is suffering from thoracolumbar pain. This was best described by Zimmerman and colleagues,[18] who reported on the relationship between radiological and scintigraphic findings in 582 horses presenting for back pain and perceived resulting poor performance. They found that only 46% of the horses examined that had radiological evidence of DSP pathology showed clinical signs of thoracolumbar pain. Similarly, only 27% of horses with evidence of increased radiopharmaceutical uptake at the level of the DSPs alone had clinical signs of

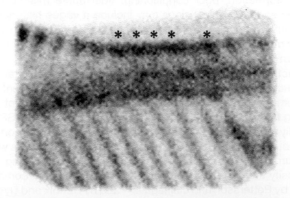

Fig. 9. Nuclear scintigraphic examination of the thoracolumbar region of an 9-year-old thoroughbred eventer. Note the focal areas of moderate-marked radiopharmaceutical uptake at the level of the caudal thoracic DSPs (*asterisks*).

thoracolumbar pain.[18] However, they found that there was an increasing correlation between the number of affected DSPs and both higher radiographic and scintigraphic scores with clinical signs of thoracolumbar pain; 83% of horses that showed a maximum radiological score of 3 and concurrently moderate or intense radiopharmaceutical uptake on scintigraphy were clinically symptomatic.[18]

Medical/Conservative Management of Overriding Dorsal Spinous Process

Historically, medical management has consisted of local injections of anti-inflammatories, physiotherapy, and/or focused extracorporeal shockwave therapy (ESWT). Although medical management can be highly successful, it is important to communicate with owners and trainers the very likely need for repeated treatment, ideally every 6 to 12 months. In a recent study, Coomer and colleagues[19] reported an 89% short-term improvement in the clinical signs of 38 horses suffering from ORDSP treated medically by means of local injections with anti-inflammatories, with a return of back pain in 56% of the horses in a median of 75 days (range 12–334 days). Conservative management by the way of rest alone can be helpful in some cases. The aim of rest in horses suffering from ORDSP is to reduce inflammation associated with the bone contact, bony remodeling, and soft tissue damage.[11] However, to effectively reduce inflammation, rest must be long enough to be beneficial, typically 3 to 9 months. This is in part (other reasons include loss of muscle mass and strength) why rest is typically combined with medical therapy or is not necessarily our first treatment choice.

Medication of the affected interspinous spaces is one of the most commonly used medical treatment modalities, consisting of injecting a combination of anti-inflammatories and analgesics. Care should be taken with regard to drug withdrawal for horses that are in active competition, as this can be highly variable among different organizations. Treatment of the affected DSPs with a course of focused ESWT consists of anywhere from 1 (for cases with only bony inflammation) to 3 to 4 (for those with bony and ligamentous injuries) treatments spaced approximately 2 to 3 weeks apart. Although the exact mechanism of action is not completely understood, its analgesic properties and proposed microtrauma effect appear to provide an environment conducive to healing. Following treatment with either interspinous injections or ESWT, these horses will be rested for a variable amount of time (1–6 weeks), except for those with ligamentous injuries in which follow-up ultrasound examinations are performed every 6 weeks until deemed appropriate to resume exercise. Once back into exercise they are typically worked on a lunge line before reintroducing them to work under saddle.

Coudry and colleagues[20] reported on the efficacy of Tildren (Tiludronate; CEVA Santé Animale, :ibourne Cedex, France) with regard to the improvement of dorsal flexibility in horses suffering from osteoarthritis of the vertebral column. They used the reported dosing regimen of 1 mg/kg intravenous as a low-rate infusion with a significant improvement in dorsal flexibility up to 60 days after treatment.[20] Although this condition is different from ORDSP, the results of this study have resulted in the use of this product in the management of horses suffering from ORDSP with no real objective evidence to date of its benefit in these patients.

Another treatment therapy that is commonly used to manage back pain with increased frequency during the past couple of years is mesotherapy. Mesotherapy relies on the concept of inhibition of nerves carrying painful information from the deep structures within a spinal segment by stimulation of nerves from more superficial structures.[11] Mesotherapy consists of a series of rows of intradermal injections of anti-inflammatories placed at the level and caudal to the source of the pain. In addition, chiropractic and manual therapies are commonly used in the management of horses suffering from ORDSP, whether as a primary means of therapy or as adjunct to other modalities. These therapies are described in more detail in this issue.

Surgical Management of Overriding Dorsal Spinous Process

Historically, horses that did not respond to medical management or those suffering from severe ORDSP are considered reasonable candidates to be managed surgically. Up to recently, surgical options consisted of partial removal of the affected DSPs using several different techniques, either through a midline or paramedian incision both under general anesthesia or standing and local sedation, or using an endoscopic approach via small incisions also under general anesthesia.[21–24]

Walmsley and colleagues[21] reported on their experience managing 215 horses suffering from ORDSP by removal of every other affected DSPs. Their results showed 81% returned to athletic use, with 72% of the cases returning to full work. A total of 13 horses (16.5%) exhibited incisional complications or infections that resolved but not without further intervention.[21] It has been our experience that horses managed in this fashion are able to return to light work at between 3 and 6 months. A similar procedure in which sections of the affected DSPs are resected but with the horse standing under light sedation also has been reported.[22] This technique has the advantage of avoiding general anesthesia; however, it can suffer from an increase in incisional complications. Desbrosse and colleagues[23] described a new technique whereby the resection of the affected DSPs was performed under general anesthesia but using a modified endoscopic technique in a minimally invasive manner. This technique showed much promise with a similar positive outcome and no reported incisional complications, but has failed to gain major popularity because of the need for extra cost and specialized instrumentation. It was not until 2014 that Jacklin and colleagues[24] reported on a modification to the subtotal DSP resection by only transecting a cranial wedge piece of the affected DSP, effectively improving on the cosmetic defect across the topline of the horse that the traditional partial ostectomy yielded (**Fig. 10**). The study reported 79% resolution of clinical signs and another 18% of the horses managed with this technique improved when compared with before surgery, with all horses found to have a good to excellent cosmetic outcome as per their owners or trainers.[24]

In 2012, Coomer and colleagues[19] described a new, minimally invasive technique that is performed with the horse standing under mild sedation and local anesthesia, which, based on their reported success, has change the way that some clinicians tackle horses suffering from ORDSP. The technique, interspinous ligament desmotomy (ISLD), consists of making a 1-cm paramedian incision on the left epaxial region, just lateral to the supraspinous ligament through which a large curved Mayo scissor or bistoury is inserted.[19] The proposed purposes of this transection are (1) to allow an increase in the interspinous space (effectively stopping the ORDSP), and (2) to relieve the tension on afferent nociceptive receptors located at the level of the insertion of the ISL, thus abolishing the sensation of pain[19] (**Fig. 11**). Following the procedure, the horses undergo an 8-week rehabilitation program consisting of stall rest with hand-walking exercise for the first month followed by another 4 weeks of limited turnout in a small paddock with lunging exercise using a Pessoa Training System. In addition, strengthening and spinal mobilization exercises, such as carrot stretches and belly pushes, are strongly recommended starting 5 days following the ISLD.[25] Coomer and colleagues[19] reported on their short-term and long-term results using this technique on 35 horses diagnosed with ORDSP. Their results showed that 95% of the horses treated by means of ISLD had a resolution of the signs of back pain and could

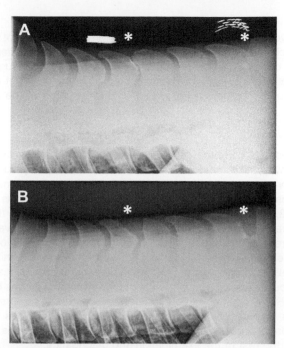

Fig. 10. Lateral radiographic projection of a horse with ORDSP before (*A*) and after cranial wedge ostectomy (*B*) at the level of the caudal thoracic DSP (*asterisks*).

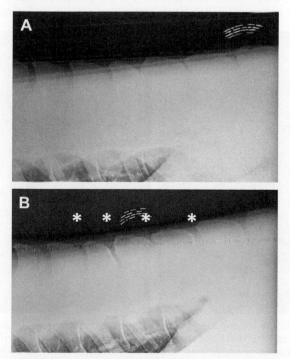

Fig. 11. Lateral radiographic projection of a horse with ORDSP before (*A*) and after (*B*) ISLD at the level of the caudal thoracic DSP (*asterisks*).

return to ridden work; when following these cases over a year, none of them showed a recurrence of back pain, although 46% of them developed other lameness problems. All but 3 of these cases were able to be managed medically and resumed athletic exercise, whether at their normal level of athletic activity (n = 10) or at a reduced level (n = 3). The 3 horses that did not have sufficient resolution of the lameness were retired.[19]

Supraspinous Desmitis

Supraspinous desmitis can be a cause for sudden onset of back discomfort and is best diagnosed with ultrasound.[26,27] Lesions within the supraspinous ligament are either anechoic or of mixed echogenicity, and cross-sectional area may be increased (**Fig. 12**). The most common location of desmitis of the supraspinous ligament is between T15 and L3.[15] In 2007, Henson and colleagues[27] reported their findings on evaluation of the supraspinous lesions up to the level of the 18th thoracic vertebra in ridden and unridden horses (39 horses total). In their study, 68% of the lesions found within the ligament were seen between T14 and T17, but there was no significance with regard to the presence of ligament pathology on ultrasound and clinical signs of back pain between groups. For this reason, and not dissimilar to what has been discussed with regard to ORDSP both on radiographs and scintigraphy, the presence of sonographic changes when evaluating the supraspinous ligament does not necessarily mean that there is clinical significance, so it is critical to evaluate this area and place it in context with the rest of the examination and diagnostics.

Osteoarthritis of the Intervertebral Facet Joints

Osteoarthritis of intervertebral facet joints of the thoracolumbar spine has been identified as a source of back pain. The intervertebral facet joints are located on the dorsal

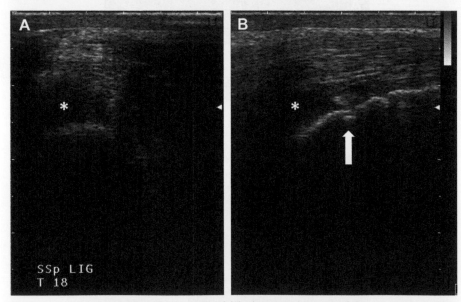

Fig. 12. Cross-sectional (A) and longitudinal (B) ultrasound image of the supraspinous ligament at the level of T18. There is a prominent anechoic region with loss of fiber alignment (*asterisks*) as well as bony irregularity (*arrow*) on T18 and overall increased cross-sectional area. E, lateral (A) and cranial (B). (*Courtesy of* Dr Katherine B. Chope, North Grafton, MA; with permission.)

aspect of the intervertebral joints and consist of the cranial articular facet of the cranial vertebra and the caudal articular facet of the caudal vertebra on either side off midline adjacent to the caudal and cranial distal aspect of the DSPs. Radiographic evaluation of these joints can be facilitated by using oblique radiographic images. In the caudal lumbar region, radiographic evaluation is difficult due to the large muscle mass overlying the region. Ultrasonographic evaluation can be done using a 3.5-MHz to 5.0-MHz transducer (**Fig. 13**). Comparison of the left and right synovial articulations of the same intertransverse joint is useful to assess size and shape. Degenerative changes of the intervertebral articulations can be detected (such as lipping and bony irregularity). However, in this author's opinion, the significance of these changes should be interpreted with caution and in conjunction with the clinical picture (as with detection of degenerative changes in any joint). Nuclear scintigraphy can be helpful in identifying abnormal bone remodeling of the intertransverse joints. Treatment of osteoarthritis of the intervertebral facet joints includes ultrasonographic-guided injection of the affected joints with a combination of corticosteroids and hyaluronic acid, systemic bisphosphonates, and mobilization exercises.

PELVIS
Sacroiliac Region/Joint

Sacroiliac joint disorders in the equine patient cause most commonly clinical signs of poor performance, lack of impulsion, and mild, chronic hind limb lameness.[28,29] Clinical evaluation may reveal sensitivity to pressure applied over the tuber sacrale and upper limb flexion tests may result in a positive response. During exercise, reduced hind limb action and shortened hind limb stride during canter (bunny hopping) may be noted. Other causes for hind limb lameness should be excluded by diagnostic analgesia. Further diagnostics include diagnostic analgesia of the sacroiliac joint, ultrasonographic evaluation of the dorsal sacroiliac ligaments, and transrectal ultrasonographic evaluation of the border of the sacroiliac joints, as well as nuclear scintigraphy. Diagnostic analgesia of the sacroiliac joint should be performed with caution because anesthesia of the sciatic nerve has been reported, which will cause hind limb weakness or non–weight bearing hind limb for up to 3 hours.

Ultrasonographically, the sacroiliac region is typically evaluated from a dorsal window, but the sacroiliac joint and ventral vertebral aspects of the sacrum can be evaluated from a rectal window.[30–32] The typical structures evaluated for the sacroiliac examination are the dorsal sacroiliac ligaments, the sacroiliac articulation, and the

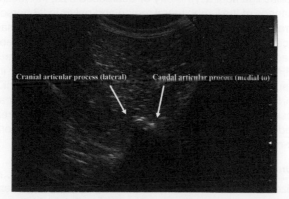

Fig. 13. Ultrasound of the intertransverse articulation between L1 and L2. E, axial. (*Courtesy of* Dr Katherine B. Chope, North Grafton, MA; with permission.)

bony surface of the sacrum and tuber sacrale. From a rectal window, the ventral aspects of the sacroiliac joint, ventral sacroiliac ligament, and caudal 2 lumbar and lumbosacral intervertebral disks can variably be appreciated. The first sacral segment is wide, flattened, and articulates with L6 by means of an intervertebral disk. Cranially, the lateral parts of the base, or wings, form the articular surface with the ilium. The sacral surface narrows caudally and is convex ventrally. The dorsal sacroiliac ligament arises as a continuation or fusion of the thoracolumbar fascia.[30–32] The width of the ventral sacroiliac joint space is reported to be 0.98 ± 0.32 cm.[31,32] The ventral sacroiliac ligament may be seen, but can be difficult to identify because of its small size of 0.34 ± 0.15 cm.[31,32] The intervertebral disks should appear as short dense bands of tissue between adjacent lumbar vertebra, similar in appearance to a meniscus. It is important to remember that normal variations in morphology can exist (ankylosis). Increases or decreases in echogenicity of the disks are abnormal, as is abnormal location (bulging). Periarticular new bone also can be identified.

Acute injuries to the dorsal sacroiliac ligaments appear enlarged, with a typical hypoechoic appearance and fiber disruption. However, Tomlinson and colleagues[32] found that the dorsal sacroiliac ligaments may be unilaterally decreased in area in chronic desmitis. This was suggested to be due to chronic instability/shearing forces, and may represent a permanent change.[32] As the sacroiliac ligaments are a paired structure, contralateral comparisons of size, shape, and appearances are recommended. Care should be taken to ensure that these comparisons are made at the same level. Engeli and colleagues[30] also reported identifying bilaterally symmetric hypoechoic lesions in the dorsal spinous ligament of clinically normal horses. On histopathology of several of these horses, fiber loss and mild degeneration, assumed to be an age-related degenerative change, was identified. Clinical significance was uncertain. In this author's experience, bilaterally symmetric mildly hypoechoic lesions with apparent fiber loss have also been identified and found to be of uncertain clinical significance, although histopathology was not performed on those cases. Caution in interpretation of this type of region is recommended, and care should be taken to assess and interpret the significance of bilateral symmetry. Marked asymmetry of the tuber sacrale may represent subluxation, although mild asymmetry is likely to be insignificant in this author's view. Changes in height or width greater than 1 cm between sides has been reported to be significant.[32]

In a study of 39 cases of lameness localized above the stifle, 20 were found to have sacroiliac pain and abnormalities of the sacroiliac region.[32] Fifteen of those had unilateral dorsal sacroiliac ligament asymmetry or decreased size. Interestingly, in a survey of pathologic changes of the lumbosacral region and pelvis in 36 horses euthanized at California racetracks, 100% had degenerative changes of the sacroiliac joint.[33] Twenty-five percent had degenerative changes of the lumbar vertebra. There were also 2 cases of acute subluxation and dorsal sacroiliac ligament tearing.[33]

Treatment of sacroiliac joint osteoarthritis consists of periarticular injection of anti-inflammatories, such as corticosteroids and a hyaluronic acid product. This treatment is typically performed, ideally ultrasound-guided, through a cranial, caudal, or medial approach. In cases of desmitis of the dorsal sacroiliac ligament, treatment options include controlled exercise programs, ESWT, and intralesional injection with biologics, such as platelet-rich plasma or mesenchymal stem cells.

Coxofemoral Joint

Lameness localized to the coxofemoral joint is relatively rare, but when present, it can be a challenge to properly diagnose and manage. Pelvic fractures that have an acetabular articular component will develop, in addition to a variable degree of significant or pronounced lameness, significant gluteal atrophy, which can make diagnosis a bit easier. However, in cases of osteoarthritis or damage to the round (accessory) ligament of the head of the femur, the lameness is usually nonspecific and highly variable. Imaging modalities, such as radiography, done either standing or under sedation, ultrasound, and nuclear scintigraphy, are critical to both make an accurate diagnosis and also rule out other areas. Diagnostic anesthesia of the coxofemoral joint can be done by palpation and use of landmarks, as described in the literature,[34] or by ultrasound guidance.[35] Both options require thorough knowledge of the anatomy of the region and a decent amount of patience.

REFERENCES

1. Carr EA, Maher O. Neurologic causes of gait abnormalities in the athletic horse. In: Hinchcliff KW, Kaneps AJ, Geor RJ, editors. Equine sports medicine and surgery. 2nd edition. Philadelphia: Saunders Elsevier; 2014. p. 503–26.
2. Dyson SJ. The cervical spine and soft tissues of the neck. In: Ross MW, Dyson SJ, editors. Diagnosis and management of lameness in the horse. 2nd edition. Philadelphia: Saunders Elsevier; 2011. p. 606–16.
3. García-López JM, Jenei T, Chope K, et al. Diagnosis and management of cranial and caudal nuchal bursitis in four horses. J Am Vet Med Assoc 2010;237:823-9.
4. Abuja GA, García-López JM, Manso-Díaz G, et al. The cranial nuchal bursa: anatomy, ultrasonography, magnetic resonance imaging and endoscopic approach. Equine Vet J 2014;46:745–50.
5. Bergren AL, Abuja GA, Bubeck KA, et al. Diagnosis, treatment and outcome of cranial nuchal bursitis in 30 horses. Equine Vet J 2017 [early view: 1–5].[Epub ahead of print].
6. Hohu KK, Lim CK, Adams SB, et al. Ultrasonographic and computed tomographic features of rice bodies in an Arabian horse with Atlantal bursitis. Vet Radiol Ultrasound 2018;1–5 [Epub ahead of print].
7. Chope K. How to perform sonographic examination and ultrasound-guided injection of the cervical vertebral facet joints in horses. AAEP Proceedings 2008;54:186.
8. Berg LC, Nielsen JV, Thoefner MB, et al. Ultrasonography of the equine cervical region: a descriptive study in eight horses. Equine Vet J 2003;35:647–55.
9. Nielsen JV, Berg LC, Thoefner MB, et al. Accuracy of ultrasound-guided intra-articular injection of cervical facet joints in horses: a cadaveric study. Equine Vet J 2003;35:657–61.
10. Birmingham SSW, Reed SM, Mattoon JS, et al. Qualitative assessment of corticosteroid cervical articular facet injection in symptomatic horses. Equine Vet Educ 2010;22:77–82.
11. Henson FM, Kidd JA. Overriding dorsal spinous processes. In: Henson FM, editor. Equine back pathology. Oxford (England): Blackwell Publishing; 2009. p. 147–56.
12. Townsend HGG, Leach DH, Doige CE, et al. Relationship between spinal biomechanics and pathological changes in the equine thoracolumbar spine. Equine Vet J 1986;18:107–12.
13. Denoix JM, Dyson SJ. Thoracolumbar spine. In: Ross MW, Dyson SJ, editors. Diagnosis and management of lameness in the horse. 2nd edition. Philadelphia: Saunders Elsevier; 2011. p. 592–605.

14. Pettersson H, Strömberg B, Myrin I. Das thorkolumbale, interspinale Syndrom (TLI) des Reitpferdes - Retriospektiver Vergleich konservativ und chirurgisch behandelter Fälle. Pferdeheilkunde 1987;3:313–9.
15. Denoix JM. Spinal biomechanics and functional anatomy. Vet Clin North Am Equine Pract 1999;15:27–60.
16. Cousty M, Retureau C, Tricaud C, et al. Location of radiological lesions of the thoracolumbar column in French trotters with and without signs of back pain. Vet Rec 2010;166:41–5.
17. Gillen A, Dyson S, Murray R. Nuclear scintigraphic assessment of the thoracolumbar synovial intervertebral articulations. Equine Vet J 2009;41:534–40.
18. Zimmerman M, Dyson S, Murray R. Close, impinging and overriding spinous processes in the thoracolumbar spine: the relationship between radiological and scintigraphic findings and clinical signs. Equine Vet J 2012;44:178–84.
19. Coomer RPC, McKane SA, Smith N, et al. A controlled study evaluating a novel surgical treatment for kissing spines in standing sedated horses. Vet Surg 2012;41:890–7.
20. Coudry V, Thibaud D, Riccio B, et al. Efficacy of tiludronate in the treatment of horses with signs of pain associated with osteoarthritic lesions of the thoracolumbar vertebral column. Am J Vet Res 2007;68:329–37.
21. Walmsley JP, Pettersson H, Winberg F, et al. Impingement of the dorsal spinous processes in two hundred and fifteen horses: case selection, surgical technique and results. Equine Vet J 2002;34:23–8.
22. Perkins JD, Schumacher J, Kelly G, et al. Subtotal ostectomy of dorsal spinous processes performed in nine standing horses. Vet Surg 2005;34:625–9.
23. Desbrosse FG, Perrin R, Launois T, et al. Endoscopic resection of dorsal spinous processes and interspinous ligament in ten horses. Vet Surg 2007;36:149–55.
24. Jacklin BD, Minshall GJ, Wright IM. A new technique for subtotal (cranial wedge) ostectomy in the treatment of impinging/overriding spinous processes: description of technique and outcome of 25 cases. Equine Vet J 2014;46:339–44.
25. Stubbs NC, Kaiser LJ, Hauptman J, et al. Dynamic mobilization exercises increase cross sectional area of musculus multifidus. Equine Vet J 2011;43:522–9.
26. Gillis C. Spinal ligament pathology. Vet Clin North Am Equine Pract 1999;15:97–101.
27. Henson FM, Lamas L, Knezevic S, et al. Ultrasonographic evaluation of the supraspinous ligament in a series of ridden and unridden horses and horses with unrelated back pathology. BMC Vet Res 2007;3:1–7.
28. Haussler KK. Diagnosis and management of sacroiliac joint injuries. In: Ross MW, Dyson SJ, editors. Diagnosis and management of lameness in the horse. 2nd edition. Philadelphia: Saunders Elsevier; 2011. p. 583–91.
29. Dyson S, Murray R. Pain associated with the sacroiliac joint region: a clinical study of 74 horses. Equine Vet J 2003;35:240–5.
30. Engeli E, Yeager AE, Hollis NE, et al. Ultrasonographic technique and normal anatomic features of the sacroiliac region in horses. Vet Radiol Ultrasound 2006;47:391–403.
31. Tomlinson JE, Sage AM, Turner TA, et al. Detailed ultrasonographic mapping of the pelvis in clinically normal horses and ponies. Am J Vet Res 2001;62:1768–75.
32. Tomlinson JE, Sage AM, Turner TA. Ultrasonographic abnormalities detected in the sacroiliac area in twenty cases of upper hind limb lameness. Equine Vet J 2003;35:48–54.
33. Haussler KK, Stover SM, Willits NH. Pathologic changes in the lumbosacral vertebrae and pelvis in Thoroughbred racehorses. Am J Vet Res 1999;60:143–53.

34. Moyer W, Schumacher J, Schumacher J. Coxofemoral joint. In: Moyer W, Schumacher J, Schumacher J, editors. Equine joint injection and regional anesthesia. Chadds Ford (PA): Academic Veterinary Solutions; 2011. p. 70–3.
35. Whitcomb MB, Vaughan B, Katzman S, et al. Ultrasound-guided injections in horses with cranioventral distension of the coxofemoral joint capsule: feasibility for a cranioventral approach. Vet Radiol Ultrasound 2016;57:199–206.

Muscle Conditions Affecting Sport Horses

Stephanie J. Valberg, DVM, PhD

KEYWORDS

- Rhabdomyolysis • Tying up • Myopathy • Polysaccharide storage • Atrophy

KEY POINTS

- Minor derangements in locomotor muscle function will impact power output, coordination, stamina, and desire to work during exercise.
- Subtle muscle atrophy reduces power output and impacts gait and athletic performance.
- Muscle strains, tears, and cramps are remarkably painful.
- Exertional myopathies such as type 1 polysaccharide storage myopathy (PSSM1), PSSM2 in Quarter horses, malignant hyperthermia, recurrent exertional rhabdomyolysis, and myofibrillar myopathy (MFM) in Arabians are characterized by rhabdomyolysis and high serum muscle enzymes.
- Other exertional myopathies, such as PSSM2 and MFM in Warmbloods, are characterized by exercise intolerance, reluctance to go forward, collect, and engage the hindquarters, and have normal serum muscle enzymes.

INTRODUCTION

Optimal function of skeletal muscle is essential for successful athletic performance. Even minor derangements in locomotor muscle function will impact power output, coordination, stamina, and desire to work during exercise. Veterinarians readily recognize signs of acute rhabdomyolysis and can confirm a diagnosis of rhabdomyolysis with assessment of serum creatine kinase (CK) and aspartate transaminase (AST) activities. Subtle muscle pain and weakness can also impact performance, but detecting their role in poor performance represents more of a diagnostic challenge because serum muscle enzyme activities are normal. Experience, select diagnostic tools, and horsemanship are often needed to determine the following:

Disclosure Statement: S.J. Valberg is one of the patent holders for the genetic test for type 1 polysaccharide storage myopathy and receives royalties from genetic testing. S.J. Valberg receives royalties from the sale of the equine feed Re-Leve designed for horses with exertional rhabdomyolysis.
Department of Large Animal Clinical Sciences, Michigan State University, McPhail Equine Performance Center, 736 Wilson Road, East Lansing, MI 48824, USA
E-mail address: valbergs@msu.edu

- The impact of muscle weakness on performance and gait
- The contributions of muscle pain, behavior, rider, or tack on poor performance
- Whether muscle pain is primarily a result of a muscle disorder or arising secondary to an underlying orthopedic disorder

In this review, the presenting clinical signs, differential diagnoses, approach to diagnostic testing, and treatment of muscle atrophy and weakness, focal muscle strain, and exertional myopathies are discussed (**Fig. 1**).

MUSCLE ATROPHY AND WEAKNESS

A marked reduction in muscle mass is readily recognized by veterinarians; however, gradual subtle changes often go unrecognized by owners and veterinarians. From an athletic perspective, even minor reductions in muscle mass will reduce power output and impact performance. Thus, owners and veterinarians involved in sports medicine are advised to routinely monitor muscle mass in sport horses and investigate causes of muscle loss at an early stage when treatment can be effective.

Loss of muscle mass can be focal or generalized. The inciting cause can be damage to the motor nerve supplying the muscle (neurogenic) or direct damage or atrophy of muscle fibers (myogenic) (see **Fig. 1**). Focal causes of muscle atrophy and a diagnostic approach are outlined in **Fig. 2**.

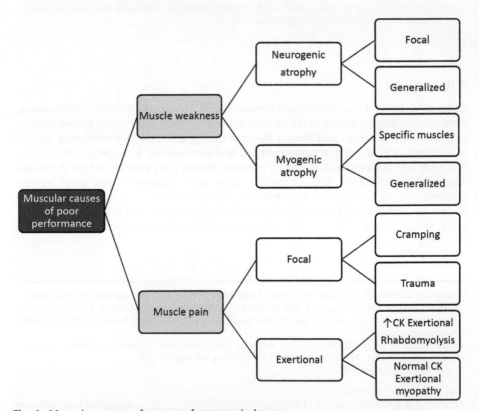

Fig. 1. Muscular causes of poor performance in horses.

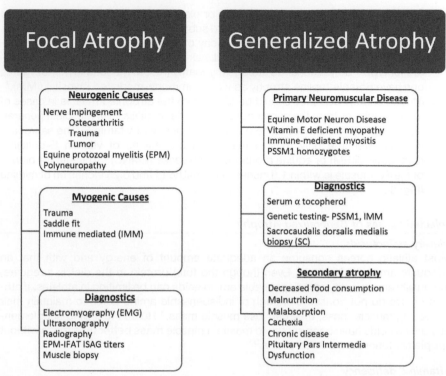

Focal Atrophy

Neurogenic Causes

Nerve Impingement
  Osteoarthritis
  Trauma
  Tumor
Equine protozoal myelitis (EPM)
Polyneuropathy

Myogenic Causes

Trauma
Saddle fit
Immune mediated (IMM)

Diagnostics

Electromyography (EMG)
Ultrasonography
Radiography
EPM-IFAT ISAG titers
Muscle biopsy

Generalized Atrophy

Primary Neuromuscular Disease

Equine Motor Neuron Disease
Vitamin E deficient myopathy
Immune-mediated myositis
PSSM1 homozygotes

Diagnostics

Serum α tocopherol
Genetic testing- PSSM1, IMM
Sacrocaudalis dorsalis medialis
biopsy (SC)

Secondary atrophy

Decreased food consumption
Malnutrition
Malabsorption
Cachexia
Chronic disease
Pituitary Pars Intermedia
Dysfunction

Fig. 2. Causes of focal and generalized muscle atrophy in horses and recommended diagnostic testing.

Diagnostic Approach to Atrophy

History

Changes in appetite, diet, supplements, access to fresh pasture, exercise routines, vaccinations, exposure to infectious diseases, and previous history of muscle atrophy or systemic disease are important to consider. Loss of muscle mass is particularly significant in horses with a normal appetite in full training.

Physical examination

Careful inspection of the horse standing perfectly square will reveal symmetric or asymmetric loss of muscle mass. Posture is important to observe because horses with weakness will have a more camped under stance and may shift weight from hind limb to alternate hind limb. Fasciculations can also indicate significant muscle weakness. Knowledge of normal muscle mass for that breed at that fitness level and the individual's previous muscle mass before poor performance is necessary to determine the significance of observations. Inspection is followed by palpation of muscle for tone, atrophy, and pain as well as completing a full physical and neurologic examination.

Differential Diagnoses and Diagnostic Tests

A list of differential diagnoses for focal and generalized muscle atrophy as well as diagnostic tests is provided in **Fig. 2**. Tests that are particularly useful to identify myogenic causes of weakness and atrophy include the following:

- *Serum vitamin E concentration:* Serum or plasma samples should be protected from light, kept cool and spun down, and submitted as soon as possible after obtaining the blood sample to prevent decay of vitamin E.
- *Genetic testing:* Depending on the breed, hair roots or EDTA blood can be submitted for type 1 polysaccharide storage myopathy (PSSM1) because homozygotes can have notable topline atrophy as well as immune-mediated myositis (IMM).[1]
- *Muscle biopsy:* Samples should be taken from the atrophied muscle in cases of focal atrophy or from the sacrocaudalis dorsalis medialis (SC) muscle if generalized atrophy is suspected to be due to a deficiency of vitamin E. The sacrocaudalis is often the only muscle that will show lesions of vitamin E–deficient myopathy (VitEM) or equine motor neuron disease (EMND).[2] The site for biopsy of the SC muscle is within 1.5 inches of the tail head and 0.25 inches off of midline (**Fig. 3**).

Selected Causes of Generalized Atrophy

Dietary amino acids

Most athletic horses consume an adequate amount of energy and with that an adequate amount of protein. Even though the total protein in the diet is adequate, the quality and quantity of indispensable amino acids can be limiting in athletes. If athletic horses do not consume enough of indispensable amino acids to maintain their increasing muscle mass, they can lose muscle mass.[3] Horses receiving supplementary amino acids have been shown to maintain muscle mass better than those without supplementation, regardless of age.[3]

Vitamin E deficiency

With the decreasing availability of fresh grass pasture, the primary source of vitamin E in a horse's diet, more horses are experiencing vitamin E (α-tocopherol) deficiency. Years of vitamin E deficiency can result in EMND characterized by dramatic muscle weakness and irreversible symmetric muscle atrophy.[2] Some horses with vitamin E deficiency develop a myopathy (VitEM) with clinical signs similar to or more subtle than EMND and atrophy that is more responsive to treatment with α-tocopherol (**Fig. 4**).[4] In many cases, diagnosis of vitamin E deficiency is based on low serum

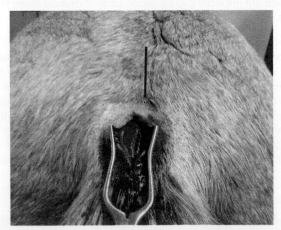

Fig. 3. The site for sacrocaudalis dorsalis muscle biopsy. The skin incision is made within 1.5 inches of the tail head, 0.25 to 0.5 inches off of midline (*vertical line*).

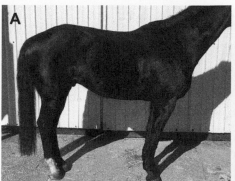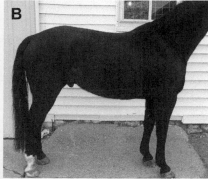

Fig. 4. (*A*) Horse with vitamin E deficiency. Note the slightly camped under stance and lack of round shape to the gluteal muscles. (*B*) The same horse after several months of supplementation with α-tocopherol. Note the increase in muscle mass over the back and hindquarters and normal stance.

α-tocopherol concentrations. Some horses with vitEM can have normal serum α-tocopherol yet low muscle α-tocopherol concentrations. In such cases, a diagnosis of vitEM is made by evaluating muscle fiber shapes and mitochondrial staining patterns in the SC.[4] EMND is typified by neurogenic angular atrophied muscle fibers, whereas vitEM shows anguloid atrophy and a moth-eaten mitochondrial staining that could represent excessive oxidative stress.

Unlike EMND, vitEM is remarkably responsive to treatment with α-tocopherol.[2,4] Before starting supplementation, serum α-tocopherol is assayed in order to monitor response to supplementation (which has individual variability). Natural-source water-dispersible forms of α-tocopherol at 10 IU/kg body weight for at least 1 month are used because they are 5 to 6 times more bioavailable than synthetic DL α-tocopherol acetate powder. Natural α-tocopheryl acetate in powdered formulations provides a good means to maintain serum α-tocopherol concentrations once in the normal range.[5] A gradual transition to powdered formulations from liquid formulations is recommended to prevent a precipitous decrease in serum α-tocopherol.[5]

Immune-mediated myositis

In contrast to vitEM, symmetric atrophy with IMM is rapid and initially primarily affects the topline muscles (**Fig. 5**).[6,7] Serum CK and AST activities are usually moderate to markedly elevated initially. Diagnosis of IMM has previously been made by identifying lymphocytic infiltrates in gluteal and epaxial muscle biopsies in early stages of atrophy. Recently, an autosomal dominant genetic mutation in *MYH1*, which encodes type 2 X myosin heavy chain, was identified in IMM horses.[1] Genetic testing will soon be available to diagnose IMM in Quarter horse–related breeds. Early identification of IMM is key to halting muscle loss through instituting treatment with dexamethasone (0.06 mg/kg) or prednisolone (1 mg/kg).[6] Doses are tapered over 4 weeks. Recurrence of atrophy is seen in at least 40% of cases.

FOCAL MUSCLE PAIN
Muscle Cramping

A muscle cramp arises from repetitive firing of a nerve and associated motor unit. Intensely painful cramps can follow forceful contraction of a shortened muscle, trauma, and marked electrolyte derangements. Most muscle cramps are also

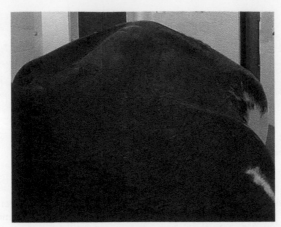

Fig. 5. Dramatic atrophy of epaxial and gluteal muscles in a horse with IMM.

accompanied by fasciculations and normal serum CK and AST activities. Mild cramps are usually self-limiting. Severe cramps of the epaxial muscles may require manipulation to release spasms. In endurance horses, cramps are part of exhaustion syndrome and require attention to dehydration, acid base, and electrolyte balance. In contrast to cramps, muscle contractures arise from direct shortening of sarcomeres without depolarization of nerves or muscle cell membranes. Contractures occur with muscle tearing and exertional rhabdomyolysis (ER), and, if sufficient muscle is damaged, are associated with high serum CK activity.

Muscle Strain

Mild muscle strains are identified as increased muscle tone and firm knots within muscles that show consistent pain upon palpation. Serum CK and AST are normal. Common sites for mild muscle strain are as follows:

- Epaxial muscles in Standardbreds, dressage, jumping horses
- Semimembranosus/semitendinosus muscles in reining, roping, cutting horses
- Pectoral muscles in event horses after cross country[8]

Muscle strain can arise from overuse, creating cramps or mild muscle damage. Potential causes include an underlying lameness that alters gait pattern and an underlying inflamed joint that induces protective, painful muscle contractions. With mild strains, serum CK and AST activities are within the normal range, and ultrasonography of the muscle shows a normal pattern.

- A detailed history, physical examination, and lameness examination are often needed to identify potential underlying causes of muscle soreness.
- Intermittent electrical stimulation can also be helpful in identifying strained muscles. The strength of stimulus necessary to induce contraction in a muscle group can be incrementally increased and compared between left and right sides. Damaged muscle tends to respond with a greater degree of pain and contraction at lower stimulus strength.[8]

The mainstays of treatment are removing inciting causes, rest, chiropractic manipulation to relieve acute muscle spasms, and treatment of any underlying lameness.

Muscle Trauma

Painful swelling and potential herniation of a muscle belly through the overlying fascia can arise from tearing of muscle fascicles due to injury. Tears result in intramuscular hemorrhage and inflammation. If tight fascia surrounds the injured muscle, swelling can result in vascular occlusion, compartment syndrome, and severe pain. Ultrasonography is very useful to determine the extent of muscle tearing. Serum CK activity is often normal unless damage is extensive. Common sites of tearing are as follows:

- In the forelimb: biceps brachii, brachiocephalicus, pectoralis, and the musculotendinous junction of the superficial digital flexor
- In the hind limb: semimembranosus and semitendinosus, adductor, gluteal and gastrocnemius muscles[8]

Diagnosis of muscle tearing can usually be achieved using palpation, thermography, and ultrasonography for superficial tears and by nuclear scintigraphy if deeper muscles are involved (**Fig. 6**).

Without quick reduction in hemorrhage and swelling, muscle repair may be impaired, resulting in chronic loss of muscle mass, fibrosis, and rarely, ossification. Chronic fibrosis of the semimembranosus/semitendinosus muscles can produce a gait abnormality termed fibrotic myopathy, whereby the anterior phase of the stride

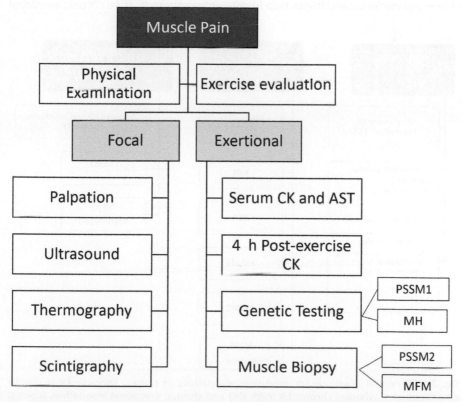

Fig. 6. Diagnostic approach to the evaluation of horses with muscle pain.

ceases abruptly, causing the leg to be pulled back before the foot suddenly slaps the ground rather than continuing its forward motion.

The initial goal of treating muscle tears is to relieve muscle spasm, decrease hemorrhage and inflammation, restore circulation, minimize scarring, and maintain range of motion. Initial treatment should focus on reducing swelling and hemorrhage with cold therapy and rest. The extent of rest depends on the degree of tearing and hemorrhage. Once swelling is reduced, other useful modalities include therapeutic ultrasound or laser therapy to promote blood flow and healing followed with massage, passive stretching, transcutaneous electrical stimulation, and a graduated, controlled exercise program. Once initiated, the exercise program must be carefully moderated according to the site of the injury, to avoid overstress in the early stages of repair, but encouraging a progressive increase in strength.

GENERALIZED EXERTIONAL MUSCLE PAIN
Diagnostic Approach

Key components of the diagnostic approach are a thorough history, physical examination, neurologic and lameness examinations, and selection of diagnostic tests (**Fig. 7**).

History
Performance level, fitness level, exercise schedule, duration, severity, and frequency of exercise intolerance/stiffness help to differentiate sporadic from chronic exertional

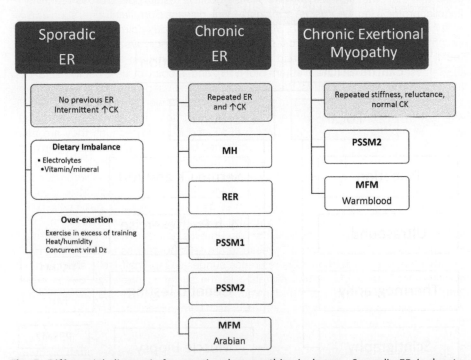

Fig. 7. Differential diagnosis for exertional myopathies in horses. Sporadic ER is due to extrinsic causes, whereas chronic ER (high CK) and chronic exertional myopathies (normal CK) are thought to result from intrinsic abnormalities in muscle structure and function.

myopathies. Changes in muscle mass and symmetry, previous lameness, changes in saddling, rider, and trainer all help to formulate a list of differential diagnoses. Time off, turn out, diet, supplements, and any factors that initiate the performance problem are essential to document in order to develop a management regimen.

Physical examination
Similar to the examination described for muscle atrophy, inspection of muscle mass with the horse standing perfectly square is important. The entire musculature is palpated for tone, heat, pain, fasciculations, and swelling or atrophy by comparing with contralateral muscle groups. Flexibility of head, neck, back, and limbs is investigated through range-of-motion evaluation. Running a blunt instrument over the lumbar and gluteal muscles should illicit extension (swayback) followed by flexion (hogback) in healthy animals. Lateral motion through the spine can be assessed by push and pull of tuber coxae and withers simultaneously. Guarding against movement may reflect abnormalities in the pelvic or thoracolumbar muscles, or pain associated with the thoracolumbar spine or sacroiliac joints. Evidence of pain or resentment should be assessed several times to ensure it is repeatable.

Blood samples should be drawn before exercise to assess serum CK and AST. At a walk, weakness is evaluated through observation of toe dragging and a shortened stride as well as through a tail pull when the hind limb is in the stance phase on the side of the examiner. The horse is then observed at a walk, trot, and canter on a lunge-line. Attention is paid to the following:

- The degree of overreach from hind hoof to fore hoof impressions
- The degree of rounding or hollowing of the back
- The degree of pushing off with the hind limbs at the trot and canter, creating either a forward thrust (normal) or a vertical thrust (abnormal)
- Reluctance to go forward causing tail swishing, bucking
- Difficulty with trot, canter transitions
- Facial expressions of pain
- Lameness

In complex cases, repeated clinical evaluations may be required, including examination of the horse under saddle. Viewing the horse under saddle with its usual rider can help to determine if saddle fit or the rider itself is contributing to muscle pain.

Lameness examination
A full lameness examination with flexion tests is part of a muscle workup because most poor performance issues in sport horses are not restricted to one body system. Use of bone scans to localize inflammation, local blocks to confirm the source of pain, and radiography and ultrasound examination to characterize lesions are often required. In addition, if horses have exercise intolerance, a standardized incremental exercise test that incorporates monitoring heart rate and blood lactate may be of value to assess horses for cardiovascular and metabolic derangements.

Exercise challenge
An exercise challenge can be helpful in detecting subclinical ER and in observing the progression of a gait abnormality with exercise. Blood samples to evaluate peak changes in CK activity should be taken before exercise and about 4 to 6 hours after, but NOT immediately after, exercise.[9]

- For unfit horses, the exercise test involves 2-minute intervals of walk and trot for up to 15 minutes. Clinical judgment should be used, and horses should not be pushed if they seem reluctant to continue to exercise. Rather, allowing a horse to stand for a minute and then asking the horse to recommence a trot often differentiates a lazy horse from one that will continue to show a stiff and stilted gait from muscle pain.
- For fit horses, the exercise test involves 4 minutes of walk and 11 minutes of continuous trot. During the test, horses should be observed carefully for exacerbation of lameness, changes in impulsion, stiffness, shortened stride, and development of a sour attitude.
- A 2- to 3-fold increase in CK indicates chronic subclinical ER.[10]
- A normal serum CK response to exercise can occur in horses with the following:
  - No muscle disease
  - PSSM1 and recurrent exertional rhabdomyolysis (RER) on well-controlled diet and exercise regimes
  - Type 2 polysaccharide storage myopathy (PSSM2), myofibrillar myopathy (MFM), and vitEM[11,12]

In addition to quantifying the extent of rhabdomyolysis during mild exercise, the exercise test can also be used to decide how rapidly to put a horse back into training. Horses with moderate to marked elevations in CK 4 hours following light exercise should be very gradually reintroduced to exercise once a therapeutic regimen is instituted.

Differential diagnoses and diagnostic tests

Differential diagnoses for exertional myopathies are shown in **Fig. 7**, and available diagnostic tests are shown in **Table 1**.

Table 1
Muscle disorders listed by breed, their primary clinical signs with recommended diagnostic tests

Breed	Primary CS	Diagnostic Test
Quarter horse, Paint, Appaloosa		
IMM	Atrophy	*MYH1* genetic test
PSSM1	ER	*GYS1* genetic test
MH	ER	*RYR1* genetic test
PSSM2	ER	CK, AST, muscle biopsy
RER (racing breeds)	ER	CK, AST, clinical signs
Thoroughbreds, Standardbreds		
RER	ER	CK, AST, clinical signs
PSSM2	ER	CK, AST, muscle biopsy
Arabians		
PSSM2	ER	CK, AST, muscle biopsy
RER	ER	CK, AST, clinical signs
MFM	ER	CK, AST, muscle biopsy
Warmbloods		
RER	ER	CK, AST, clinical signs
PSSM1	ER	*GYS1* genetic test
PSSM2	EI/ER	Muscle biopsy
MFM	EI/ER	Muscle biopsy

Abbreviations: CS, clinical signs; EI, exercise intolerance; ER, exertional rhabdomyolysis; *MYH1*, myosin heavy chain 1.

- Serum α tocopherol and whole blood selenium concentrations are measured in horses from areas of known deficiency.
- Genetic testing for malignant hyperthermia (MH) and PSSM1 is indicated in Quarter horse–related breeds.[13,14] PSSM1 is also present in a small percentage of Warmbloods and at least 20 other breeds.[15,16] Light breeds, such as Arabian, Thoroughbred, and Standardbred horses, do not appear to possess the MH or PSSM1 mutations.
- Muscle biopsy is indicated if genetic testing is negative, if chronic muscle pain impedes performance, or if horses are not responding to changes in diet and exercise management.
  - Gluteal or semimembranosus biopsies are preferred.
  - A portion fixed in formalin and a portion fresh placed in a hard container on ice packs are sent to specialized laboratories.

A muscle should only be biopsied in the face of a high degree of suspicion of clinical muscle disease after lameness has been thoroughly investigated. Recommendations for selective use of muscle biopsy arise because, for disorders such as PSSM2, assessment of glycogen stains has relatively low sensitivity and specificity.

Classification of Exertional Myopathies

Exertional myopathies are defined by muscle pain and impaired performance apparent during or after exercise. ER represents a subset of exertional myopathies characterized by elevations in serum CK and AST activity. Some exertional myopathies are not characterized by elevations in serum muscle enzymes or by very rare elevations in muscle enzymes (see **Fig. 7**). Rider, tack, behavioral, and orthopedic causes of decreased performance need to be ruled out before investigating a primary exertional myopathy.

Exertional Rhabdomyolysis

Overt ER can arise as a sporadic event because of extrinsic factors, such as exercise in excess of training, nutritional imbalances, or exercise during viral illness. ER can also occur as a chronic disease because of intrinsic abnormalities in muscle function. Acute clinical signs of ER are very similar across the spectrum of causes.
  Clinical signs include the following:

- Muscle stiffness, shortened hind limb stride, reluctance to move
- Firm, painful hindquarter muscles
- Anxiety, pain, sweating, increased respiratory rate

Cause of Sporadic Exertional Rhabdomyolysis

Sporadic forms of ER develop from the following:

- Exercise in excess of training, identified by comparing the intensity of the instigating exertion with the horse's foundation of training. ER, for example, affects up to 9% of US polo horses, with most of these horses only having one episode of ER early in the polo season.[17]
- Dietary imbalances, including high nonstructural carbohydrate (NSC) content and low forage content, deficiencies in electrolytes.[18,19] ER may be exacerbated by inadequate selenium and vitamin E.
- Exhaustion in endurance or sport horses exercising in hot, humid weather. In addition to signs of ER, horses have hyperthermia (105°F–108°F), weakness, ataxia, rapid breathing, and, in severe cases, collapse. Muscles are frequently

not firm on palpation, although serum CK activity can be markedly elevated and myoglobinuria may be noted with exhaustion.[20,21]

Chronic Exertional Rhabdomyolysis

Chronic forms of ER appear to develop in horses because of intrinsic abnormalities in muscle function. In some cases, muscle dysfunction is attributed to a single gene defect.[13,14,22,23] In other cases, there may be multiple genes impacting muscle dysfunction or posttranslational modifications of gene products that arise under certain environmental stimuli.

Recurrent exertional rhabdomyolysis

RER describes a subset of ER that is thought to be due to an abnormality in the regulation of muscle contraction and relaxation.[10,24–26] Research into RER has primarily been performed in Thoroughbreds and to a lesser extent in Standardbred horses.[24,27–29] There are reports of ER in racing Quarter horses, Arabian, and Warmblood horses[30] that may have the same underlying cause as based on the overlapping histories, clinical signs, muscle biopsy findings, and response to management (see **Table 1**).

Prevalence The prevalence of RER in Thoroughbred and standard racehorses is remarkably similar around the world with estimates ranging from 4.9% in the United States,[27] 5.4% in Australia,[31] 6.7% in the United Kingdom,[32,33] and 6.4% in Sweden.[34] Standardbred trotters with a history of RER have faster racing times from a standstill start than those without a history of RER, suggesting the trait may have beneficial as well as deleterious effects.[34] A genetic susceptibility to RER has been postulated but not proven in Thoroughbred horses with RER.[35,36] Mares more commonly have RER than males; however, no general correlation has been observed between episodes of ER and stages of the estrus cycle.[37] Nervous horses, particularly nervous fillies, have a higher incidence of ER than calm horses.[27,33,34] Diet also has an impact with Thoroughbred horses fed more than 2.5 kg of grain being more likely to show signs.[38]

In Standardbreds, ER commonly begins after 15 to 30 minutes of jogging at 5 m/s, although clinical signs may not be apparent until after exercise.[28] In Thoroughbreds at the racetrack, ER occurs commonly when horses are held back to a paced gallop.[27] During eventing, ER commonly occurs after the excitement of the steeplechase or early in the cross-country phase when horses are held to a predetermined speed.[33] ER rarely occurs when horses are allowed to achieve maximal exercise speeds, such as racing. A day or more of rest before this type of exercise results in higher serum CK activity after exercise.

Pathogenesis Rhabdomyolysis is triggered suddenly during exercise in RER horses resulting in a sharp increase in serum myoglobin and CK activity.[9] Clinically, the triggering event is often associated with excitement in a horse that already has an underlying nervous temperament.[27,32] Serum cortisol concentrations are higher in RER horses than normal horses before exercise and increase during an episode of ER.[9] Serum concentrations of epinephrine and norepinephrine are normal before an episode but increase dramatically in horses with marked elevations in serum CK activity.[9] Research suggests that horses with RER may have an inherent abnormality in intramuscular calcium regulation that is intermittently manifested during exercise.[26,39] Myoplasmic calcium concentrations are tightly controlled by channels and pumps in the sarcoplasmic reticulum and usually unaffected by normal serum calcium concentrations. Basal muscle intracellular calcium concentrations in RER horses are similar to healthy horses based on assays in muscle cell cultures.[39] Higher intracellular calcium concentrations have been measured in horses of unspecified breeds during an episode of ER; however, this also could be secondary to any insult that impairs energy generation or cell membrane integrity.[40] Muscle contracture testing, calcium imaging in muscle cell cultures, and calcium release by isolated muscle membrane preparations have been evaluated in RER horses. These studies support an abnormality in intracellular calcium regulation in the Thoroughbred or Standardbred horses studied, but none have conclusively identified a specific defect in muscle excitation-contraction coupling.

Diagnosis A presumptive diagnosis of RER is based on clinical signs of exertional muscle pain and the presence of risk factors commonly associated with RER. Serum CK and AST activities serve as the basis for detecting muscle degeneration, and they often show intermittent abnormal elevations that return to normal relatively quickly during the course of training. Muscle histopathology is nonspecific in RER horses: either no abnormalities or evidence of centrally located nuclei in mature fibers and potentially waves of myofiber degeneration or regeneration is found.[10] There is a notable absence of abnormal amylase-resistant polysaccharide, although increased subsarcolemmal amylase–sensitive glycogen may be present.[41] The value of a muscle biopsy as a diagnostic tool in horses with suspected RER is largely confined to particularly recurrent unmanageable cases whereby a need arises to rule in or out other forms of ER.

Malignant hyperthermia
MH caused by an autosomal dominant mutation in the skeletal muscle ryanodine receptor 1 gene (*RYR1*) occurs in less than 1% of Quarter horses and Paint horses.[13,42] Horses with MH can be asymptomatic or intermittently show signs of ER and elevated body temperature.[42] The *RYR1* mutation lowers the activation and heightens the deactivation threshold of the ryanodine receptor, which intermittently can result in a drastic efflux of calcium from the sarcoplasmic reticulum, increasing myoplasmic calcium and producing a contracture.[43] Anaerobic glycogen metabolism is activated; lactate is produced, and excessive heat is generated while massive muscle necrosis ensues. Some MH affected horses have died suddenly after an episode of ER.

Genetic testing is recommended in Quarter horses and Paint horses with severe ER or ER associated with elevated body temperature (see **Table 1**). A subset of horses with MH also has the *GYS1* mutation associated with PSSM1. Such horses have more severe episodes of ER, higher serum CK activity after exercise, and a more moderated response to the diet and exercise regimes recommended for PSSM1.[44]

Polysaccharide storage myopathy
Several acronyms are used for polysaccharide storage myopathy besides PSSM,[45] including EPSM (equine polysaccharide storage myopathy)[18] and EPSSM.[46] Considerable controversy existed as to whether these acronyms encompassed one muscle condition.[18,19,47] In 2008, a H309G mutation in the glycogen synthase 1 gene (*GYS1*) was found to be highly associated with the presence of amylase-resistant polysaccharide in skeletal muscle.[14] Genetic testing of hundreds of horses previously diagnosed with PSSM by muscle biopsy revealed that most cases of PSSM characterized by amylase-resistant polysaccharide in skeletal muscle had the *GYS1* genetic mutation. Normal glycogen is readily digested by the enzyme amylase, whereas abnormal polysaccharides are resistant to amylase digestion. Some cases previously diagnosed with PSSM by muscle biopsy, particularly those with excessive amylase-sensitive glycogen, did not possess the genetic mutation. These findings suggested that there

are at least 2 forms of PSSM.[14,22] For clarity, the form of PSSM caused by a *GYS1* mutation is termed type 1 (PSSM1), whereas the form or forms of PSSM not caused by the *GYS1* mutation and whose origins are yet unknown are termed type 2 (PSSM2).[22] PSSM1 is likely the same disorder described as "Azoturia" or "Monday morning disease" in work horses in the nineteenth and twentieth centuries.

Type 1 polysaccharide storage myopathy PSSM1 is caused by an autosomal dominant gain-of-function mutation in *GYS1* that results in elevated glycogen synthase activity and greater than 1.5-fold higher muscle glycogen concentrations in skeletal muscle.[14] The enzyme mutation enhances synthesis of glycogen and appears to disrupt metabolism of this energy substrate.

Prevalence More than 20 breeds possess the *GYS1* mutation responsible for PSSM1 with the highest prevalence in draft horses derived from Continental European breeds.[15,23,48,49] Six percent to 10% of Quarter horses, American Paint horses, and Appaloosa horses possess the *GYS1* mutation with the highest frequency in halter Quarter horses (28% affected) and the lowest frequency in racing Quarter horses.[50] PSSM1 affects a small proportion of warmblood horses. The prevalence of PSSM1 is very low to nonexistent in light horse breeds, such as Arabians, Standardbreds, and Thoroughbreds.

Clinical signs The severity of clinical signs of PSSM1 can vary widely from asymptomatic to severe incapacitation. The most common trigger for ER is less than 20 minutes of light exercise, particularly if the horse has been rested for several days before exercise or is unfit. Diets high in NSC also increase the risk of muscle pain and stiffness in PSSM1 horses.[51]

- Acute clinical signs resemble those of other forms of ER.
- Chronic clinical signs include a lack of energy under saddle, reluctance to move forward, stopping and stretching out as if to urinate, and a sour attitude toward exercise.[30,52]
- Dressage and show jumpers can present with chronic back pain, failure to round over fences, and fasciculations or pain upon palpation of lumbar muscles.[41]

Diagnostic testing
- Serum CK activities are often elevated in unmanaged horses, even when horses are rested.[53]
- If horses have normal serum muscle enzymes at rest, an exercise test consisting of a maximum of 15 minutes lunging at a walk and trot often show a greater than 3-fold elevation in CK activity 4 hours after exercise in unmanaged PSSM1 cases.
- The gold standard for diagnosis of PSSM1 is genetic testing for the *GYS1* mutation performed on whole blood or hair root samples (see **Table 1**).
- Muscle biopsies of horses greater than 2 years of age will contain amylase-resistant polysaccharide.

Type 2 polysaccharide storage myopathy PSSM2 is a histopathologic designation that indicates the presence of abnormal-appearing amylase-sensitive or amylase-resistant polysaccharide in muscle biopsies of horses lacking the *GYS1* mutation. Importantly, the term PSSM2 does not indicate a specific cause because no specific genetic mutations or biochemical aberrations have been described in these horses as of yet. A designation of moderate PSSM2 indicates one or more of the following: a dark periodic acid Schiff's (PAS) stain for glycogen, larger amounts of cytoplasmic aggregates of glycogen, amylase-resistant polysaccharide. A designation of mild PSSM2 indicates the presence of cytoplasmic aggregates of amylase-sensitive glycogen. The assessment of amylase-sensitive aggregates of glycogen is subjective and impacted by tissue handling, leaving considerable room for false positive diagnoses and overlap with a diagnosis of RER.[23,46,47] Thus, cases diagnosed with mild PSSM in particular should receive a full physical and lameness examination to ensure that there are no other underlying causes for poor performance.

Prevalence In the United Kingdom, approximately 35% of PSSM cases diagnosed by muscle biopsy would be classified as PSSM2.[23] Approximately 28% of cases of PSSM diagnosed by muscle biopsy in Quarter horse–related breeds would be classified as PSSM2.[54] PSSM2 seems to be common in both high-performance Quarter horse types, such as barrel racing, reining and cutting horses as well as pleasure and halter horses. About 80% of Warmblood horses diagnosed with PSSM by muscle biopsy are classified as PSSM2.[54]

Clinical signs
- In Quarter horses and light breeds, chronic ER is the predominant clinical sign.[22]
  - Elevations in CK and AST are common.
- In Warmblood horses, by 10 years of age horses show signs of sore muscles, an undiagnosed lameness, poor performance, reluctance to go forward under saddle, reluctance to collect, and in some cases, slow onset of topline atrophy, particularly if taken out of work.
  - Postexercise increase in serum CK activity is absent to infrequent in Warmbloods.

Diagnosis In Quarter horses, dark PAS staining, amylase-resistant, and amylase-sensitive abnormal polysaccharide are common diagnostic features (**Fig. 8**B). Standardbreds, Thoroughbreds, Arabians, and Warmbloods usually demonstrate an increase in anguloid myofiber atrophy, centrally displaced myonuclei, and increased subsarcolemmal or cytoplasmic aggregates of amylase-sensitive polysaccharide (**Fig. 8**C).[22]

Myofibrillar myopathy
MFM is a recently identified disorder in horses presenting with exercise intolerance or intermittent ER that is defined by specific histopathology.[12,55] First and foremost, MFM horses have cytoplasmic aggregates of the cytoskeletal protein desmin in scattered muscle fibers (see **Fig. 8**D). Desmin functions to align sarcomeres at the Z-disc and tether them to the cell membrane. Other ultrastructural derangements evident in electron microscopy include disrupted myofibrillar alignment, ectopic accumulation of cytoskeletal proteins, and Z-disc degeneration. In some cases, MFM is also characterized by cytoplasmic aggregates of glycogen similar to PSSM2. Glycogen aggregates likely form because pools of glycogen accumulate within disrupted myofibrils. MFM may represent a more extreme subset of PSSM2. Muscle glycogen concentrations in horses with MFM are similar to controls.

Warmbloods Warmblood horses diagnosed with MFM have an insidious onset of exercise intolerance notable by 6 to 8 years of age characterized by a lack of stamina, unwillingness to go forward, inability to collect, abnormal canter transitions, and inability to sustain a normal canter.[12] Unresolved hind limb lameness, stiffness, muscle pain, and, rarely, an episode of ER are reported. Serum CK and AST activities are usually within normal limits unless samples are taken in conjunction with ER.

Arabians Arabian endurance horses diagnosed with MFM usually have a history of intermittent elevations in serum CK activity after endurance rides (>10,000 U/L) or

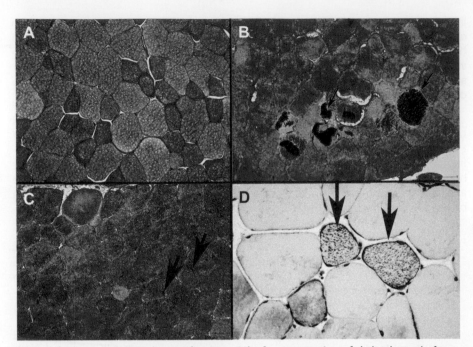

Fig. 8. (*A*) PAS stain (original magnification ×20) of a cross-section of skeletal muscle from a normal horse. (*B*) PAS stain (original magnification ×20) of a cross-section of skeletal muscle showing the presence of amylase-resistant polysaccharide (*arrows*) in a few fibers in a Quarter horses diagnosed with PSSM2. (*C*) PAS stain (original magnification ×20) of a cross-section of skeletal muscle showing the presence of small amylase-sensitive aggregates of glycogen (*arrows*) in a warmblood horse diagnosed with PSSM2. (*D*) Desmin immunohistochemical stain (original magnification ×40) of a cross-section of skeletal muscle from an Arabian horse showing 2 muscle fibers with abnormal desmin positive cytoplasmic aggregates (*arrows*).

during exercise that follows a week or more of rest.[55] Horses do not necessarily always show the same degree of pain, sweating, and reluctance to move as is frequently seen in other forms of acute ER. Myoglobinuria can be observed in horses with only mild muscle stiffness. Between episodes, the heart rate, lactate, CK, and AST responses to exercise are normal.

Transcriptomic and proteomic analyses of muscle biopsies obtained before and 3 hours after exercise in Arabian horses with MFM suggest that there may be a relationship between oxidant stress and MFM (Stephanie J. Valberg, Submitted for publication).

TREATMENT OF ACUTE EXERTIONAL RHABDOMYOLYSIS

Treatment of acute ER is aimed at relieving anxiety and muscle pain as well as correcting fluid deficits. Acepromazine (0.04–0.07 mg/kg) and xylazine (0.4-0.8 mg/kg) are among the most effective means of providing pain relief in mild to moderate cases. In more painful horses, detomidine (0.02-0.04 μg/kg) combined with butorphanol (0.01–0.04 mg/kg) provides excellent analgesia. Nonsteroidal anti-inflammatory drugs (NSAIDs), such as phenylbutazone (2.2–4.4. mg/kg) or flunixine meglumine (1.1 mg/kg), can provide additional pain relief but are not as effective in initially managing pain as sedatives. Muscle relaxants such as methocarbamol (5–22 mg/kg, intravenous [IV] slowly) seem to produce variable results possibly depending on the dosage used. Most horses are relatively pain free after an episode of ER within 18 to 24 hours.

For horses with ongoing rhabdomyolysis and extreme pain and distress, a constant rate infusion of detomidine (0.22 μg/kg IV followed by 0.1 μg/kg/min IV), lidocaine (1.3 mg/kg IV followed by 0.05 mg/kg/min IV), or butorphanol (13 μg/kg/h) can make the difference between adequate time for recovery and euthanasia. In addition, the administration of dantrium sodium (2–4 mg/kg orally) repeated in 4 to 6 hours can decrease ongoing rhabdomyolysis through its ability to decrease release of calcium from the sarcoplasmic reticulum, which further aggravates muscle contracture and necrosis. Caution is advised when administering dantrium to horses with HYPP (hyperkalemic periodic paralysis) because it can elevate serum K concentrations and precipitate an episode of fasciculations. Severe rhabdomyolysis can lead to renal compromise because of the ischemic and the combined nephrotoxic effects of myoglobinuria, dehydration, and NSAIDs. In such cases, IV fluid therapy using balanced polyionic electrolyte is advised. Affected animals are usually alkalotic, making bicarbonate therapy inappropriate.

Exercise

Following acute episodes of ER, horses can be stall confined for up to 48 hours if they are reluctant to move and have muscle stiffness. Usually within 48 hours, stiffness has resolved, and horses can be turned out in small turnout areas initially graduating to larger pastures over time.

MANAGEMENT OF CHRONIC EXERTIONAL MUSCLE DISORDERS

Altering diet and exercise regimes to compensate for underlying defects is often the best available strategy to assist horses with exertional myopathies. Identifying and eliminating any known factors that trigger ER are also important to preventing further episodes. Controlled treatment trials have been performed to validate management strategies for RER and PSSM1.[51,56,57] There is less evidenced-based information with regard to management of PSSM2 and MFM, and recommendations are based largely on retrospective studies or clinical impressions.[30]

Diet

A nutritionally balanced diet and appropriate caloric intake and adequate vitamins and minerals are the core elements of treating all forms of exertional myopathies (**Table 2**).

Forage
Forage is recommended at a rate of 1.5% to 2% of body weight.

- Hay with less than 12% NSC has been shown to prevent insulin release, a desirable effect in PSSM1 horses because insulin stimulates the already overactive glycogen synthase enzyme.[57]
- Grazing muzzles are recommended for PSSM1 horses when lush grass has particularly high sugar content.
- PSSM2 horses are currently managed similar to PSSM1; however, there is no published research to determine if this is the best strategy for these horses.

Concentrates
Concentrates with a restricted amount of starch and sugar and supplemental calories supplied with fat are commonly used to manage RER, PSSM1, and PSSM2. The current recommendations in terms of percentage of digestible energy to provide for horses with RER, PSSM1, PSSM2, and MFM are provided in **Table 2** with principles provided below:

- RER: A low to moderate dietary NSC decreases excitability with calories replaced by fat supplementation to prevent weight loss.[56] The challenge in many racehorses

Table 2
Treatments used to manage horses with various exertional myopathies

Treatment	RER	PSSM1 and PSSM2 Quarter Horses	PSSM2, Other Breeds	MFM
Diet				
NSC	<20% of DE	<10% of DE	15%–20%[a]	15%–20%[a]
Fat	15%–20% of DE	15%–20% of DE	If needed for weight	If needed for weight
Amino acids	Branched chain-NE[a]	NE	Whey protein if atrophy[a]	Whey protein[a]
Vitamin E and selenium or other antioxidants	If deficient	If deficient	If deficient	Yes
Exercise				
Turnout	Maximal	Maximal	Maximal	Maximal
Long-low lunge	No	No	Yes	Yes
Mounted 5–7 d/wk	Yes	Yes	Yes	Yes
Medication				
Low-dose acepromazine	Yes	No	No	No
Dantrolene, 2–4 mg/kg 60 min preexercise	Yes	If ER not controlled by diet	No	No

References provided where trials have been performed.
Abbreviations: DE, digestible energy; NE, no evidence.
[a] Current recommendations lacking research.

with RER is finding a highly palatable feed that will meet energy demands. Some racehorse trainers using low-starch fat-supplemented concentrates add a titrated amount of grain 3 days before a race to increase their horse's energy level.

- PSSM1: A low NSC concentrate decreases insulin release and stimulation of glycogen synthase.[51] Fat supplements provide a needed alternative energy source to glycogen. The challenge for PSSM1 horses is preventing excessive weight gain while still supplementing the diet with a fat source.
- PSSM2: Quarter horses with ER respond well to low NSC diets (Stephanie J. Valberg, Personal observation, 2017). Warmbloods with PSSM2 or MFM are fed similar NSC to PSSM1; however, there is less evidence that very low NSC or high-fat diets are the most effective means to manage these disorders.

Protein
For horses with symmetric topline muscle atrophy and horses with MFM, amino acid supplements are currently recommended (see **Table 2**).[3,12] Whey-based proteins are rich in cysteine. Cysteine is a key component of many antioxidants, and Arabian horses with MFM appear to have an increased cysteine requirement following exercise (Stephanie J. Valberg and colleagues, Submitted for publication). There is an increasing number of whey-based amino acid supplements on the market for horses.

Electrolyte supplementation
Horses require daily dietary supplementation with sodium and chloride in the form of either loose salt (30–50 g/d), a salt block, or specific supplements. Additional electrolyte supplementation is indicated in hot humid conditions.

Other dietary supplements

Several supplements are sold that are purported to decrease lactic acid buildup in skeletal muscle of ER horses. These supplements include sodium bicarbonate, B vitamins, branched chain amino acids, and dimethylglycine. Because lactic acidosis is no longer implicated as a cause for ER, it is difficult to find a rationale for their use. Acetyl L carnitine is recommended by some veterinarians for horses with PSSM1 and PSSM2 with the thought that it will promote transport of fat into mitochondria for metabolism. A deficiency in acetyl L carnitine has not been demonstrated in PSSM horses, and no clinical trials have been performed with regard to its efficacy in PSSM.

Rest

Prolonged stall rest is not recommended for any exertional myopathies because movement is essential for normal muscle function. In fact, prolonged confinement of PSSM1 horses will result in persistently elevated serum CK activity. Daily turnout for as long as possible is recommended as part of the management of EM in order to decrease anxiety in RER horses and enhance energy metabolism in PSSM1 and PSSM2 horses.

Exercise

The foundation for managing most ER horses is regular daily exercise.

Recurrent exertional rhabdomyolysis

Mild, calm, low-intensity daily exercise (<15 minutes) is recommended after an episode of ER in racehorses until serum CK is less than 1500 U/L.

- Thoroughbred racehorses often develop rhabdomyolysis when riders fight to keep horses at a slower speed (gallop exercise), and therefore, this type of exercise is best avoided in RER-prone horses.
- Standardbreds often develop ER after 15 to 30 minutes of submaximal jogging, and therefore, interval training and reduction of jog miles to no more than 15 minutes per session are recommended.
- Event horses may require training that incorporates calm exposure to speed work to prevent ER as well as interval training at the speeds achieved during competitions.

Excitement is a common triggering factor for RER, and thus avoiding this trigger is recommended.[27] Many horses respond to a regular routine, including feeding before other horses and training first before other horses, especially if the horse becomes impatient while waiting. Housing next to calm companionable horses in an area of the barn where horses are not always walking past can decrease excitement. The use of hot walkers, exercise machines, and swimming pools should be evaluated on an individual basis, because some horses develop rhabdomyolysis when using this type of equipment and others find it beneficial. Horses that develop ER at specific events, such as horse shows, may need to be reconditioned to decrease the stress level associated with such events.

Polysaccharide storage myopathy 1

The objective of the exercise regime in PSSM1 horses is to enhance oxidative metabolism and facilitate the metabolism of fat as an energy substrate. Exercise needs to be much more gradually reintroduced in PSSM1 horses than horses with RER following time off or introduction to a new diet.

- Successive daily addition of 2-minute intervals of walk and trot beginning with only 4 minutes of exercise, working up to 30 minutes after 3 weeks is recommended after which mounted exercise can resume.

- Advancing the horse too quickly often results in poor adaptation or an episode of ER and repeated frustration for the owner.
- Subclinical elevations in serum CK activity are common when exercise is reintroduced in PSSM1 horses, and a return to normal levels often requires 4 to 6 weeks of gradual exercise. Therefore, reevaluating serum CK activity is not recommended for the first 4 to 6 weeks unless a PSSM1 horse has an overt episode of ER.

Polysaccharide storage myopathy 2 and myofibrillar myopathy

At present, no controlled clinical trials have been performed for PSSM2 and MFM; however, regular exercise is considered to be important. Before mounted exercise, a relaxed warmup period in a long, low frame may help relieve tension in topline muscles. Aids such as Vienna reins, Pessoa, or neck stretchers can assist with achieving this frame during lunging. A gradually accelerating exercise program that adds 2-minute intervals of trot and canter or collection to the initial relaxed warmup period is recommended to get horses back into work. Rest periods that allow horses to relax and stretch their muscles between 2- and 5-minute periods of collection under saddle are recommended.

Medications

Recurrent exertional rhabdomyolysis

- Low doses of acepromazine before exercise have been used in RER horses prone to excitement. A dose of 7 mg IV 20 minutes before exercise is reported to make horses more relaxed and manageable. Reserpine and fluphenazine, which have a longer duration of effect, are also used for this purpose. Horses given fluphenazine may occasionally exhibit bizarre extrapyramidal behavior. Use of tranquilizers may only be necessary when horses are in their initial phase of training and accommodation to a new environment because they obviously cannot compete on these medications.
- Dantrolene sodium acts to decrease release of calcium from the calcium release channel in skeletal muscle, which can be of benefit to horses with RER, MH, or acute ER.[58,59] Recommended doses range from 800 mg per horse to 4 mg/kg orally 1 hour before exercise.
- Phenytoin (1.4–2.7 mg/kg orally twice a day) acts on several ion channels within muscle and nerves and has been used to manage horses with RER. Therapeutic levels vary, so oral doses are adjusted by monitoring serum levels to achieve 8 μg/mL and not to exceed 12 μg/mL.[60] Drowsiness and ataxia are evidence that the dose of phenytoin is too high, and the dose should be decreased by half. Initial dosages start at 6 to 8 mg/kg orally twice a day for 3 to 5 days. If the horse is still experiencing rhabdomyolysis but is not drowsy, the dose can be increased by 1-mg/kg increments every 3 to 4 days.

Some mares appear to exhibit signs of ER during estrus, and it may well be of benefit in these horses to suppress estrus behavior using progesterone injections. Testosterone and anabolic steroids have been used at racetracks to prevent signs of RER, but they are now prohibited.

Adjunct therapies

Massage, myofascial release, mesotherapy, stretching, and hot/cold therapy performed by experienced therapists may be of benefit in individual cases of ER.

Expectations

Most horses with chronic forms of ER will always have an underlying predilection for muscle soreness. Many horses with RER can be managed using the described recommendations and have successful careers unimpeded by occasional episodes of ER. A few RER horses are extremely difficult to manage and may be retired from racing. At least 70% of horses with PSSM1 and PSSM2 show notable improvement in clinical signs, and many return to acceptable levels of performance with adherence to both diet and exercise recommendations.[18,30,52] PSSM1 horses that also have the mutation for MH do not respond as well to diet and exercise recommendations and may continue to develop ER with the possibility of a fatal episode.[44] Most PSSM1 and PSSM2 horses can be successful pleasure and trail horses, but they may not achieve success in upper levels of dressage or fast-paced activities like barrel racing. Arabians horses with MFM can have very successful endurance careers when carefully managed. Warmblood horses with MFM can improve with management, but they often do not achieve the owners desired level of performance.[12]

REFERENCES

1. Finno CJ, Gianino G, Perumbakkam S, et al. A missense mutation in MYH1 is associated with susceptibility to immune-mediated myositis in quarter horses. Skelet Muscle 2018;8(1):7.
2. Divers TJ, Mohammed HO, Cummings JF, et al. Equine motor neuron disease: findings in 28 horses and proposal of a pathophysiological mechanism for the disease. Equine Vet J 1994;26:409–15.
3. Graham-Thiers PM, Kronfeld DS. Amino acid supplementation improves muscle mass in aged and young horses. J Anim Sci 2005;83:2783–8.
4. Bedford HE, Valberg SJ, Firshman AM, et al. Histopathologic findings in the sacrocaudalis dorsalis medialis muscle of horses with vitamin E-responsive muscle atrophy and weakness. J Am Vet Med Assoc 2013;242:1127–37.
5. Brown JC, Valberg SJ, Hogg M, et al. Effects of feeding two RRR-alpha-tocopherol formulations on serum, cerebrospinal fluid and muscle alpha-tocopherol concentrations in horses with subclinical vitamin E deficiency. Equine Vet J 2017;49:753–8.
6. Lewis SS, Valberg SJ, Nielsen IL. Suspected immune-mediated myositis in horses. J Vet Intern Med 2007;21:495–503.
7. Hunyadi L, Sundman EA, Kass PH, et al. Clinical implications and hospital outcome of immune-mediated myositis in horses. J Vet Intern Med 2017;31:170–5.
8. Valberg SJD, SJ. Skeletal muscle and lameness. In: Ross MWD, Dyson SJ, editors. Lameness in the horse. St Louis (MO): Elsevier; 2011. p. 818–38.
9. Valberg S, Haggendal J, Lindholm A. Blood chemistry and skeletal muscle metabolic responses to exercise in horses with recurrent exertional rhabdomyolysis. Equine Vet J 1993;25:17–22.
10. Valberg SJ, Mickelson JR, Gallant EM, et al. Exertional rhabdomyolysis in quarter horses and thoroughbreds: one syndrome, multiple aetiologies. Equine Vet J Suppl 1999;(30):533–8.
11. Lewis SS, Nicholson AM, Williams ZJ, et al. Clinical characteristics and muscle glycogen concentrations in warmblood horses with polysaccharide storage myopathy. Am J Vet Res 2017;78:1305–12.
12. Valberg SJ, Nicholson AM, Lewis SS, et al. Clinical and histopathological features of myofibrillar myopathy in warmblood horses. Equine Vet J 2017;49(6):739–45.
13. Aleman M, Riehl J, Aldridge BM, et al. Association of a mutation in the ryanodine receptor 1 gene with equine malignant hyperthermia. Muscle Nerve 2004;30: 356–65.
14. McCue ME, Valberg SJ, Miller MB, et al. Glycogen synthase (GYS1) mutation causes a novel skeletal muscle glycogenosis. Genomics 2008;91:458–66.

15. McCue ME, Anderson SM, Valberg SJ, et al. Estimated prevalence of the type 1 polysaccharide storage myopathy mutation in selected North American and European breeds. Anim Genet 2010;41(suppl 2):145–9.

16. Baird JD, Valberg SJ, Anderson SM, et al. Presence of the glycogen synthase 1 (GYS1) mutation causing type 1 polysaccharide storage myopathy in continental European draught horse breeds. Vet Rec 2010;167:781–4.

17. McGowan CM, Posner RE, Christley RM. Incidence of exertional rhabdomyolysis in polo horses in the USA and the United Kingdom in the 1999/2000 season. Vet Rec 2002;150:535–7.

18. Valentine BA, Van Saun RJ, Thompson KN, et al. Role of dietary carbohydrate and fat in horses with equine polysaccharide storage myopathy. J Am Vet Med Assoc 2001;219:1537–44.

19. Valentine BA, Hintz HF, Freels KM, et al. Dietary control of exertional rhabdomyolysis in horses. J Am Vet Med Assoc 1998;212:1588–93.

20. Carlson GP. Medical problems associated with protracted heat and work stress in horses. Proceedings of the Fifth Annual Meeting of the Association of Equine Sports Medicine. Reno, Nevada, December 1985. p. 84–99.

21. Foreman JH. The exhausted horse syndrome. Vet Clin North Am Equine Pract 1998;14:205–19.

22. McCue ME, Armien AG, Lucio M, et al. Comparative skeletal muscle histopathologic and ultrastructural features in two forms of polysaccharide storage myopathy in horses. Vet Pathol 2009;46:1281–91.

23. Stanley RL, McCue ME, Valberg SJ, et al. A glycogen synthase 1 mutation associated with equine polysaccharide storage myopathy and exertional rhabdomyolysis occurs in a variety of UK breeds. Equine Vet J 2009;41:597–601.

24. Beech J, Lindborg S, Fletcher JE, et al. Caffeine contractures, twitch characteristics and the threshold for Ca(2+)-induced Ca2+ release in skeletal muscle from horses with chronic intermittent rhabdomyolysis. Res Vet Sci 1993;54:110–7.

25. Beech J. Chronic exertional rhabdomyolysis. Vet Clin North Am Equine Pract 1997;13:145–68.

26. Lentz LR, Valberg SJ, Balog EM, et al. Abnormal regulation of muscle contraction in horses with recurrent exertional rhabdomyolysis. Am J Vet Res 1999;60:992–9.

27. MacLeay JM, Sorum SA, Valberg SJ, et al. Epidemiologic analysis of factors influencing exertional rhabdomyolysis in thoroughbreds. Am J Vet Res 1999;60:1562–6.

28. Valberg S, Jonsson L, Lindholm A, et al. Muscle histopathology and plasma aspartate aminotransferase, creatine kinase and myoglobin changes with exercise in horses with recurrent exertional rhabdomyolysis. Equine Vet J 1993;25:11–6.

29. Lindholm A, Johansson HE, Kjaersgaard P. Acute rhabdomyolysis ("tying-up") in standardbred horses. A morphological and biochemical study. Acta Vet Scand 1974;15:325–39.

30. Hunt LM, Valberg SJ, Steffenhagen K, et al. An epidemiological study of myopathies in Warmblood horses. Equine Vet J 2008;40:171–7.

31. Cole FL, Mellor DJ, Hodgson DR, et al. Prevalence and demographic characteristics of exertional rhabdomyolysis in horses in Australia. Vet Rec 2004;155:625–30.

32. McGowan CM, Fordham T, Christley RM. Incidence and risk factors for exertional rhabdomyolysis in thoroughbred racehorses in the United Kingdom. Vet Rec 2002;151:623–6.

33. Upjohn MM, Archer RM, Christley RM, et al. Incidence and risk factors associated with exertional rhabdomyolysis syndrome in National Hunt Racehorses in Great Britain. Vet Rec 2005;156:763–6.

34. Isgren CM, Upjohn MM, Fernandez-Fuente M, et al. Epidemiology of exertional rhabdomyolysis susceptibility in standardbred horses reveals associated risk factors and underlying enhanced performance. PLoS One 2010;5:e11594.

35. Dranchak PK, Valberg SJ, Onan GW, et al. Inheritance of recurrent exertional rhabdomyolysis in thoroughbreds. J Am Vet Med Assoc 2005;227:762–7.

36. MacLeay JM, Valberg SJ, Sorum SA, et al. Heritability of recurrent exertional rhabdomyolysis in thoroughbred racehorses. Am J Vet Res 1999;60:250–6.

37. Fraunfelder HC, Rossdale PD, Rickets SW. Changes in serum muscle enzyme levels associated with training schedules and stages of oestrus cycle in thoroughbred racehorses. Equine Vet J 1986;18:371–4.

38. MacLeay JM, Valberg SJ, Pagan JD, et al. Effect of ration and exercise on plasma creatine kinase activity and lactate concentration in thoroughbred horses with recurrent exertional rhabdomyolysis. Am J Vet Res 2000;61:1390–5.

39. Lentz LR, Valberg SJ, Herold LV, et al. Myoplasmic calcium regulation in myotubes from horses with recurrent exertional rhabdomyolysis. Am J Vet Res 2002;63:1724–31.

40. Lopez JR, Linares N, Cordovez G, et al. Elevated myoplasmic calcium in exercise-induced equine rhabdomyolysis. Pflugers Arch 1995;430:293–5.

41. Quiroz-Rothe E, Novales M, Guilera-Tejero E, et al. Polysaccharide storage myopathy in the M. longissimus lumborum of showjumpers and dressage horses with back pain. Equine Vet J 2002;34:171–6.

42. Aleman M, Nieto JE, Magdesian KG. Malignant hyperthermia associated with ryanodine receptor 1 (C7360G) mutation in quarter horses. J Vet Intern Med 2009;23:329–34.

43. Mickelson JR, Louis CF. Malignant hyperthermia: excitation-contraction coupling, Ca2+ release channel, and cell Ca2+ regulation defects. Physiol Rev 1996;76:537–92.

44. McCue ME, Valberg SJ, Jackson M, et al. Polysaccharide storage myopathy phenotype in quarter horse-related breeds is modified by the presence of an RYR1 mutation. Neuromuscul Disord 2009;19:37–43.

45. Valberg SJ, MacLeay JM, Billstrom JA, et al. Skeletal muscle metabolic response to exercise in horses with 'tying-up' due to polysaccharide storage myopathy. Equine Vet J 1999;31:43–7.

46. Valentine BA, McDonough SP, Chang YF, et al. Polysaccharide storage myopathy in Morgan, Arabian, and standardbred related horses and Welsh-cross ponies. Vet Pathol 2000;37:193–6.

47. Valentine BA, Cooper BJ. Incidence of polysaccharide storage myopathy: noo ropsy study of 225 horses. Vet Pathol 2005;42:823–7.

48. McGowan CM, Menzies-Gow NJ, McDiarmid AM, et al. Four cases of equine polysaccharide storage myopathy in the United Kingdom. Vet Rec 2003;152:109–12.

49. McGowan CM, McGowan TW, Patterson-Kane JC. Prevalence of equine polysaccharide storage myopathy and other myopathies in two equine populations in the United Kingdom. Vet J 2009;180:330–6.

50. Tryon RC, Penedo MC, McCue ME, et al. Evaluation of allele frequencies of inherited disease genes in subgroups of American quarter horses. J Am Vet Med Assoc 2009;234:120–5.

51. Ribeiro WP, Valberg SJ, Pagan JD, et al. The effect of varying dietary starch and fat content on serum creatine kinase activity and substrate availability in equine polysaccharide storage myopathy. J Vet Intern Med 2004;18:887–94.
52. Firshman AM, Valberg SJ, Bender JB, et al. Epidemiologic characteristics and management of polysaccharide storage myopathy in quarter horses. Am J Vet Res 2003;64:1319–27.
53. Valberg SJ, MacLeay JM, Mickelson JR. Polysaccharide storage myopathy associated with exertional rhabdomyolysis in horses. Comp Cont Educ Pract 1997; 19(9):1077–86.
54. McCue ME, Ribeiro WP, Valberg SJ. Prevalence of polysaccharide storage myopathy in horses with neuromuscular disorders. Equine Vet J Suppl 2006;36:340–4.
55. Valberg SJ, McKenzie EC, Eyrich LV, et al. Suspected myofibrillar myopathy in Arabian horses with a history of exertional rhabdomyolysis. Equine Vet J 2016; 48:548–56.
56. McKenzie EC, Valberg SJ, Godden SM, et al. Effect of dietary starch, fat, and bicarbonate content on exercise responses and serum creatine kinase activity in equine recurrent exertional rhabdomyolysis. J Vet Intern Med 2003;17:693–701.
57. Borgia L, Valberg S, McCue M, et al. Glycaemic and insulinaemic responses to feeding hay with different non-structural carbohydrate content in control and polysaccharide storage myopathy-affected horses. J Anim Physiol Anim Nutr (Berl) 2011;95:798–807.
58. McKenzie EC, Valberg SJ, Godden SM, et al. Effect of oral administration of dantrolene sodium on serum creatine kinase activity after exercise in horses with recurrent exertional rhabdomyolysis. Am J Vet Res 2004;65:74–9.
59. Edwards JG, Newtont JR, Ramzan PH, et al. The efficacy of dantrolene sodium in controlling exertional rhabdomyolysis in the thoroughbred racehorse. Equine Vet J 2003;35:707–11.
60. Beech J, Fletcher JE, Lizzo F, et al. Effect of phenytoin on the clinical signs and in vitro muscle twitch characteristics in horses with chronic intermittent rhabdomyolysis and myotonia. Am J Vet Res 1988;49:2130–3.

Neurologic Conditions Affecting the Equine Athlete

Daniela Bedenice, Dr med vet[a],*, Amy L. Johnson, BA, DVM[b]

KEYWORDS

- Equine herpes virus (EHV-1) myeloencephalopathy (EHM)
- Equine protozoal myeloencephalitis (EPM)
- Equine degenerative myeloencephalopathy (EDM)
- Cervical vertebral stenotic myelopathy (CVSM)

KEY POINTS

- Equine protozoal myeloencephalitis, cervical vertebral stenotic myelopathy, and equine degenerative myeloencephalopathy are 3 of the most common neurologic diseases in US horses, with the latter 2 conditions being most prevalent in young horses. Furthermore, horses competing at shows and performance events are at greater risk of exposure to highly contagious, neurologic equine herpes virus-1 outbreaks.
- Horses with mild or early clinical signs of neurologic gait deficits often present for performance-related concerns that can be difficult to discern from a lameness condition. Horses with unspecific gait changes should therefore undergo a complete neurologic examination.
- A diagnosis of neurologic disease should always start with a detailed clinical examination and not be based on diagnostic imaging or serologic testing of prevalent disease conditions alone.

INTRODUCTION

Neurologic disease can often mimic or be mistaken for an orthopedic condition when horses present for performance-related concerns. A careful history, clinical examination, appropriate diagnostic testing, and interpretation are thus essential for an accurate diagnosis. A thorough history includes the duration and extent of the problem, a change or progression of clinical abnormalities over time, response to analgesia, events of tripping or falling, and exacerbation of clinical signs during specific activities or movements.

[a] Department of Clinical Sciences, Cummings School of Veterinary Medicine at Tufts University, 200 Westboro Road, North Grafton, MA 01536, USA; [b] Department of Clinical Studies, University of Pennsylvania, School of Veterinary Medicine, New Bolton Center, 382 West Street Road, Kennett Square, PA 19348, USA
* Corresponding author.
E-mail address: daniela.bedenice@tufts.edu

Vet Clin Equine 34 (2018) 277–297
https://doi.org/10.1016/j.cveq.2018.04.006
0749-0739/18/© 2018 Elsevier Inc. All rights reserved.

vetequine.theclinics.com

In general, lame horses are more commonly reluctant to work or to continue to work than ataxic horses. However, both conditions may lead to premature exhaustion or exercise intolerance due to inefficiency of locomotion, especially if ataxia is associated with weakness. Most orthopedic conditions are affected by the level and duration of exercise; whereas osteoarthritis may improve after the horse has warmed up, lameness associated with acute arthritis will likely become more severe during increasing exercise. These effects are not commonly noted in ataxic horses.[1] Similarly, most causes of neurologic disease do not induce pain, with the notable exception of some forms of cervical vertebral stenotic myelopathy (CVSM) or other vertebral arthropathies. Perineural and/or intrasynovial (local) anesthesia may thus help in the differentiation of lameness and ataxia. Systemic analgesia (a single intravenous (IV) dose of phenylbutazone) may lead to a more obvious response in lameness reduction for patients with acute single-limb lameness, than in the typical clinical patient with chronic multilimb lameness. The latter more consistently show a general increase in willingness to work with nonsteroidal anti-inflammatory drugs (NSAIDs), whereas no such change is usually expected in pain-free ataxic horses. In contrast, ataxia is usually exacerbated after sedation (eg, for obtaining radiographs of the cervical spine).[1]

It is important that the diagnosis of neurologic disease always starts with a detailed clinical examination and is not based on diagnostic imaging or serologic testing of prevalent disease conditions alone. There is generally little disagreement between clinicians when assessing the presence or absence of neurologic signs in moderately to severely affected horses. However, considerable interobserver variability exists in both the recognition and grading of neurologic abnormalities, especially when the clinical signs in the horse are subtle.[2,3] Athletes, such as hunters, jumpers, and dressage horses, with mild neurologic disease can often meet performance expectations to a certain point, or complete their existing job quite well (until their disease progresses or confounding conditions, such as lameness, develop). The true onset of their neurologic signs can thus be difficult to ascertain.

The current article focuses on the clinical recognition, diagnosis, and management of the 3 most commonly reported neurologic conditions in US horses (equine protozoal myeloencephalitis [EPM], CVSM, and equine degenerative myeloencephalopathy [EDM]); in addition to equine herpes virus-1 (EHV-1) myeloencephalopathy as a highly contagious infectious disease of increasing importance at performance venues and large equestrian farms.[4] Many additional neurologic disorders exist that may result in gait deficits or performance problems, but are beyond the scope of this review.

CERVICAL VERTEBRAL STENOTIC MYELOPATHY

CVSM is almost certainly one of the most common causes of ataxia in sport horses. Its etiology is complicated, and CVSM is widely considered to be a developmental abnormality modulated by genetic predispositions and environmental influences, including diet, rate of growth, workload, and trauma. The pathophysiology of the disease involves spinal cord compression due to malformation, malarticulation, instability, and soft tissue or bony changes of the cervical vertebrae, their articulations, and associated soft tissue structures. Various investigators have attempted to categorize CVSM based on the structural abnormalities. Rooney[5] described 3 types: type I, a fixed flexural deformity of the neck that usually occurs at C2-C3 and is present at birth; type II, symmetric overgrowth of the articular processes causing spinal cord compression during neck flexion, usually occurring in the mid-cervical region of foals and weanlings; and type III, asymmetrical overgrowth of 1 articular process that compresses the spinal cord directly by bony proliferation or indirectly by associated soft tissue hypertrophy, usually affecting caudal cervical vertebrae of mature horses.[5] More recently, CVSM has been divided into 2 broad categories: 1 affecting young horses (type I, similar to Rooney's type II), and 1 affecting older horses (type II, similar to Rooney's type III).[6,7] Type I generally affects young horses, particularly thoroughbreds, manifesting as developmental abnormalities, such as malformation of the vertebral canal, enlargement of the physes, extension of the dorsal aspect of the vertebral arch, angulation between adjacent vertebrae, and malformation and osteochondrosis of the articular processes.[8] Type II generally affects older horses of all breeds and involves osteoarthritic changes of the articular processes.[8,9] There is substantial overlap between types, and older horses can have developmental abnormalities despite a late onset of clinical disease, whereas very young horses can have osteoarthritic changes that contribute to their clinical signs. Additionally, older horses frequently develop cervical osteoarthritis in the absence of spinal cord disease.

Clinical Signs

CVSM is characterized by general proprioceptive ataxia and weakness caused by disruption of the upper motor neuron and general proprioceptive tracts within the cervical spinal cord, and sometimes the lower motor neurons and nerve roots of the cervical intumescence. Most commonly, horses with cervical spinal cord disease due to CVSM have general proprioceptive deficits in all 4 limbs. Horses with mild lesions can appear to be unaffected in the thoracic limbs, with mild signs in the pelvic limbs, and it is common for deficits in the hindlimbs to be more obvious than those in the forelimbs. A long-strided spastic gait characteristic of upper motor neuron paresis is generally seen in all 4 limbs. However, caudal cervical disease can cause lower motor neuron signs in the thoracic limbs. These signs include a short-strided, choppy forelimb gait, limb buckling at rest or during movement, and muscle atrophy. Signs are generally symmetric or mildly asymmetric, although occasional horses have marked asymmetry.

Signs of neck pain are inconsistently present. Young horses with malformations frequently do not appear uncomfortable, whereas older horses with caudal cervical arthritis can show mild to severe signs of discomfort. These signs include abnormal head and neck posture, most commonly carrying the head lower than normal, or decreased range of motion when asked to bend laterally or raise and lower the head. More severely affected horses rarely bend their necks, even when asked to circle, and display a rigid "weathervane" posture when moving. If nerve root compression is occurring, the horse might show thoracic limb lameness or even a "root signature," during which the affected thoracic limb is raised and held off the ground. Rarely, a horse will become "stuck" with the head and neck held in an abnormal position, often lowered. Abnormal musculature might be evident; some horses have poorly developed cervical musculature, others seem to have poor topline muscling that extends to their rumps, and some have neurogenic muscle atrophy, most commonly of the caudal neck and thoracic limbs.

Not every horse with CVSM shows overt signs of neurologic disease or neck pain. In some cases, the first sign of the problem is a behavior change under saddle, such as bucking, bolting, rearing, or stopping at fences. The horse might be resistant when working in one direction, reluctant to move forward, reluctant to bring its head and neck up into a frame, or just lose enthusiasm for its job. Difficulty with bending or lateral work, often worse in one direction, and mild thoracic limb lameness can be observed. The rider might notice an occasional stumble, or the horse might have fallen under circumstances in which it was not expected. Some horses have difficulty traversing hills, but work well in other situations. The rider might comment that the horse feels lame, or different, but no apparent lameness is present. Recently, investigation of a hoppinglike forelimb lameness syndrome in ridden horses suggested that cervical abnormalities might sometimes be responsible for the unusual gait deficit.[10] Obviously many other orthopedic or even systemic problems can cause similar signs and poor performance. In summary, many performance problems as noted by the rider could stem from CVSM, and horses without an obvious lameness or other explanation should be assessed carefully for neurologic disease and neck pain.

Diagnosis and Differential Diagnosis

The basis for diagnosis should be a comprehensive history and neurologic evaluation, followed by appropriate imaging.

History
Clinical signs as described previously can become apparent at any age, depending on severity of spinal cord compression and demands placed on the horse. Many cases are recognized when training or competitions begin or when workload and demands increase. The recognized problem might have an acute onset, such as occurs after a fall or other trauma, or the clients might have noticed more subtle abnormalities over a prolonged period. As described in the Clinical Signs section, horses with CVSM can have performance problems due to behavioral changes or pain, and clinicians should consider the possibility of CVSM even if neurologic disease is not the presenting complaint. Adequate or even superior performance results, particularly at lower levels, do not exclude the possibility of CVSM; horses can frequently compensate for mild neurologic deficits.

Clinical examination
Thorough neurologic evaluation, with special focus on the gait examination, is essential for diagnosis. The horse should be observed for signs of proprioceptive deficits, ataxia, and weakness while moving in hand at the walk and trot, both in a straight line and circling. Additional maneuvers performed at the walk can include moving in a serpentine, walking with head elevation, walking tail pull, tight circles, backing, and walking up and down hills with the head in a neutral and elevated position. The horse is asked to bend laterally for a food reward and touch its nose to its flank bilaterally; normal horses accomplish this easily and bend fairly evenly throughout the length of their neck, while abnormal horses cannot or will not reach back to their flank. They might try to reach the food reward by twisting their head and bending only the cranial aspect of their neck. The horse is also asked to reach up in the air and down to the ground for food or observed grazing. Hesitation in lowering the head or abnormal limb position while grazing with thoracic limbs widely spread can be observed in horses with neck pain. Ridden examination is not performed if neurologic deficits are clearly identified while the horse is in hand. However, evaluation under saddle can be informative for horses with very subtle or equivocal deficits; some horses show a marked change in gait when ridden with their head and neck in a tighter (upright, flexed) frame compared with a lower, more relaxed position or when ridden in one direction compared with the other.

Imaging
Cervical radiography is usually the first imaging pursued when CVSM is suspected. Some practitioners also use sonography to evaluate the vertebral column, particularly the articular process joints. Depending on findings, more advanced imaging, such as myelography, computed tomography (CT), or MRI might be warranted.

A complete cervical radiographic series should include views from the occiput to the first thoracic vertebra, such that all articulations (atlanto-occipital through C7-T1) are included, with each articulation relatively centered in at least one view. True laterolateral projections should be obtained such that the transverse processes for any given vertebra and the paired synovial articulations (articular process joints [APJs]) are superimposed. When indicated, oblique views of the APJs can allow more accurate assessment of asymmetric pathology; techniques for obtaining and interpreting oblique projections have been described.[11]

Radiographic assessment should begin with assessment of study quality, including completeness and laterality. Radiographs with mild obliquity can be assessed, but true lateral projections are necessary to obtain accurate and repeatable minimum sagittal diameter ratio measurements. The examiner should systematically assess the alignment and shape of the vertebrae, particularly the vertebral canal and articular processes, as well as the intervertebral foramina and intervertebral disk spaces. Determining the clinical relevance of bony changes can be difficult because age-related remodeling of the APJs is common in horses and not necessarily indicative of an abnormality. A grading system for bony enlargement of the APJs has been described[12] but is not widely used.

After subjective assessment of the vertebral column, more objective assessment should be undertaken using measurement software. The minimum intravertebral sagittal diameter ratio is obtained by dividing the smallest height of the vertebral canal by the largest height of the corresponding vertebral body at its cranial aspect. The minimum intervertebral sagittal ratio is obtained by dividing the smallest dorsoventral measurement between 2 adjacent vertebrae (from the caudodorsal arch of the cranial vertebra to the craniodorsal aspect of the caudal vertebral body, or from the caudodorsal aspect of the epiphysis of the cranial vertebral body to the craniodorsal aspect of the arch of the caudal vertebra) by the largest height of the caudal vertebral body at its cranial aspect (**Fig. 1**).

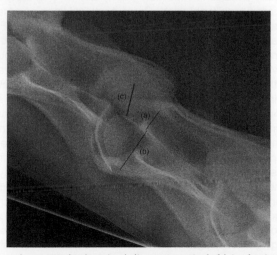

Fig. 1. The minimum intravertebral sagittal diameter ratio (a/b) is obtained by dividing the smallest height of the vertebral canal (a) by the largest height of the corresponding vertebral body at its cranial aspect (b). The minimum intervertebral sagittal ratio (c/b) is obtained by dividing the smallest dorsoventral measurement between two adjacent vertebrae (c) (from the caudodorsal arch of the cranial vertebra to the craniodorsal aspect of the caudal vertebral body) by the largest height of the caudal vertebral body at its cranial aspect (b).

Radiographic diagnosis of CVSM is usually achieved by documenting both subjective abnormalities and abnormal minimum sagittal ratio measurements. More subjective radiographic indicators include subluxation (dorsal angulation of the more caudal vertebra), physeal enlargement with dorsal projection of the caudal physis, osteoarthritis and bony proliferation of the articular processes, osteochondrotic changes at the articular processes, and caudal extension of the dorsocaudal vertebral arch over the cranial physis of the adjacent vertebrae.[8] Both intravertebral and intervertebral minimum sagittal ratios have been described.[9,13] Published cutoffs for intravertebral ratios are 0.52 for C4, C5, and C6, and 0.56 for C7.[9] Ratios below the cutoffs indicate an increased risk of having CVSM but do not confirm the diagnosis, nor do they accurately indicate the site of compression. Intravertebral measurements $\leq$0.485 identified all 8 cases of CVSM in a more recent study of 26 horses.[13]

Cervical vertebral anomalies contributing to CVSM are less frequently discussed by clinicians but should not be overlooked. Anomalous C6 vertebrae appear to be common, particularly in warmblood breeds.[10] In a population of 100 horses, 24% had anomalous C6, with either asymmetric or symmetric absence of the ventral lamina of the transverse process. Preliminary research suggests that anomalous C6 might be associated with increased perceived cervical pain as well as decreased size of the vertebral canal as assessed by minimum intravertebral sagittal ratio.[10] Other cervical vertebral anomalies are uncommon but often significant when present. Examples include block vertebrae and anomalous or transitional vertebrae.

Plain radiography is insufficient for confirming spinal cord compression. Myelography is often considered the most accurate antemortem test for CVSM, but in the future might be supplanted by CT myelography or MRI. Somewhat surprisingly, the diagnostic criteria for myelography have not been definitively established.[14] The most commonly used criteria include $\geq$50% reduction of the dorsal myelographic column and $\geq$20% reduction of the total height of the dural sac, although subjective evaluation by an experienced observer might be more accurate than either of those methods.

One of the primary limitations with radiography and myelography in horses is that only lateral views are typically obtained. Cross-sectional imaging obtained with CT or MRI is the standard for spinal cord evaluation in smaller species. For decades, CT and MRI size limitations precluded imaging the caudal equine neck. However, the availability of large-bore and robotic CTs for clinical use will revolutionize our understanding of the equine cervical vertebral column and its pathology. Major advantages of these systems include the ability to image the neck in multiple planes, detection of lateral or dorsolateral spinal cord compression, and, with some systems, the ability to perform studies in the standing horse. Although these systems will likely improve sensitivity and specificity of diagnosis, we still have much to learn, and the agreement between traditional myelography and CT myelography is unknown. Many people prefer to avoid anesthesia when possible but there are safety concerns with performing myelographic studies in nonanesthetized horses using standing systems. Additionally, dynamic views (flexion and extension) are more difficult to obtain in the standing horse.

Cervical vertebral canal endoscopy has been described as a diagnostic test but is rarely used.[15] Nuclear scintigraphy does not lead to a specific diagnosis but might serve to exclude other potential causes of poor performance. Likewise, cerebrospinal fluid (CSF) cytology generally yields normal or nonspecific results, but analysis of CSF can allow exclusion of other potential diseases, such as EPM.

Treatment

Horses with CVSM can be treated medically or surgically. The mainstays of medical treatment involve rest or reduction in exercise and systemic or local anti-inflammatory treatment. Young horses are also sometimes treated with dietary modifications to reduce rate of growth.[16,17] There are no controlled studies to evaluate the efficacy of the "paced growth" diet or any anti-inflammatory protocol. Horses with arthritis of the APJs are frequently treated with intraarticular injections of corticosteroids, hyaluronan, or autologous protein solution. Theoretically, these injections might reduce inflammatory mediators and pain, reduce soft tissue swelling, and stabilize or prevent bone proliferation. Subjectively, horses with ataxia due to spinal cord compression rarely show prolonged improvement in their neurologic grade post injection.

Surgical treatment generally entails vertebral fusion with the goal of eliminating movement at the affected articulation. If the horse has dynamic compression, with increased spinal cord compression in flexion or extension, fixation of the affected articulation will immediately reduce damage to the spinal cord. If the horse has static compression, with spinal cord compression in all neck positions, stabilization can lead to clinical improvement due to gradual decompression. Sequential radiographs as well as postmortem evaluations performed months to years after cervical fixation will demonstrate atrophy and remodeling of the articular soft tissue and bony structures, generally causing enlargement of the vertebral canal.

The most common surgical technique uses a partially or fully threaded cylindrical implant (Kerf cut cylinder [KCC]) placed ventrally into 2 adjacent vertebrae with an autologous bone graft. The implant markedly reduces but does not totally eliminate movement of the vertebrae, although subsequent osseous fusion should lead to complete fixation. This procedure is performed by a limited number of surgeons at a limited number of facilities, and critical evaluation in the literature is currently lacking. However, experts estimate that the procedure has been performed on more than 2000 horses and long-term survival is more than 80%.[18]

Other surgical procedures have been described in the literature, including a subtotal dorsal decompressive laminectomy and locking compression plate fixation.[19,20] The former procedure provides immediate decompression of the spinal cord but is not routinely used because of its technical demands and a high risk of life-threatening complications. Locking compression plate fixation has been shown in vivo to have superior mechanical properties to KCC fixation[21] and has been used in a limited number of adult horses with success, but formal evaluation is currently unavailable.

Prognosis

Factors that influence prognosis include age of the horse, severity of neurologic deficits, duration of neurologic signs, and owner expectations for performance. Most horses with CVSM do not have life-threatening ataxia, although some horses become fully recumbent or demonstrate such severe ataxia that safety concerns warrant euthanasia. Without treatment, prognosis for substantial improvement in neurologic function is generally poor, as the underlying malformation, instability, or bony proliferation will continue to damage the spinal cord. Additionally, sudden deterioration in neurologic status can occur following trauma, as a horse with a stenotic vertebral canal has little ability to compensate or avoid further injury to the cord when trauma occurs.

Medical treatment alone is unlikely to lead to long-term improvement in ataxia, although improvement in comfort can be observed. If acute spinal cord damage has occurred, initial response to medical therapy with anti-inflammatory drugs is often good. However, without removing the inciting cause of spinal cord damage, neurologic deficits are likely to remain or reoccur in the future. A low-protein, low-energy "paced" diet has been described in the treatment of young horses (<12 months) with a presumptive diagnosis of CVSM; 83% improved and had at least 1 racing start.[8] This uncontrolled study evaluated a small number of horses that did not undergo myelography for confirmation, and whether diet or time was the primary factor responsible for the perceived improvement is unclear. A different population of young thoroughbreds (1–2 years of age) with CVSM that received only medical treatment showed less success, with only 30% having at least 1 racing start.[22] If arthritis is present, articular joint injections with corticosteroids or other anti-inflammatory substances might relieve discomfort or reduce soft tissue impingement on nervous structures. However, improvement is often transient and repeated injections might be necessary.[23]

Surgical stabilization provides the best long-term prognosis despite short-term risk. If owners are willing to consider surgical stabilization, this course should be pursued as soon as feasible after diagnosis to reduce cumulative injury to the spinal cord. Published studies estimate that approximately 75% of horses improved, and 45% to 60% achieved athletic function.[24] Anecdotally (Reed S, personal communication), current success rates have slightly improved, with clinical improvement in approximately 80% of horses and 63% of horses returning to athletic function. Subjectively, the author feels like sport horses undergoing cervical fusion often can be ridden at equivalent or lower levels but rarely if ever continue to progress in their training so that they successfully compete at higher levels postoperatively.

EQUINE PROTOZOAL MYELOENCEPHALITIS

EPM is one of the most commonly diagnosed infectious neurologic conditions in horses of North America. The protozoan parasites *Sarcocystis neurona* and *Neospora hughesi* are the 2 known causative agents of EPM, although most cases are caused by central nervous system (CNS) infection with *S neurona*.[25] The latter has a 2-host life cycle that alternates between the definitive host (the opossum *Didelphis virginiana* in North America), and any of several mammal intermediate hosts, including skunks, raccoons, armadillos, and cats. Horses are infected with *S neurona* through the consumption of food or water contaminated with opossum feces containing sporocysts. In contrast, *S neurona* is not transmitted horizontally between horses, nor can it be transmitted to horses from the intermediate hosts. Because mature sarcocysts are not typically found in equids, the horse is unlikely to support completion of the *S neurona* life cycle.[25]

Although all horses are considered susceptible to the development of EPM, some epidemiologic studies have shown that racehorses and show horses had a higher risk of developing EPM compared with breeding and pleasure horses.[26,27] Similarly, the annual incidence of EPM in the United States was estimated to be highest among horses used for racing, showing, or competition.[28] However, these data could be biased, as performance horses may be more likely to be diagnosed as having neurologic deficits, as they undergo more strenuous activities and closer observation. However, stresses associated with competition and transport might predispose to the development of clinical disease.[27] Horses of all breeds appear to be affected by EPM and there is no apparent gender bias. Standardbred, thoroughbred, and quarter horses have been overrepresented in some EPM studies,[29,30] but this likely reflects a selection bias that is further influenced by breed prevalence, breed-specific uses, or management factors that increase infection risk. It has been shown that stressful events (including high-intensity training, heavy exercise, transport, or injury) or advanced age may predispose to the development of EPM via immune suppression. However, most studies suggest that EPM is more common in young to middle-aged horses, with the highest disease risk found in 1-year-old to 5-year-old horses by Saville and colleagues,[26] whereas others report a higher incidence in 3-year-old to approximately 15-year-old horses. Because most competition and show horses are young to middle-aged, the age-related risk may be based on their use and performance.

Clinical Signs

The protozoan merozoites may affect any part of the CNS, leading to highly variable multifocal or focal signs of neurologic disease involving the brain, brainstem, or spinal cord. Spinal cord symptoms often predominate, leading to general proprioceptive (spinal) ataxia as well as evidence of lower motor neuron weakness or muscle atrophy that is often asymmetric. Early signs of asymmetric gait deficits may be noted under saddle as an uneven stride, stumbling, tripping, interference between limbs, or difficulties changing leads, and can initially be confused with lameness. Clinical signs vary from acute to chronic with insidious onset, and subsequently progress slowly or rapidly. EPM infection can thus mimic a variety of other neurologic diseases and can rarely be discounted based on clinical signs alone, although infected horses are typically not painful or febrile unless comorbidities exist. Brainstem involvement may manifest as depression and cranial nerve deficits. The latter more commonly manifest in dysphagia, but can also be associated with vestibular abnormalities, wasting of the temporalis and masseter muscles, facial nerve paralysis, and evidence of upper airway dysfunction.[31,32]

Diagnosis and Differential Diagnosis

Despite decades of research, a definitive diagnosis of EPM remains diagnostically challenging. Almost all clinical signs found in other neurologic equine conditions also can be present in EPM-affected horses. Therefore, a presumptive antemortem diagnosis of EPM is considered most accurate if all of the following 3 criteria are fulfilled: compatible clinical signs consistent with CNS disease (most commonly related to spinal cord and brain stem dysfunction); exclusion of other likely diseases; and confirmation of exposure to S neurona or N hughesi by immunologic testing.[25,31]

In areas where S neurona and opossums are common, there is extensive exposure of horses to the protozoa. The reported seroprevalence of S neurona in horses from the United States thus varies widely, and ranges from as low as 15% to as high as 89%, depending on geographic region.[25] Because EPM occurs only in a small percentage of horses infected with S neurona, it is extremely important that an EPM diagnosis is not merely based on seroconversion, as many horses will falsely be considered positive.

Diagnostic Testing

A variety of immunologic tests are currently in use for the diagnosis of EPM and are based on the identification of antibodies in serum or CSF. However, the test interpretation can be confounded by various factors: (1) exposure to S neurona in the absence of CNS infection (ie, exposed but not infected animals), (2) blood contamination of a CSF sample, and (3) natural diffusion of antibodies from blood into CSF (which may be exacerbated in patients with nonspecific CNS inflammation).

The Western blot, a semiquantitative test for antibodies against merozoite lysate, is the oldest available diagnostic test. Although the sensitivity of the Western blot is high (approximately 80%–90%), the specificity is low (approximately 40%), and minimal blood contamination of CSF may lead to false-positive results.[33,34] However, the presence of a negative Western blot would make a diagnosis of EPM unlikely, because the probability of a false-negative test result is low. Some commercial laboratories no longer offer this test.

The indirect fluorescent antibody test (IFAT) is a quantitative test for antibodies against whole merozoites,[35] with a reported test sensitivity of 65% to 100% and specificity of 90% to 99% for CSF samples, based on 3 independent studies using the currently laboratory-recommended positive CSF cutoff ($\geq$1:5).[36–38] As an important clinical consideration when submitting CSF samples, the IFAT is more resilient to blood contamination than the Western blot, with no reported false-positive results at contamination levels as high as 10,000 red blood cells/μL CSF.[39] The currently reported test sensitivity for IFAT serum samples ranges between 59% and 94%, with a specificity of 71% to 100%, depending on which serum cutoff was used and in which geographic region the samples were collected.[14,35,37] Serum IFAT titers have been used to predict the likelihood of EPM, with higher titers suggesting greater probability of disease. However, these predictions are likely less accurate in geographic regions with high EPM seroprevalence and should be interpreted with caution.

Surface antigen (SAG) enzyme-linked immunosorbent assays (ELISAs) are the most recently developed, commercially available quantitative tests based on immunodominant *S neurona* surface antigens. *S neurona* expresses multiple surface antigens (SnSAGs) that serve as virulence factors for the parasite but are immunogenic to the host. SnSAGs-2, 3, and 4 appear to be well-conserved among *S neurona* strains, and recently marketed EPM tests use monovalent and polyvalent ELISAs to detect antibodies against these 3 antigens (SnSAG-2, 4/3 ELISA). An ELISA combining SnSAG-1, 5, and 6 is also currently offered, although no published reports describe the validation of this assay to date. SnSAG-1 is not expressed by all strains of *S neurona*,[25] thereby reducing its utility for serologic detection. Two independent studies of a commercial SnSAG-2, 4/3 ELISA showed that testing serum alone yielded less accurate results than CSF testing alone or a serum-to-CSF titer ratio. For serum SnSAG-2, 4/3 ELISA analysis, the currently reported test sensitivity is 71% to 86%, with a specificity of 37% to 50%, using a positive serum cutoff $\geq$1:500.[38,40] Based on the low specificity, serum testing alone will lead to a high number of false-positive results, which should be considered when performing EPM testing merely on blood samples. In contrast, both studies demonstrated the highest overall accuracy for the SAG2, 4/3 ELISA serum-to-CSF titer ratio as compared with any other diagnostic test (Western blot, IFAT, and SAG-1 ELISA). The reported test sensitivity ranged between 88% and 93%, with a specificity of 83% to 100%, using a positive serum-to-CSF ratio cutoff $\leq$1:100.[38,40] The available evidence therefore suggests that measuring specific antibodies in both serum and CSF to allow calculation of a serum-to-CSF ratio is the most accurate means of diagnosis. In general, antibodies are partitioned between blood and CSF at a relatively constant ratio (>100:1), based on the restriction coefficient of the blood-brain barrier. Infection of the CNS leads to intrathecal antibody production and a decrease in this ratio, which is useful in the clinical diagnosis of EPM.[31,41]

The detection of serum antibodies against *N hughesi* in neurologic horses has a higher positive predictive value for EPM than positive serology against *S neurona*. The latter is based on the overall low seroprevalence of *N hughesi* in horses (with some geographic differences), which has also impaired the ability to fully validate the *N hughesi* IFAT and *N hughesi* SAG-1 ELISA to date.[25]

Treatment

Three treatments are currently approved by the US Food and Drug Administration (FDA) for EPM, and available on the US market (3/2018): a combination of sulfadiazine and pyrimethamine, ponazuril, and diclazuril; with apparently similar efficacy across therapies.

ReBalance (PRN Pharmacal, Pensacola, FL) is an approved combined EPM treatment of sulfadiazine at 20 mg/kg and pyrimethamine at 1 mg/kg daily given orally for a minimum of 90 days. Both sulfadiazine and pyrimethamine inhibit an enzyme in the folic acid pathway, thereby impeding thymidine synthesis. Although the combined use of trimethoprim and pyrimethamine has been suggested in the past, this combination is no longer recommended, as trimethoprim reduces the efficacy of pyrimethamine in inhibiting dihydrofolate reductase.[42] A field study performed during the approval process of ReBalance resulted in successful outcomes in 61.5% (16/26) of horses, based on 2 or more improvement grades in the overall neurologic function or reversion to a CSF-negative status.[43] Bone marrow suppression (mild anemia, leukopenia, neutropenia, and/or thrombocytopenia) was the most common adverse effect. Additional reported side effects may include gastrointestinal complications (anorexia, depression, glossitis, or diarrhea) and reproductive problems (abortions, changes in copulation or ejaculation, and congenital defects).[31] Folate supplementation is not thought to be beneficial and may increase the risk of toxicity.[25]

Marquis (Merial, Duluth, GA) is a 15% wt/wt ponazuril paste (a triazinetrione antiprotozoal drug) that is labeled for use at a loading dose of 15 mg/kg orally on day 1 (in an effort to achieve therapeutic concentrations more quickly), followed by 5 mg/kg given daily by mouth for the following 27 days. A field study performed during the drug approval process described a 60% (28/47) success rate, based on an improvement in neurologic score by at least 1 grade (on a 0–5 scale) or CSF conversion to negative status on Western blot for *S neurona* antibodies, following a 28-day course of 5 mg/kg ponazuril given orally daily.[44] No adverse effects were noted. Data have shown that the concurrent administration of vegetable oil (1/2 cup) may increase the bioavailability of the FDA-approved ponazuril product up to 15%.[25]

Protazil (Merck Animal Health, Kansas City, KS) is marketed as a pelleted (alfalfa-based) oral antiprotozoal medication, containing 1.56% diclazuril (a triazinetrione antiprotozoal agent similar to ponazuril) and administered as a daily top-dress at 1.0 mg/kg for 28 days. A field study performed during the approval process described an efficacy similar to the other products, with 67% (28/42) of horses being considered treatment successes after 28 days of drug therapy, based on an improvement in neurologic score by at least 1 grade or CSF conversion to negative status on Western blot. Successful treatment was confirmed in 10 (42%) of 24 horses based on independent expert evaluation of masked videotape analysis. The latter study did not identify a clinical difference in success rates among horses treated with 1, 5, or 10 mg/kg diclazuril, and no important adverse reactions were reported.[45] Based on the data, a loading dose for the FDA-approved diclazuril product is not required and the use of vegetable oil has not been shown to increase its bioavailability.[25]

Both FDA-approved triazine antiprotozoal agents have been shown to be safe at higher doses. As such, ponazuril is used frequently in extralabel dosing regimens, often at significantly higher dosages or for a longer duration.[31,46] The duration of treatment should be based on neurologic improvement and thus depend on the clinical response to antiprotozoal administration. Antibody retesting in blood, CSF, or both is currently not recommended to determine discontinuation of antiprotozoal drug administration.[25]

Supportive Medical Management

Ancillary treatments for EPM may include a short course of nonsteroidal anti-inflammatory medications or corticosteroids (and/or dimethyl sulfoxide) in an attempt to control the inflammatory response and prevent potential worsening of neurologic signs during the early antiprotozoal treatment phase in moderately to severely affected horses. Additionally, natural vitamin E formulations (eg, 10–20 IU/kg orally per day) are often supplemented as an adjunct antioxidant treatment, because the damaged CNS is susceptible to oxidant injury. Immunomodulators also have been used anecdotally by some, based on the assumption that horses develop EPM in association with immune compromise. These drugs may include mycobacterial wall extract (Equimune IV; Bioniche Animal Health Vetoquinol, Belville, ON, Canada), inactivated parapox ovis virus (Zylexis; Zoetis, Florham Park, NJ), killed *Propionibacterium acnes* (Eqstim; Neogen, Lansing, MI), transfer factor (4Life Transfer Factor; 4LifeResearch, Sandy, UT), and levamisole (1 mg/kg orally every 12 hours for the first 2 weeks of antiprotozoal treatment and for the first week of each month thereafter).[25] However, no studies have been conducted to evaluate the efficacy of these medications or supplements in horses with EPM. Decoquinate in combination with the immunomodulator levamisole is available as a compounded combination product for a 10-day treatment of EPM, but is not currently approved by the FDA. Levamisole can be metabolized to aminorex, a CNS stimulant that is banned in performance horses. The use of levamisole in performance horses may thus give rise to the possibility of regulatory concerns if subjected to drug testing.[46,47]

Prognosis

Approximately 60% of EPM-affected horses are expected to improve at least 1 grade with treatment regardless of type, while a smaller percentage (10%–20%) may return to normal athletic performance (recover completely). However, it is reasonable to estimate that 10% to 20% of successfully treated horses will suffer at least 1 relapse within 1 to 3 years after discontinuation of treatment. The outlook for mildly affected horses (grade 1) may be considerably better, and early recognition and treatment will likely result in the best outcome.[48]

Prevention

Preventive approaches to EPM are generally directed at decreasing stress in performance horses, along with reducing contamination of feeds and environment by *S neurona* sporocysts from feces of opossums. This may be accomplished by providing individual (separate) fresh water sources for horses, not feeding from the ground, and limiting opossum access to the barnyard and feed sources. The utility of controlling intermediate hosts in an effort to reduce environmental sporocyst load remains controversial.[48] The daily administration of low-dose diclazuril (as pellet topdressing) was shown to significantly reduce the monthly seroprevalence to *S neurona* in healthy foals with a high exposure risk to the parasite.[49] However, future longitudinal studies will be required to evaluate potential benefits of preventive strategies, and must consider the risk of facilitating drug resistance.

EQUINE DEGENERATIVE MYELOENCEPHALOPATHY

EDM is a diffuse neurodegenerative condition in young horses that is predominantly characterized by a symmetric general proprioceptive ataxia. EDM is considered a pathologically more advanced form of neuroaxonal dystrophy (NAD). Clinically, EDM and NAD are indistinguishable from one another, but are differentiated histologically.[50] Both familial (genetic) and environmental factors are believed to play a role in the pathophysiology of EDM. As such, low dietary vitamin E (α-tocopherol) levels with resultant oxidative damage to selected neurons contribute to the disease pathogenesis.

Studies have also shown that vitamin E supplementation decreased the prevalence of EDM in genetically predisposed horses.[51] In a retrospective case-control study, the reported risk factors for EDM included housing on dirt lots, and exposure of young foals to insecticides and wood preservatives; whereas housing in green pasture (as a source of natural vitamin E) was considered protective.[52] EDM has been recognized in most sport-horse breeds with reports of familial disease in appaloosas, Morgans, standardbreds, Mongolian wild horses, quarter horses, and Lusitano horses.[4,50]

Clinical Signs

EDM may either have an acute or insidious onset of bilaterally symmetric ataxia, with proprioceptive deficits and weakness, where the forelimbs can be equally or less severely affected than the hindlimbs. Horses also may appear "clumsy," show a 2-beat "pacing" gait at walking speed, a truncal sway, base-wide stance, or notable spasticity (hypometria) in the affected limbs. Neurogenic muscle atrophy is not seen in horses with EDM. Clinical symptoms can thus be similar to those of cervical vertebral malformation (CVM). However, a dull mentation, inconsistent menace response, and reduced laryngeal adductor (slap) or cutaneous trunci responses may be observed in a subset of affected horses. Pigment retinopathy also has been reported in a small number of EDM-affected warmblood horses with α-tocopherol deficiency, and related to oxidative damage to photoreceptors.[53] The clinical signs of EDM typically develop between 1 and 12 months of age and can remain unchanged, or progress for days to months before stabilizing. Mild cases may therefore present for performance-related concerns and can be difficult to discern from a lameness condition. EDM sometimes remains undetected for years unless the horse specifically undergoes a neurologic examination.[4,54] Personal experience (unpublished results) has shown that late-onset EDM may also be recognized in older horses (often 6–12-year-old warmbloods or less frequently thoroughbreds) that initially present with behavior changes (altered personality, loss of work ethic, bolting, refusing fences) and subsequent ataxia, where a diagnosis of EDM can ultimately be confirmed on necropsy.

Diagnosis and Differential Diagnosis

A definitive antemortem diagnosis of EDM is not possible, but is clinically suspected based on patient signalment, suggestive clinical findings and exclusion of alternate diagnoses in young horses. Early onset (<2 years) of symmetric limb ataxia, coupled with confirmed EDM in the bloodlines of affected horses, a low or marginal serum vitamin E level (≤2.0 μg/mL) or deficient dietary vitamin E is strongly suggestive of the disease. Serum samples submitted for vitamin E analysis must not be visibly hemolyzed, should remain protected from light, and be stored so that the blood is not in contact with the rubber stopper.[54] Because dietary and serum vitamin E levels are not always abnormal, a deficiency in a metabolic pathway or function of vitamin E cannot be ruled out in affected horses.[4]

Differential diagnoses of the clinical signs of EDM include conditions associated with spinal cord compression (CVM), vertebral trauma, and inflammatory or ischemic spinal cord diseases.[54] A postmortem diagnosis of EDM is commonly based on histopathologic findings of diffuse neuronal fiber degeneration of the white matter of the spinal cord, and some brainstem nuclei.[4,55]

Treatment

Vitamin E supplementation is the treatment of choice, but is unlikely to result in significant improvement of clinically affected horses. However, in susceptible families, vitamin E supplementation of breeding stock and young horses can decrease the incidence and severity of developing disease.[50] Natural vitamin E (RRR-α-tocopherol) has a notably higher bioavailability and potency than synthetic vitamin E (all rac-α-tocopherol acetate or d,l-α-tocopherol)[56] and is commonly supplemented at 10 to 20 IU/kg orally per day in deficient horses (5000–10,000 IU per horse). Dietary fat is required for enteric absorption, so vitamin E should be given with feed or vegetable oil.[54]

Prognosis

The prognosis for recovery is poor in affected horses, which generally stabilize over time without improvement in their neurologic signs or performance. Rare reports of clinical improvement exist following supplementation with natural vitamin E.[4]

Prevention

Preventive measures should focus on maintaining adequate dietary vitamin E levels in breeding stock and young horses. Natural sources of vitamin E include access to green pasture and fresh, well-cured hays.[4] Specific dietary vitamin E supplementation is therefore recommended in circumstances of familial predisposition, use of processed feed, lack of pasture access, and exposure to insecticides or wood preservatives. Both genetic and nutritional management are expected to significantly reduce the incidence of EDM.[54]

EQUINE HERPES VIRUS-1 MYELOENCEPHALOPATHY

EHV-1 infection has received significant attention in the past decade because of several high-profile disease outbreaks, state-mandated quarantines, and recognition of a neuropathogenic strain (D752 genotype). Primary infection with the ubiquitous alpha-herpesvirus EHV-1 occurs by the respiratory tract, leading to fever, inappetence, and nasal discharge in young horses. Secondary disease manifestations also include abortions, neonatal death, chorioretinopathy, and neurologic disease, known as EHM. Although the EHV-1 D752 genotype viruses (containing a point-mutation within the virus' DNA polymerase) are more commonly associated with Equine Herpes Virus Myeloencephalopathy (EHM), the N752 genotype (wild-type) is responsible for approximately 15% to 26% of neurologic EHV-1 outbreaks.[57] Latent infections involving the trigeminal ganglia and respiratory tract lymph nodes are common, and stressful events may trigger virus reactivation. As such, horses returning from shows, competitions, or extended travel may experience recrudescence of latent infection, resulting in active viral shedding and transmission to naive horses.[31] Currently, it is estimated that up to 80% of all horses are latently infected with EHV-1.[31,57]

Disease is spread via aerosolization of respiratory secretions or direct contact with infected horses or fomites. Virus moves from respiratory epithelial cells to regional lymph nodes to peripheral blood leukocytes, inducing a cell-associated viremia. When the virus subsequently crosses from leukocytes into CNS endothelial cells, it causes vasculitis, with hemorrhage and thrombosis. The latter results in tissue hypoxia and ischemia in surrounding CNS tissue and manifests in EHM.[31] However, EHM merely develops in a proportion of viremic horses (10% to 40%), with older animals considered at increased risk. Additionally, robust small pony breeds are less likely to develop EHM when compared with large-breed performance horses (standardbred, thoroughbred, various warmblood breeds, quarter and draft horses).[58]

Clinical Signs

Clinical signs of ataxia and weakness due to spinal cord damage can be mild to severe, asymmetrical or symmetric, and lead to recumbency (paralysis or tetraplegia) in severe cases. Usually, the pelvic limbs are more severely affected than the thoracic limbs, resulting in more notable hind limb weakness, bladder dysfunction with urine dribbling, sensory deficits in the perineal area, and decreased tail and anal tone with fecal retention.[31] Less frequently, horses with EHM can develop cortical, brainstem, or vestibular disease characterized by depression, head tilt, ataxia, and cranial nerve dysfunction. Neurologic signs generally develop 6 to 10 days after the initial EHV-1 infection (1–3 days after resolution of a fever) and typically reach peak severity within 2 to 3 days.[57]

Diagnosis and Differential Diagnosis

Quantitative polymerase chain reaction (qPCR) testing of nasopharyngeal secretions and uncoagulated whole blood is recommended at the appropriate time(s) within an affected group of horses, to assess viral load and differentiate neuropathogenic from non-neuropathogenic EHV-1 strains. Viral shedding through nasal secretions typically persists for 10 to 14 days (up to 21 days in some horses) following infection, but is usually highest during the first 5 days and is considered the best time to collect nasal swabs for PCR. During disease outbreaks, it is therefore important to sample in-contact horses that are febrile, but may not show any other clinical signs. Viremia classically occurs between days 4 and 10 postinfection, which makes this the most suitable time to collect whole blood samples (±10 mL per horse in EDTA tubes) for PCR testing. Because the postexposure temporal profiles of EHV-1 in nasal secretions and leukocytes do not overlap completely, it is possible for one test to be positive while the other is negative. Therefore, both samples (blood and nasal swabs) are usually collected from suspect cases. CSF collection would be appropriate between days 7 and 16 postinfection in horses with EHM, for the detection of virus or viral nucleic acid, if indicated.[59] CSF cytology can also be supportive of infection, but is not specific for EHV-1; changes are consistent with a vasculopathy and typically consist of a normal to mildly elevated white cell count with increased total protein (albuminocytologic dissociation with xanthochromia). Virus isolation or paired serum neutralization titers obtained 7 to 21 days apart are less frequently used in the clinical setting since the widespread availability of PCR testing. A postmortem diagnosis of EHM is obtained with a combination of histology and confirmatory immunohistochemistry or PCR.[31]

Treatment

The treatment of EHM-affected horses is challenging and often focuses on appropriate supportive care, with specific attention to hydration, nutrition, rectal evacuation of retained manure, sling support, and bladder care (catheterization and treatment of cystitis as warranted). Supportive drug therapy focuses on reducing inflammation and preventing thromboembolic sequelae. Anti-inflammatory drugs are also thought to downregulate the expression of cellular adhesion molecules, thereby decreasing the rate of EHV-1 infection of CNS endothelial cells.[60] Flunixin meglumine is commonly indicated for the treatment of CNS vasculitis, and the control of fever. Similarly, Firocoxib may be used at the first detection of a fever and continued for an additional 3 to 5 days once the fever has resolved.[60] This preferential COX-2 inhibitor shows a sparing effect on gastrointestinal mucosa, with convenient once-daily administration. For severely affected animals, a short course of corticosteroid treatment with prednisolone acetate or dexamethasone for 2 to 3 days, is frequently recommended.[57] The latter should be given at judicious doses ($\leq$0.05 mg/kg dexamethasone once to twice daily) and not in combination with an NSAID.[60] Additionally, several drugs have been empirically used to help avert thromboembolic events related to vasculitis, including dimethyl sulfoxide, aspirin, unfractionated or low-molecular-weight heparin, and pentoxifylline.[57] Heparin anticoagulants have actually been shown to inhibit EHV-1–induced platelet activation in vitro.[61] During a natural disease outbreak, heparin treatment (25,000 IU per horse subcutaneously every 12 hours for 3 days) was also associated with a lower EHM incidence (1/31 [3.2%]) than observed in untreated horses (7/30 [23.3%]; P = .03). However, variations in immune status or virus load in EHV-1–exposed horses may have influenced the reported results.[62]

Antiviral agents are often used to reduce the magnitude of viremia and thus limit the extent of CNS endothelial cell infection. As such, early antiviral treatment with oral valacyclovir has been shown to significantly decrease viral replication, viral dissemination, and severity of clinical disease in older, experimentally EHV-1–infected horses.[63] Valacyclovir administration within 2 days after viral inoculation had favorable effects by reducing viral shedding, viremia, pyrexia, clinical score, and severity (but not incidence) of ataxia. The protective effects were greatest when treatment was initiated before viral inoculation and maintained for 2 weeks, but still remained significant when treatment was delayed until the first onset of fever (day 2). During an outbreak of EHM, antiviral treatment may thus be initiated in horses at various stages of infection, including horses that have not yet developed clinical signs of viral disease.[63]

Valacyclovir is a prodrug of acyclovir that has considerably better (41%–60%) oral bioavailability than acyclovir, and is not significantly affected by prior feeding.[64,65] However, tablets should not be dissolved and stored before administration, as the ester bond of valacyclovir is subject to degradation in neutral to alkaline aqueous solutions.[66] One proposed treatment protocol involves the use of a loading-dose regimen of 27 mg/kg orally every 8 hours for the first 2 days, followed by 18 mg/kg orally every 12 hours,[63] which is sometimes rounded to 30 mg/kg and 20 mg/kg orally, respectively, for convenience. The proposed dose regimen appears to reach effective concentrations in most horses, but a higher dose may be required in some animals due to wide interindividual pharmacokinetic variability.[63,65] A higher valacyclovir dosing regimen of 40 mg/kg every 8 hours has also been proposed and was able to maintain acyclovir concentrations above a goal of 1.7 to 3.0 µg/mL for more than half of the dosing interval.[64] Hematological monitoring of renal and complete blood count parameters should be considered during prolonged use of higher doses. Intravenously administered ganciclovir is more potent than acyclovir, but at the recommended loading dose of 2.5 mg/kg IV 3 times a day for 2 days, followed by 2.5 mg/kg twice a day, it is currently cost-prohibitive for most cases.[67]

Biosecurity

When EHV-1 infection is suspected, particularly if 1 or more horses show signs of neurologic disease, immediate steps to prevent spread of infection are warranted.[68] EHV-1 is a reportable disease, and the state veterinarian should be informed of any potential cases. Early diagnosis of infection is imperative and is best based on real-time PCR testing. Affected horses should be isolated, the facility quarantined, and biosecurity protocols instituted under guidance of the state veterinarian. Temperatures should be monitored twice daily in all affected and in-contact horses following identification of an index case. Febrile horses must be assumed infected and separated accordingly to minimize virus transmission. Unfortunately, recent EHV-1 outbreaks have shown that even extensive barrier precautions are potentially ineffective in preventing spread of infection when EHM cases are housed in the same building as other horses, and therefore an isolation facility is recommended. In general, 21-day to 28-day quarantine periods are elected. Alternatively, shorter 14-day quarantine periods can be used if followed by testing of all horses with quantitative real-time PCR analysis for 2 to 4 consecutive days before releasing the quarantine.[31,69]

EHV-1 does not survive well outside of the horse, but remains stable and infectious for approximately 1 week under normal conditions (up to 1 month under selected conditions).[57] In experimental studies, the virus survived for up to a week at ambient temperatures when dried onto paper, wood, or rope, and up to 35 days on horsehair or burlap. Herpes viruses are susceptible to many disinfectants used for cleaning of buildings and equipment. In general, a 1:10 dilution of bleach to water is effective against EHV-1. However, both alcohol and bleach are inactivated by organic matter, such as manure and soil. Before disinfection, all areas must therefore be thoroughly cleaned with soap or detergent to decrease the organic matter present. In barn environments, it is advisable to use a disinfectant that retains activity in the presence of organic matter because it cannot be completely eliminated. Phenolics, such as 1Stoke Environ or SynPhenol-3, and accelerated hydrogen peroxide products, such as Virkon and Accel, retain activity in the face of residual organic matter better than most other disinfectants.[70] It is important to follow manufacturer recommendations and label instructions for individual products.

Prognosis

The prognosis for EHM-affected horses is highly variable and dependent on disease severity. Mildly affected horses have a fair to good chance for a full recovery and return to athletic performance.[31] Improvement is often apparent within 5 to 7 days after the peak of clinical disease severity. However, recumbent horses usually do not fully recover and may be left with permanent residual neurologic deficits, even after extended recovery periods. Horses should, therefore, be reevaluated in several weeks to months for chronic-persistent signs of EHM, after the initial diagnosis.[60] Cumulative data from 6 US neurologic EHV-1 outbreaks (2001–2005) showed a 33% incidence of EHM in 403 EHV-1–infected horses, with a mean case fatality rate of 40%.[71] In contrast, other reports have documented that approximately 5% to 15% of infected horses will die or require euthanasia.[70]

Prevention

Appropriate biosecurity measures and management protocols of horses entering the premises are essential to prevent introduction and spread of EHV-1 at equine facilities. Routine vaccination of horses is indicated to maximize herd immunity, to reduce viral shedding in the event of exposure to EHV-1.[68] However, booster vaccination of horses that are likely to have been exposed during an active EHV-1 outbreak is not recommended.[57]

No commercial vaccines are labeled for the prevention of neurologic disease. Preliminary research suggested that use of a modified-live virus vaccine (Rhinomune; Boehringer Ingelheim Vetmedica, St Joseph, MO) was more protective against EHM than use of an inactivated vaccine.[72] However, this study used a small number of horses and induced only mild signs of neurologic disease. A more recent study compared the modified-live vaccine Rhinomune to the high-antigen-load killed vaccine Pneumabort-K (Pfizer Animal Health, New York, NY) in a pony challenge model.[73] Both vaccines reduced clinical signs of respiratory disease and nasal viral shedding, and the killed vaccine reduced the number of days of viremia. Despite the use of an optimized vaccination regime, neither vaccine prevented viremia, which may lead to EHM.[31]

REFERENCES

1. Licka TF. Differentiation of ataxic and orthopedic gait abnormalities in the horse. Vet Clin North Am Equine Pract 2011;27:411–6.
2. Olsen E, Dunkel B, Barker WH, et al. Rater agreement on gait assessment during neurologic examination of horses. J Vet Intern Med 2014;28:630–8.
3. Saville WJA, Reed SM, Dubey JP, et al. Interobserver variation in the diagnosis of neurologic abnormalities in the horse. J Vet Intern Med 2017;31:1871–6.
4. Carr EA, Maher O. Neurologic causes of gait abnormalities in the athletic horse. In: Hinchcliff KW, Kaneps A, Geor R, editors. Equine sports medicine and surgery. 2nd edition. St Louis (MO): Elsevier; 2014. p. 503–26.
5. Rooney JR. Disorders of the nervous system. In: Biomechanics of lameness in horses. Baltimore (MD): The Williams & Wilkins Company; 1969. p. 219–33.
6. Van Biervliet J. An evidence-based approach to clinical questions in the practice of equine neurology. Vet Clin North Am Equine Pract 2007;23:317–28.
7. Oswald J, Love S, Parkin TD, et al. Prevalence of cervical vertebral stenotic myelopathy in a population of thoroughbred horses. Vet Rec 2010;166:82–3.
8. Mayhew IG, Donawick WJ, Green SL, et al. Diagnosis and prediction of cervical vertebral malformation in thoroughbred foals based on semi-quantitative radiographic indicators. Equine Vet J 1993;25:435–40.
9. Moore BR, Reed SM, Biller DS, et al. Assessment of vertebral canal diameter and bony malformations of the cervical part of the spine in horses with cervical stenotic myelopathy. Am J Vet Res 1994;55:5–13.
10. DeRouen A, Spriet M, Aleman M. Prevalence of anatomical variation of the sixth cervical vertebra and association with vertebral canal stenosis and articular process osteoarthritis in the horse. Vet Radiol Ultrasound 2016;57:253–8.
11. Withers JM, Voute LC, Hammond G, et al. Radiographic anatomy of the articular process joints of the caudal cervical vertebrae in the horse on lateral and oblique projections. Equine Vet J 2009;41:895–902.
12. Down SS, Henson FM. Radiographic retrospective study of the caudal cervical articular process joints in the horse. Equine Vet J 2009;41:518–24.
13. Hahn CN, Handel I, Green SL, et al. Assessment of the utility of using intra- and intervertebral minimum sagittal diameter ratios in the diagnosis of cervical vertebral malformation in horses. Vet Radiol Ultrasound 2008;49:1–6.
14. Van Biervliet J, Scrivani PV, Divers TJ, et al. Evaluation of decision criteria for detection of spinal cord compression based on cervical myelography in horses: 38 cases (1981-2001). Equine Vet J 2004;36:14–20.
15. Prange T, Carr EA, Stick JA, et al. Cervical vertebral canal endoscopy in a horse with cervical vertebral stenotic myelopathy. Equine Vet J 2012;44:116–9.
16. Donawick W, Mayhew I, Galligan D, et al. Early diagnosis of cervical vertebral malformation in young thoroughbred horses and successful treatment with restricted, paced diet and confinement. 35th Annual American Association of Equine Practitioners Convention. Proc Am Assoc Equine Pract, 1989. p. 525–8.
17. Kronfeld DS, Meacham TN, Donoghue S. Dietary aspects of developmental orthopedic disease in young horses. Vet Clin North Am Equine Pract 1990;6: 451–65.
18. Johnson A, Reed S. Cervical vertebral stenotic myelopathy. In: Furr M, RS, editors. Equine neurology. 2nd edition. Ames (IA): Wiley-Blackwell; 2015. p. 349–67.
19. Nixon A, Stashak T. Dorsal laminectomy in the horse I. Review of the literature and description of a new procedure. Vet Surg 1983;12:172–6.

20. Reardon R, Kummer M, Lischer C. Ventral locking compression plate for treatment of cervical stenotic myelopathy in a 3-month-old warmblood foal. Vet Surg 2009;38:537–42.
21. Reardon RJ, Bailey R, Walmsley JP, et al. An in vitro biomechanical comparison of a locking compression plate fixation and kerf cut cylinder fixation for ventral arthrodesis of the fourth and the fifth equine cervical vertebrae. Vet Surg 2010; 39:980–90.
22. Hoffman CJ, Clark CK. Prognosis for racing with conservative management of cervical vertebral malformation in thoroughbreds: 103 cases (2002-2010). J Vet Intern Med 2013;27:317–23.
23. Birmingham S, Reed S, Mattoon J, et al. Qualitative assessment of corticosteroid cervical articular facet injection in symptomatic horses. Equine Vet Educ 2010;22:77–82.
24. Walmsley J. Surgical treatment of cervical spinal cord compression in horses: a European experience. Equine Vet Educ 2005;17:39–43.
25. Reed SM, Furr M, Howe DK, et al. Equine protozoal myeloencephalitis: an updated consensus statement with a focus on parasite biology, diagnosis, treatment, and prevention. J Vet Intern Med 2016;30:491–502.
26. Saville WJ, Reed SM, Morley PS, et al. Analysis of risk factors for the development of equine protozoal myeloencephalitis in horses. J Am Vet Med Assoc 2000;217: 1174–80.
27. Cohen ND, Mackay RJ, Toby E, et al. A multicenter case-control study of risk factors for equine protozoal myeloencephalitis. J Am Vet Med Assoc 2007;231:1857–63.
28. APHIS, USDA. EPM: EPM in the US National Animal Health Monitoring System. Veterinary Services. 2001. Available at: https://www.aphis.usda.gov/animal_health/ nahms/equine/downloads/equine98/Equine98_dr_EPM.pdf. Accessed March 15, 2018.
29. Fayer R, Mayhew IG, Baird JD, et al. Epidemiology of equine protozoal myeloencephalitis in North America based on histologically confirmed cases. A report. J Vet Intern Med 1990;4:54–7.
30. Pusterla N, Tamez-Trevino E, White A, et al. Comparison of prevalence factors in horses with and without seropositivity to *Neospora hughesi* and/or *Sarcocystis neurona*. Vet J 2014;200:332–4.
31. Johnson AL. Update on infectious diseases affecting the equine nervous system. Vet Clin North Am Equine Pract 2011;27:573–87.
32. Furr M, Rowe DK. Equine protozoal myeloencephalitis. In: Furr M, Reed S, editors. Equine neurology. 2nd edition. Ames (IA): Wiley-Blackwell; 2015. p. 285–305.
33. Daft BM, Barr BC, Gardner IA, et al. Sensitivity and specificity of western blot testing of cerebrospinal fluid and serum for diagnosis of equine protozoal myeloencephalitis in horses with and without neurologic abnormalities. J Am Vet Med Assoc 2002;221:1007–13.
34. Miller MM, Sweeney CR, Russell GE, et al. Effects of blood contamination of cerebrospinal fluid on western blot analysis for detection of antibodies against *Sarcocystis neurona* and on albumin quotient and immunoglobulin G index in horses. J Am Vet Med Assoc 1999;215:67–71.
35. Duarte PC, Daft BM, Conrad PA, et al. Comparison of a serum indirect fluorescent antibody test with two Western blot tests for the diagnosis of equine protozoal myeloencephalitis. J Vet Diagn Invest 2003;15:8–13.
36. Duarte PC, Daft BM, Conrad PA, et al. Evaluation and comparison of an indirect fluorescent antibody test for detection of antibodies to *Sarcocystis neurona*, using serum and cerebrospinal fluid of naturally and experimentally infected, and vaccinated horses. J Parasitol 2004;90:379–86.

37. Johnson AL, Burton AJ, Sweeney RW. Utility of 2 immunological tests for ante-mortem diagnosis of equine protozoal myeloencephalitis (*Sarcocystis neurona* infection) in naturally occurring cases. J Vet Intern Med 2010;24:1184–9.

38. Johnson AL, Morrow JK, Sweeney RW. Indirect fluorescent antibody test and sur-face antigen ELISAs for antemortem diagnosis of equine protozoal myeloence-phalitis. J Vet Intern Med 2013;27:596–9.

39. Finno CJ, Packham AE, David Wilson W, et al. Effects of blood contamination of cerebrospinal fluid on results of indirect fluorescent antibody tests for detection of antibodies against *Sarcocystis neurona* and *Neospora hughesi*. J Vet Diagn Invest 2007;19:286–9.

40. Reed SM, Howe DK, Morrow JK, et al. Accurate antemortem diagnosis of equine protozoal myeloencephalitis (EPM) based on detecting intrathecal antibodies against *Sarcocystis neurona* using the SnSAG2 and SnSAG4/3 ELISAs. J Vet Intern Med 2013;27:1193–200.

41. Furr M, Howe D, Reed S, et al. Antibody coefficients for the diagnosis of equine protozoal myeloencephalitis. J Vet Intern Med 2011;25:138–42.

42. Dirikolu L, Foreman JH, Tobin T. Current therapeutic approaches to equine proto-zoal myeloencephalitis. J Am Vet Med Assoc 2013;242:482–91.

43. Animal-Health-Pharmaceuticals. Freedom of information summary, NADA 141–240. REBALANCE Antiprotozoal Oral Suspension (sulfadiazine and pyrimeth-amine) for the treatment of horses with equine protozoal myeloencephalitis (EPM) caused by *Sarcocystis neurona*. St Joseph (MT), 2004. Available at: http://www.epmhorse.org/images/Rebalance.pdf.

44. Furr M, Kennedy T, MacKay R, et al. Efficacy of ponazuril 15% oral paste as a treatment for equine protozoal myeloencephalitis. Vet Ther 2001;2:215–22.

45. Schering-Plough-Animal-Health-Corporation. Freedom of information summary, NADA 141–268. PROTAZIL anti-protozoal pellets (1.56% diclazuril) for the treat-ment of equine protozoal myeloencephalitis (EPM) caused by *Sarcocystis neu-rona* in horses. Langehorne (PA), 2007. Available at: http://www.epmhorse.org/images/Diclazuril.pdf.

46. Pusterla N, Tobin T. Therapeutics for equine protozoal myeloencephalitis. Vet Clin North Am Equine Pract 2017;33:87–97.

47. Gutierrez J, Eisenberg RL, Koval NJ, et al. Pemoline and tetramisole 'positives' in English racehorses following levamisole administration. Ir Vet J 2010;63:498–500.

48. MacKay R. Equine protozoal myeloencephalitis: treatment, prognosis, and pre-vention. Clin Tech Equine Pract 2006;5:9–16.

49. Pusterla N, Packham A, Mackie S, et al. Daily feeding of diclazuril top dress pel-lets in foals reduces seroconversion to *Sarcocystis neurona*. Vet J 2015;206:236–8.

50. Finno CJ, Higgins RJ, Aleman M, et al. Equine degenerative myeloencephalop-athy in Lusitano horses. J Vet Intern Med 2011;25:1439–46.

51. Mayhew IG, Brown CM, Stowe HD, et al. Equine degenerative myeloencephalop-athy: a vitamin E deficiency that may be familial. J Vet Intern Med 1987;1:45–50.

52. Dill SG, Correa MT, Erb HN, et al. Factors associated with the development of equine degenerative myeloencephalopathy. Am J Vet Res 1990;51:1300–5.

53. Finno CJ, Kaese HJ, Miller AD, et al. Pigment retinopathy in warmblood horses with equine degenerative myeloencephalopathy and equine motor neuron dis-ease. Vet Ophthalmol 2017;20:304–9.

54. MacKay R. Neurodegenerative disorders. In: Furr M, Reed S, editors. Equine neurology. 2nd edition. Ames (IA): Wiley-Blackwell; 2015.

55. Mayhew IG, deLahunta A, Whitlock RH, et al. Spinal cord disease in the horse. Cornell Vet 1978;68:207.
56. Finno CJ, Valberg SJ. A comparative review of vitamin E and associated equine disorders. J Vet Intern Med 2012;26:1251–66.
57. Pusterla N, Hussey GS. Equine herpesvirus 1 myeloencephalopathy. Vet Clin North Am Equine Pract 2014;30:489–506.
58. Goehring LS, van Winden SC, van Maanen C, et al. Equine herpesvirus type 1-associated myeloencephalopathy in The Netherlands: a four-year retrospective study (1999-2003). J Vet Intern Med 2006;20:601–7.
59. Balasuriya UB, Crossley BM, Timoney PJ. A review of traditional and contemporary assays for direct and indirect detection of equid herpesvirus 1 in clinical samples. J Vet Diagn Invest 2015;27:673–87.
60. Goehring LS. Equid herpesvirus-associated myeloencephalopathy. In: Furr M, Reed S, editors. Equine neurology. 2nd edition. Ames (IA): Wiley-Blackwell; 2015.
61. Stokol T, Serpa PBS, Zahid MN, et al. Unfractionated and low-molecular-weight heparin and the phosphodiesterase inhibitors, IBMX and cilostazol, block ex vivo equid herpesvirus type-1-induced platelet activation. Front Vet Sci 2016;3:99.
62. Walter J, Seeh C, Fey K, et al. Prevention of equine herpesvirus myeloencephalopathy—is heparin a novel option? A case report. Tierarztl Prax Ausg G Grosstiere Nutztiere 2016;44:313–7.
63. Maxwell LK, Bentz BG, Gilliam LL, et al. Efficacy of the early administration of valacyclovir hydrochloride for the treatment of neuropathogenic equine herpesvirus type-1 infection in horses. Am J Vet Res 2017;78:1126–39.
64. Garre B, Shebany K, Gryspeerdt A, et al. Pharmacokinetics of acyclovir after intravenous infusion of acyclovir and after oral administration of acyclovir and its prodrug valacyclovir in healthy adult horses. Antimicrob Agents Chemother 2007;51:4308–14.
65. Maxwell LK. Antiherpetic drugs in equine medicine. Vet Clin North Am Equine Pract 2017;33:99–125.
66. Granero GE, Amidon GL. Stability of valacyclovir: implications for its oral bioavailability. Int J Pharm 2006;317:14–8.
67. Carmichael RJ, Whitfield C, Maxwell LK. Pharmacokinetics of ganciclovir and valganciclovir in the adult horse. J Vet Pharmacol Ther 2013;36:441–9.
68. Lunn DP, Davis-Poynter N, Flaminio MJ, et al. Equine herpesvirus-1 consensus statement. J Vet Intern Med 2009;23:450–61.
69. Goehring LS, Landolt GA, Morley PS. Detection and management of an outbreak of equine herpesvirus type 1 infection and associated neurological disease in a veterinary teaching hospital. J Vet Intern Med 2010;24:1176–83.
70. CDFA. Equine herpesvirus-1: neuropathogenic strain frequently asked questions. California Department of Food and Agriculture. 2012. Available at: http://selectequine.com/clients/19834/documents/EHV-1NeuropathogenicStrain%20FAQ.pdf Accessed March 15, 2018.
71. APHIS, USDA. Equine herpesvirus myeloencephalopathy: a potentially emerging disease: centers for epidemiology and animal health. Veterinary Services, 2007. USDA-APHIS Online Report Available at: https://www.aphis.usda.gov/animal_health/emergingissues/downloads/ehv1final.pdf.
72. Goodman LB, Wagner B, Flaminio MJ, et al. Comparison of the efficacy of inactivated combination and modified-live virus vaccines against challenge infection with neuropathogenic equine herpesvirus type 1 (EHV-1). Vaccine 2006;24:3636–45.
73. Goehring LS, Wagner B, Bigbie R, et al. Control of EHV-1 viremia and nasal shedding by commercial vaccines. Vaccine 2010;28:5203–11.

Endocrine Disorders of the Equine Athlete

Nicholas Frank, DVM, PhD

KEYWORDS

- Adiposity • Equine metabolic syndrome • Insulin dysregulation • Laminitis
- Pituitary pars intermedia dysfunction

KEY POINTS

- Laminitis poses the greatest threat to the health of the athletic horse and insulin dysregulation (ID) is an important risk factor for this condition.
- ID is likely to have a genetic basis, and exacerbating factors include obesity, age, lack of exercise, systemic disease, pituitary pars intermedia dysfunction (PPID), and corticosteroid administration.
- Mild ID is managed by lowering the nonstructural carbohydrate content of the diet, reducing body fat mass, and increasing exercise, but medical treatments such as metformin may be required for managing severe ID.
- PPID is a cause of poor performance in athletic horses and may also result in loss of topline muscle mass and delayed shedding of the winter hair coat.
- Pergolide is an effective medical treatment of PPID in horses but may not be permitted during competitions.

INTRODUCTION

Equine athletes are affected by the same endocrine and metabolic disorders as other horses, but conditions affecting performance are of particular concern. Laminitis poses the greatest threat to performance because of the damage that it causes to hoof structures and the pain associated with lengthening and separation of dermal and epidermal laminae. There is mounting evidence that *insulin dysregulation (ID)* is an important cause of laminitis in horses, and this highlights the need for screening tests to identify at-risk horses. This article includes an in-depth discussion of ID and other risk factors for laminitis that are grouped together as *equine metabolic syndrome (EMS)*. As horses age, the risk of *pituitary pars intermedia dysfunction (PPID)* increases, and this endocrine disorder may exacerbate preexisting ID and further increase the risk of laminitis. This form of hyperadrenocorticism also weakens tissues and may increase susceptibility to tendon and ligament injury. Equine athletes that

Department of Clinical Sciences, Cummings School of Veterinary Medicine at Tufts University, 200 Westboro Road, North Grafton, MA 01536, USA
E-mail address: nicholas.frank@tufts.edu

Vet Clin Equine 34 (2018) 299–312
https://doi.org/10.1016/j.cveq.2018.04.003
0749-0739/18/© 2018 Elsevier Inc. All rights reserved.

vetequine.theclinics.com

develop PPID may be presented because of poor performance and loss of muscle along the topline, and medical treatment with pergolide allows activity levels to increase and muscle mass to return. Use of corticosteroids for the treatment of musculoskeletal problems or medical conditions such as equine asthma may exacerbate ID and increase the likelihood of laminitis developing in high-risk horses.

INSULIN DYSREGULATION IN THE EQUINE ATHLETE

ID manifests as fasting hyperinsulinemia, excessive insulin responses to oral sugars, or insulin resistance in horses,[1] and this endocrine disorder is a major health concern because of its association with laminitis. Insulin became the focus of intense research when laminitis was experimentally induced in healthy ponies and Standardbred horses by infusing insulin intravenously,[2,3] and excessive insulin responses to oral sugars have been detected in equids with naturally occurring laminitis.[4,5] ID is the central feature of EMS, a collection of risk factors for endocrinopathic laminitis that also includes increased adiposity, dyslipidemia, hypertension, and adipokine alterations.[1,6–8]

Genetics are thought to play a major role in ID, but only a few studies have examined this relationship to date. Jeffcott and colleagues[9] detected differences in glucose tolerance and insulin sensitivity between ponies and standardbred horses and attributed this to genetic variability among breeds. Fat and laminitic ponies showed more modest responses to exogenous insulin, indicating that insulin sensitivity was lower in these animals. Treiber and colleagues,[4] also detected familial associations after performing pedigree analysis on a group of ponies with laminitis from a closed herd. Differences in postprandial insulin responses to meals have also been detected among standardbred horses, mixed-breed ponies, and Andalusian cross horses, and this provides further evidence of breed-related variability in glucose and insulin dynamics.[10] A more detailed examination of genetics has been performed in Arabian horses using genome-wide association, and an EMS locus has been identified.[11] All of these findings are relevant to equine athletes because Arabians, Morgans, Paso Finos, ponies, and warmbloods appear to be genetically susceptible to ID, and they are often used as performance horses. ID is exacerbated by obesity, age, lack of exercise, systemic disease, PPID, and corticosteroid administration, and these risk factors are discussed later.

Obesity

This problem occurs in athletic horses when they are placed on diets that provide more energy than required. Athletic horses commonly receive grain or other concentrates in their diet because it assumed that additional energy is required to meet the demands of exercise. A diet should ideally be formulated for the individual horse, with body condition scoring performed regularly to assess body fat mass. Unfortunately, this is not always the case, and performance horses become obese as a result of overfeeding. Interestingly, obesity is more difficult to assess through visual examination in performance horses, and increased fat mass is sometimes mistaken for increased muscle mass. In the author's experience, this occurs more frequently in warmblood horses because of their larger stature. Palpation is required to assess body condition score in these animals, or ultrasound examination can be performed to measure the depth of subcutaneous or abdominal fat. Plasma leptin concentrations correlate with body fat mass,[12] and it is sometimes useful to measure this adipokine to convince owners that their horse is obese. Because obesity exacerbates ID and therefore raises the risk of laminitis, all horse owners should be strongly advised to manage obesity in athletic horses.

Some affected horses develop regional adiposity and accumulate fat in the neck region, and this may be referred to as a "cresty neck." Fat may also accumulate in the tail head, prepuce, or mammary gland regions, and subcutaneous fat masses sometimes appear in random locations. The neck should be palpated as part of routine physical examinations, and a cresty neck scoring system can be used to measure of adiposity in this region.[13] A horse with an enlarged neck crest is displayed in **Fig. 1**.

Age

Racehorses tend to be younger in age, but athletic horses used for other disciplines such as dressage remain in competition until they reach middle age. Age-related insulin resistance may occur in horses as it does in other species,[14] and the risk of PPID developing increases with age. If a horse is already genetically susceptible to ID, then these factors may raise blood insulin concentrations even further and increase the risk of laminitis developing.

Exercise

ID may be exacerbated when horses are laid up because of injuries and kept on a high-energy diet. Fat accumulates in adipose, muscle, and hepatic tissues and lowers insulin sensitivity, which raises insulin concentrations and increases the risk laminitis of laminitis occurring. Accumulation of fat within the liver decreases insulin clearance from the portal blood and causes plasma insulin concentrations to rise. More than 70% of the insulin secreted by pancreatic beta cells is cleared from the portal blood by the liver, so conditions that compromise liver function increase insulin concentrations within the peripheral blood.[15] The risk of hyperinsulinemia is highest in horses and ponies that are genetically predisposed to ID, so it is imperative that at-risk animals be placed on diets that are low in energy and nonstructural carbohydrates (NSC) whenever they are taken out of work.

Systemic Disease

Athletic horses travel more than other horses because they compete at different events, and their risk of acquiring infectious diseases is higher as a result. The stress associated with travel, housing in unfamiliar environments, and competition further increases the risk of infectious disease, and the combination of increased stress hormones and systemic inflammation may increase the risk of laminitis. When considering this group of risk factors, it is important to return to the concept of genetic susceptibility to ID because a Welsh pony with systemic inflammation may be more likely to develop laminitis than a thoroughbred with the same condition.

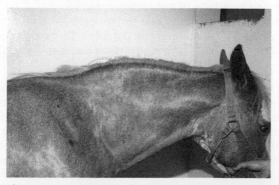

Fig. 1. Enlarged neck crest as an example of regional adiposity in a horse.

Pituitary Pars Intermedia Dysfunction

The risk of this endocrinopathy developing increases with age, and horses older than 10 years of age should be observed closely for clinical signs of muscle loss and delayed shedding of the winter hair coat. Development of PPID in a horse with preexisting ID is more worrisome than the same disease occurring in a horse with normal insulin status, and it is important to consider the breed of the horse being examined. Concurrent ID and PPID raises the risk of laminitis, and Mastro and colleagues[16] reported that some horses with PPID suffer from ID, whereas others have normal insulin sensitivity. Laminitis risk is more closely tied to ID than PPID status. As discussed in greater detail in later discussion, PPID can be seen in middle-aged athletic horses and negatively impacts performance. It is also a concern when managing ID because PPID appears to exacerbate ID and raise the risk of laminitis developing.

Corticosteroids

This controversial topic has been discussed in several articles, and debate continues about the risk of laminitis developing after corticosteroid administration.[17–19] An important piece of evidence was recently provided by an epidemiologic study of pasture- and endocrinopathy-associated laminitis, where an odds ratio of 10 was reported for laminitis developing after corticosteroid administration.[20] In the author's experience, the risk of laminitis after intra-articular or systemic administration of corticosteroids depends on multiple factors, and care should be taken to fully assess the patient before administering these drugs. If the horse has a higher risk of ID because of its breed, and exacerbating factors, such as obesity or systemic inflammation, are also noted, then there is a higher risk of laminitis developing after corticosteroid administration. Other exacerbating factors such as recent reduction in exercise, stall confinement, or the pain of lameness must also be considered. A high-grain diet also increases the risk of laminitis in horses receiving corticosteroid injections, and owners should be advised to lower NSC intake when these drugs are being administered. Corticosteroids lower tissue insulin sensitivity and raise blood insulin concentrations,[21–24] and marked hyperinsulinemia can induce laminitis.

Diagnostic Testing for Insulin Dysregulation

Diagnostic tests for ID are described in **Table 1**. The oral sugar test (OST) is preferred because stimulating insulin release from the pancreas allows mild ID to be detected. If owners raise concerns about inducing or exacerbating laminitis by performing the OST, then resting glucose and insulin concentrations should be measured first. However, it is still important to proceed with the OST if resting concentrations are normal because of the limited sensitivity of this resting measure.

Radiographs of the feet are a diagnostic test for EMS because laminitis may occur at a subclinical level before lameness is first detected. Divergent hoof rings ("founder lines") and widening of the white line are also clues that laminitis has been occurring.

Oral sugar test

This dynamic test assesses the magnitude of postprandial hyperinsulinemia in equids[6] and is a more sensitive diagnostic test than resting insulin concentrations. The test is performed by withholding feed for approximately 6 hours before administering corn syrup (Karo Light; ACH Food Companies, Inc, Cordova, TN, USA) at a dosage of 0.15 mL/kg (75 mL for a 500-kg horse) by mouth. Leave only one flake of hay with the horse after 10 PM and perform the test the next morning, or feed as normal in the morning and then fast the horse for 4 to 6 hours before performing the test in the afternoon. Corn syrup is given by mouth using 60-mL catheter-tip syringes, and

Table 1
Recommended diagnostic tests for insulin dysregulation

Oral Sugar Test

Normal	Mild ID	Marked ID
Insulin	Insulin	Insulin
<45 µU/mL	45–60 µU/mL	>60 µU/mL
(radioimmunoassay) at 60	(radioimmunoassay) at 60	(radioimmunoassay)
and 90 min	or 90 min	at 60 or 90 min

Excessive glucose response if glucose concentration
>125 mg/dL at 60 or 90 min

Resting (fed) insulin concentration

Negative	Mild ID	Marked ID
Insulin	Insulin	Insulin
<20 µU/mL	20–50 µU/mL	>50 µU/mL
(radioimmunoassay)	(radioimmunoassay)	(radioimmunoassay)

Adapted from the 2016 equine endocrinology group recommendations on diagnosis and management of equine metabolic syndome in horses. Available at: http://sites.tufts.edu/equineendogroup. Accessed May 23, 2018; with permission.

blood samples are collected for glucose and insulin measurements 60 and 90 minutes later. Owners can administer corn syrup themselves so that the veterinarian needs only to arrive in time to collect blood at 60 and 90 minutes.

Resting insulin concentrations were previously recommended for assessing insulin status in horses, and this test can still be used to confirm the diagnosis of ID in severely affected animals.[3] Blood is collected under fed conditions with horses having access to hay or grass, but grain must not be fed for 6 hours before blood is collected.

Other diagnostic tests for EMS include measurement of plasma leptin concentrations to assess internal and external fat depots (normal <10 ng/mL; Cornell Animal Health Diagnostic Center). Plasma high-molecular-weight adiponectin concentrations have also been measured in research studies, and it is hoped that diagnostic laboratories will start offering this test soon.[25,26] High-molecular-weight adiponectin concentrations decrease as ID gets worse. An octreotide response test for diagnosing ID is being developed,[27] but additional research is required.

Management of Insulin Dysregulation

When making recommendations for horses with ID, it is important to first assess the severity of ID. OST insulin concentrations greater than 60 µU/mL define marked ID, and patients with values in this range require more intensive management than those with OST insulin values in the 45- to 60-µU/mL range (mild ID). It has recently been shown that oral glucose test results predict the risk of laminitis in ponies,[20] so it can be assumed that animals with severe ID are at high risk for developing laminitis if they are left untreated.

Dietary management of mild insulin dysregulation

When OST insulin results fall within the 45- to 60-µU/mL range, it can be assumed that risk of laminitis is high, and steps should immediately be taken to lower insulin concentrations. Insulin concentrations increase after feeding, and postprandial hyperinsulinemia may induce laminitis, so the main goal of dietary management is to decrease stimulation of insulin release from the pancreas; this is achieved by reducing simple sugars in the diet. As previously mentioned, many athletic horses are on high-NSC diets because it is assumed that they have a higher energy requirement than other horses. If high-NSC sweet feeds or other grain mixtures are being fed, they should be discontinued right away and replaced with hay. If hay does not provide enough energy to meet the demands of the horse, as determined by body condition scoring, then additional calories can be added in the form of vegetable oil (1–2 cups per day). Low-NSC pelleted feeds are another option, and a wide array of products are available. Horses on hay-only diets require a vitamin-mineral supplement, and some owners provide a ration balancer containing additional protein, although care must be taken to select one with low-NSC content. Access to pasture should be restricted until insulin concentrations return to normal, and this is achieved by placing the horse and a companion in a small (150 ft × 150 ft) grass paddock or enclosed section of the pasture. A grazing muzzle can also be used to limit the amount of grass consumed. It is not necessary to eliminate access to grass altogether when only mild ID is detected, but care must be taken to limit intake because pasture grass is the most variable source of sugars and amino acids in the horse's diet.

Dietary management of severe insulin dysregulation

Horses, ponies, miniature horses, and donkeys with markedly increased insulin concentrations require more intensive dietary management. In these situations, all components of the horse's diet must be closely scrutinized to determine the amounts of sugars and amino acids that are being ingested. A hay diet is recommended, and it is important to analyze the hay that is fed to severely affected horses. Hay samples should be sent to a commercial laboratory for measurement of NSC content, and the greater the severity of ID, the more important it is to feed hay with a low-NSC value. An NSC (water-soluble carbohydrates + starches) value of less than 10% has been previously recommended for horses with ID,[6] but this cutoff value was not determined by research studies. Blood insulin responses to hay are determined by the feed itself, and also the severity of ID in the individual horse, and this can be investigated further by measuring the patient's insulin concentrations 2 and 4 hours after feeding the hay. It is also advisable to soak hay in cold water for 30 to 60 minutes to remove some of the simple sugars, although results vary according to the type of hay selected.[29] Severely affected horses must be removed from pasture and placed in dirt paddocks, but it may be possible to permit grazing again in the future if insulin concentrations return to normal or fall back into the range for mild ID. If hay is not providing enough energy for exercise and the horse is losing body condition, fat or a low-NSC pelleted feed can be added to the diet. Feeding horses smaller amounts of hay more frequently is recommended if ID is severe, and this can be achieved by using slow-feeder bags.

Management of obesity in the horse with mild insulin dysregulation

Increased adiposity manifests as generalized obesity or more subtle expansion of subcutaneous or visceral fat stores. Lipid may also accumulate within the liver, and mildly increased plasma Gamma Glutamyl Transferase activities are sometimes noted in these cases. If increased adiposity is a detected through body condition scoring, ultrasound examination, or measurement of plasma leptin concentrations, then a weight loss plan is required. This plan should consist of decreasing the amount of energy provided in the diet, while increasing exercise to accelerate energy consumption. Energy intake should be incrementally decreased using a stepwise reduction in the amounts of concentrates (grain, pelleted feed, or fat/oil supplement) provided. If obesity persists once concentrates are removed from the diet, hay amounts should be incrementally decreased at 2-week intervals. One approach is to first lower the amount of hay provided to the amount equivalent to 1.5% of current body weight. If the horse has not started to lose weight after 2 weeks, the amount of hay provided should be lowered to 1.5% of ideal body weight. A further reduction to 1% of ideal body weight can be considered if the horse is still not losing weight after 2 weeks.

Exercise increases consumption of energy, which helps to address the problem of obesity and improve insulin sensitivity,[30,31] and moderate-intensity exercise is recommended whenever possible. As previously mentioned, ID may develop when athletic horses are forced to rest because of lameness or other medical problems. Immediate adjustments in diet are required in these cases, and the horse should be encouraged to exercise if permitted, even when training has been halted. Placing the horse in a small paddock with a companion is one approach, and another strategy is to place feed in different locations within the paddock to encourage exercise. Swimming is an effective form of exercise, and a recent article described the positive effects of swimming on insulin dynamics in horses.[31]

Management of obesity in the horse with severe insulin dysregulation
A more intensive approach is required when ID is severe because the risk of laminitis remains high for as long as insulin concentrations stay elevated. Levothyroxine sodium (Thyro L, Lloyd, Inc, Shenandoah, IA, USA) can be administered at high doses to accelerate weight loss in severely affected horses, and this treatment is also selected for horses that remain obese, even after all diet and exercise strategies have been attempted. The goal of levothyroxine treatment is to induce mild subclinical hyperthyroidism and increase metabolic rate, and a starting dosage of 0.1 mg/kg body weight every 24 hours orally is selected, which is equivalent to approximately 48 mg (4 teaspoons) levothyroxine powder per day for a 500-kg horse, given by mouth or mixed in a handful of low-NSC pellets. Levothyroxine is administered until body fat mass decreases or for a maximum of 6 months, and then the dose is incrementally lowered over 2 weeks before treatment is discontinued. Dietary recommendations must be followed at the same time that levothyroxine is administered; otherwise, horses consume additional feed to compensate for the increase in metabolic rate.

Medical management of the horse with severe insulin dysregulation
Metformin hydrochloride is commonly prescribed for the management of diabetes mellitus in humans, and this drug can be used to manage postprandial hyperinsulinemia in horses. Although metformin is an effective antidiabetic drug in humans, oral bioavailability is low for the formulations of metformin that are currently available for use in horses. Hustace and colleagues[32] reported only 7% oral bioavailability for metformin in horses when feed is withheld, and this value decreased to 4% when the same horses were fed before the drug was administered. Results of one study suggest that metformin administered at a dose of 15 mg/kg every 12 hours orally improves insulin sensitivity in horses and ponies with ID,[33] but in a subsequent study of insulin-resistant ponies, metformin had no effect on insulin dynamics.[34] Another study showed that metformin (30 mg/kg) administered 1 hour before an oral glucose test lowered blood glucose and insulin concentrations, and this suggests that the drug affects glucose absorption from the intestine.[35] On the basis of these results, owners are instructed to administer metformin 30 to 60 minutes before feeding when the drug is prescribed for horses with severe ID. A starting dosage of 30 mg/kg every 8 to 12 hours orally is currently recommended when using metformin in horses, and the author has extended the dose range to 50 mg/kg every 8 to 12 hours orally in some cases. Current formulations of metformin may cause oral irritation when administered at high doses, so horses on treatment should be monitored

closely. Rinsing the mouth with water after administering metformin helps to reduce oral irritation and prevent ulcers from forming. Responses to metformin appear to vary among horses with severe ID, and it is therefore ideal to assess the individual horse by measuring postprandial insulin concentrations 2 hours after the horse is fed, before and after initiating metformin treatment.

Management of refractory insulin dysregulation in horses

Unfortunately a small number of patients with severe ID fail to respond to the management strategies outlined above, and it is possible that they have a different manifestation of ID than other affected animals. All attempts should be made to manage these cases, but only partial responses to management changes may be seen. New antidiabetic drugs are being developed for use in humans and sodium-glucose cotransporter 2 inhibitors show promise as drugs for managing severe ID in horses. These drugs are expensive at present but may be worth considering for short-term management of ID when severely affected horses enter an acute crisis, for example, when a horse with ID is accidentally fed grain, breaks into the feed room, or escapes from its paddock and grazes on pasture. Canagliflozin belongs to this class of drugs, and it is administered orally on a once-daily basis.

PITUITARY PARS INTERMEDIA DYSFUNCTION IN THE EQUINE ATHLETE

Middle-aged (10–20 years) and aged (>20 years) horses are at risk for developing PPID, and this is a relatively common cause of poor performance in athletic horses that fall within these age ranges. Owners may report decreased performance during training sessions and say that affected horses seem duller than normal or lethargic. These signs are subtle to begin with, and it is difficult for the veterinarian to appreciate the shifts in behavior that the owner or trainer is noting. Occasionally, owners report that a horse with a history of being difficult to ride is calmer than before. Over time, horses with PPID show decreased epaxial muscle mass along the topline, and owners report a decrease in body condition, even though exercise and feeding regimens have remained the same. Muscle loss is sometimes attributed to the horse growing older, but aging changes are gradual and muscle loss associated with PPID occurs more rapidly. Delayed shedding of winter hair may also be noted. One of the first signs of PPID in show horses is the need for clipping to be performed more frequently.

Presenting complaints for *early PPID* include the detection of longer hair in certain regions of the body, such as the palmar/plantar aspects of the legs, and this is referred to as regional hypertrichosis. The hair coat may appear duller and feel coarser or thicker than normal, and owners may not have noticed these abnormalities because of their gradual onset. Reproductive performance might also be affected by PPID because dopamine inhibition is involved in regulation of the seasonal anovulatory period,[36] although definitive studies are lacking in this area.

Advanced PPID is easily recognized, and a presumptive diagnosis is reached by taking a history and performing a physical examination. As PPID progresses, horses show year-round retention of the winter hair coat and generalized hypertrichosis. The long curly hair coat detected in horses with advanced disease was previously referred to as hirsutism, and it is sometimes considered a pathognomonic clinical sign for PPID. Other clinical findings of advanced PPID include rounding of the abdomen, polyuria/polydipsia, recurrent bacterial infections, persistent neutrophilia and lymphopenia, infertility, and inappropriate lactation. Sole abscesses occur with greater frequency in horses with PPID, and this problem may be noted in performance horses that are shod on a regular basis.

Suspensory Ligament Degeneration

Older horses with PPID have a higher incidence of suspensory ligament injury, and there is evidence to suggest that increased tissue-specific cortisol action is responsible for weakening these structures.[37,38] Wellness examinations in middle-aged performance horses should therefore include PPID testing, and those with positive test results should be placed on pergolide treatment to prevent further degeneration of suspensory ligaments.

Diagnostic Testing for Pituitary Pars Intermedia Dysfunction

Diagnostic tests for PPID are outlined in **Table 2**, and it is important to select the correct test for the stage of disease and time of the year when testing is performed. The thyrotropin-releasing hormone (TRH) stimulation test is recommended for the diagnosis of early PPID because resting adrenocorticotropic hormone (ACTH) concentrations often fall within reference interval at this stage of the disease. To perform this test, first collect a preinjection baseline blood sample and then administer 1.0 mg TRH (1 mL) via intravenous injection. Compounding pharmacies now supply TRH, and their product elicits the same responses as TRH prepared in research laboratories.[39] A second blood sample is collected 10 minutes later, and both samples are submitted for measurement of ACTH. TRH stimulates ACTH secretion, and higher concentrations are detected in horses with PPID, compared with healthy horses.[40] Melanotrophs possess TRH receptors, and more ACTH is released when hyperplastic or neoplastic cells within the pars intermedia are stimulated. There are some short-term side effects of TRH administration, including yawning and nonproductive coughing, but these problems resolve within a few minutes and are not a major concern.[41] One limitation of the TRH stimulation test is that seasonally adjusted reference intervals have not been established for the late summer and fall, so these times should be avoided until further research is performed.

As PPID advances, resting ACTH concentrations rise above reference interval, and this test becomes more useful. However, ACTH concentrations normally increase in the late summer and fall as animals prepare for winter, so seasonally adjusted

Table 2
Recommended diagnostic tests for pituitary pars intermedia dysfunction

Early PPID	TRH stimulation test			
	Non-Fall	Negative	Equivocal	Positive
	Mid-November to mid-July	Plasma ACTH <110 pg/mL at 10 min	Plasma ACTH 110–200 pg/mL at 10 min	Plasma ACTH >200 pg/mL at 10 min
	Fall Mid-July to mid-November	Reference intervals not available at this time		
Advanced PPID	Resting ACTH concentration			
	Non-Fall	Negative	Equivocal	Positive
	Mid-November to mid-July	Plasma ACTH <30 pg/mL	Plasma ACTH 30–50 pg/mL	Plasma ACTH >50 pg/mL
	Fall Mid-July to mid-November	Negative Plasma ACTH <50 pg/mL	Equivocal Plasma ACTH 50–100 pg/mL	Positive Plasma ACTH >100 pg/mL

Adapted from the 2017 equine endocrinology group recommendations on diagnosis and management of pituitary pars intermedia dysfunction in horses. Available at: http://sites.tufts.edu/equineendogroup. Accessed May 23, 2018; with permission.

reference intervals must be applied when interpreting results during these seasons. It was previously thought that the late summer and fall should be avoided when testing horses for PPID, but the opposite approach is now recommended. Measuring plasma ACTH concentrations when hormonal systems are stimulated increases the likelihood of detecting PPID.

Management of Pituitary Pars Intermedia Dysfunction

Managing pituitary pars intermedia dysfunction to lower laminitis risk in horses with insulin dysregulation

As previously discussed, laminitis is one of the greatest threats to the health of the athletic horse. PPID may exacerbate ID in horses, and this is an important consideration when assessing the risk of laminitis in an individual patient. High insulin concentrations are detected in some, but not all horses and ponies with PPID,[42–44] and laminitis is more closely associated with ID than PPID.[1,43,45] Other risk factors, such as systemic inflammation or corticosteroid administration, are a greater concern in horses with concurrent ID and PPID, and the risk of laminitis is high in these animals.

Medical management of pituitary pars intermedia dysfunction

Pergolide is recommended for the treatment of PPID in horses at an initial dosage of 0.002 mg/kg, and it is available as 1-mg tablets (Prascend; Boehringer Ingelheim Vetmedica Inc, St. Joseph, MO, USA). This ergot alkaloid dopamine receptor agonist is administered to restore dopaminergic inhibition of melanotrophs, and its interaction with D2 receptors inhibits hormone secretion. It has not been determined if pergolide treatment also inhibits the development of pituitary hyperplasia or reduces the size of pituitary adenomas, but these beneficial effects are plausible considering its mechanism of action. Pergolide was available in the past as Permax (previously manufactured by Eli Lilly Co), and it was used in humans for the treatment of Parkinson disease. However, this product was voluntarily withdrawn from the market in March 2007 after the US Food and Drug Administration (FDA) issued a warning that pergolide was associated with increased incidence of valvular regurgitation in people.[46,47] Cardiac problems have not been encountered in horses, and Prascend was introduced in December 2011 as an FDA-approved drug for the treatment of PPID in horses.

If the horse is concurrently affected by ID and PPID, insulin concentrations typically decrease in response to pergolide treatment, and this lowers the likelihood of laminitis reoccurring. Horses with ID can be monitored by measuring resting insulin concentrations under fed conditions or by performing an OST. If insulin concentrations do not decrease after administering pergolide for 2 weeks at the dosage level selected, consider increasing the dose by 0.5 mg/d, even if ACTH concentrations have normalized.

When plasma ACTH concentrations do not decrease in response to pergolide treatment, the drug formulation and dose must be considered. If compounded pergolide is being administered, it may not be effective because of quality control issues and lack of stability. Davis and colleagues[48] demonstrated that pergolide is unstable over a 35-day period when prepared as an aqueous suspension, with higher temperatures and exposure to light-enhancing degradation. The dosage level selected is very important, and the dose should be appropriate for the stage of disease. For example, horses with PPID that have generalized hypertrichosis and muscle wasting may require 3 mg/d pergolide before plasma ACTH concentrations significantly decrease.

Cyproheptadine is also used for the management of PPID, but the author reserves this drug for horses with advanced PPID that are on higher doses of pergolide. This drug inhibits the action of serotonin, an excitatory transmitter that stimulates melanotrophs. Consider adding cyproheptadine at a dosage of 0.25 mg/kg orally every 12 hours or 0.50 mg/kg every 24 hours orally once the 3-mg pergolide/d level is reached.

Dietary management of pituitary pars intermedia dysfunction

Recommendations should be based on the body condition score of the horse, and glucose and insulin results. If a high OST insulin response is detected or resting hyper-insulinemia (>50 mU/L) is detected, care must be taken to select low-NSC feeds. Commercial low-NSC/low-starch pelleted feeds are recommended, or molasses-free beet pulp can be fed with vegetable oil added as a more economical alternative. Hay with low-NSC content should be provided. It is also important to note that many horses with PPID do not suffer from ID. They are not genetically predisposed to ID and have not suffered from laminitis in the past. Horses in this group have normal OST insulin responses and can be fed senior feeds with higher NSC content.

Medical Treatments and Drug Regulations

Fédération Equestre Internationale (FEI) regulations and rules set by other governing bodies for competitions must be reviewed before drugs recommended in this article are administered. Attempts are being made to have pergolide approved by the FEI for use in horses with documented PPID, but at the time of writing, this drug is still listed as a prohibited substance, and appropriate withdrawal times are required.

SUMMARY

ID and PPID are important endocrine/metabolic disorders in athletic horses because they are associated with laminitis, a condition of the equine foot that significantly impacts performance. Horses that are genetically predisposed to ID as a result of their breed and exhibit regional adiposity should undergo diagnostic testing to assess insulin status and their risk of laminitis. Those with clinical signs of PPID should be tested and placed on long-term pergolide treatment.

REFERENCES

1. Frank N, Tadros EM. Insulin dysregulation. Equine Vet J 2014;46:103–12.
2. Asplin KE, Sillence MN, Pollitt CC, et al. Induction of laminitis by prolonged hyper-insulinaemia in clinically normal ponies. Vet J 2007;174:530–5.
3. de Laat MA, McGowan CM, Sillence MN, et al. Equine laminitis: induced by 48 h hyperinsulinaemia in Standardbred horses. Equine Vet J 2010;42:129–35.
4. Treiber KH, Kronfeld DS, Hess TM, et al. Evaluation of genetic and metabolic pre-dispositions and nutritional risk factors for pasture-associated laminitis in ponies. J Am Vet Med Assoc 2006;228:1538–45.
5. Frank N, Elliott SB, Brandt LE, et al. Physical characteristics, blood hormone concentrations, and plasma lipid concentrations in obese horses with insulin resistance. J Am Vet Med Assoc 2006;228:1383–90.
6. Frank N, Geor RJ, Bailey SR, et al. Equine metabolic syndrome. J Vet Intern Med 2010;24:467–75.
7. Bailey SR, Habershon-Butcher JL, Ransom KJ, et al. Hypertension and insulin resistance in a mixed-breed population of ponies predisposed to laminitis. Am J Vet Res 2008;69:122–9.
8. Wooldridge AA, Edwards HG, Plaisance EP, et al. Evaluation of high-molecular weight adiponectin in horses. Am J Vet Res 2012;73:1230–40.

9. Jeffcott LB, Field JR, McLean JG, et al. Glucose tolerance and insulin sensitivity in ponies and Standardbred horses. Equine Vet J 1986;18:97–101.

10. Bamford NJ, Baskerville CL, Harris PA, et al. Postprandial glucose, insulin, and glucagon-like peptide-1 responses of different equine breeds adapted to meals containing micronized maize. J Anim Sci 2015;93:3377–83.

11. Lewis SL, Holl HM, Streeter C, et al. Genomewide association study reveals a risk locus for equine metabolic syndrome in the Arabian horse. J Anim Sci 2017;95: 1071–9.

12. Gentry LR, Thompson DL Jr, Gentry GT Jr, et al. The relationship between body condition, leptin, and reproductive and hormonal characteristics of mares during the seasonal anovulatory period. J Anim Sci 2002;80:2695–703.

13. Carter RA, Geor RJ, Burton Staniar W, et al. Apparent adiposity assessed by standardised scoring systems and morphometric measurements in horses and ponies. Vet J 2009;179:204–10.

14. Yang Y, Dong R, Chen Z, et al. Endothelium-specific CYP2J2 overexpression attenuates age-related insulin resistance. Aging Cell 2018;17(2).

15. Toth F, Frank N, Martin-Jimenez T, et al. Measurement of C-peptide concentrations and responses to somatostatin, glucose infusion, and insulin resistance in horses. Equine Vet J 2010;42:149–55.

16. Mastro LM, Adams AA, Urschel KL. Pituitary pars intermedia dysfunction does not necessarily impair insulin sensitivity in old horses. Domest Anim Endocrinol 2015;50:14–25.

17. Bailey SR, Elliott J. The corticosteroid laminitis story: 2. Science of if, when and how. Equine Vet J 2007;39:7–11.

18. Bailey SR. Corticosteroid-associated laminitis. Vet Clin North Am Equine Pract 2010;26:277–85.

19. Johnson PJ, Slight SH, Ganjam VK, et al. Glucocorticoids and laminitis in the horse. Vet Clin North Am Equine Pract 2002;18:219–36.

20. Coleman M, Belknap J, Bramlage L, et al. Case control study of pasture and endocrinopathy-associated laminitis in horses. Proceedings of the Havemeyer International Equine Endocrinology Summit 2017. Coral Gables, FL, January 4-6, 2017. p. 25.

21. Freestone JF, Wolfsheimer KJ, Ford RB, et al. Triglyceride, insulin, and cortisol responses of ponies to fasting and dexamethasone administration. J Vet Intern Med 1991;5:15–22.

22. Tiley HA, Geor RJ, McCutcheon LJ. Effects of dexamethasone administration on insulin resistance and components of insulin signaling and glucose metabolism in equine skeletal muscle. Am J Vet Res 2008;69:51–8.

23. Haffner JC, Eiler H, Hoffman RM, et al. Effect of a single dose of dexamethasone on glucose homeostasis in healthy horses by using the combined intravenous glucose and insulin test. J Anim Sci 2009;87:131–5.

24. French K, Pollitt CC, Pass MA. Pharmacokinetics and metabolic effects of triamcinolone acetonide and their possible relationships to glucocorticoid-induced laminitis in horses. J Vet Pharmacol Ther 2000;23:287–92.

25. Wooldridge AA, Taylor DR, Zhong Q, et al. High molecular weight adiponectin is reduced in horses with obesity and inflammatory disease [abstract]. J Vet Intern Med 2010;24:781.

26. Frank N, Walsh DM. Repeatability of oral sugar test results, glucagon-like peptide-1 measurements, and serum high-molecular-weight adiponectin concentrations in horses. J Vet Intern Med 2017;31:1178–87.

27. Frank N, Hermida P, Sanchez-Londono A, et al. Blood glucose and insulin concentrations after octreotide administration in horses with insulin dysregulation. J Vet Intern Med 2017;31:1188–92.
28. Meier AD, de Laat MA, Reiche DB, et al. The oral glucose test predicts laminitis risk in ponies fed a diet high in nonstructural carbohydrates. Domest Anim Endocrinol 2018;63:1–9.
29. Longland AC, Barfoot C, Harris PA. Effects of soaking on the water-soluble carbohydrate and crude protein content of hay. Vet Rec 2011;168:618.
30. Powell DM, Reedy SE, Sessions DR, et al. Effect of short-term exercise training on insulin sensitivity in obese and lean mares. Equine Vet J Suppl 2002;(34):81–4.
31. Bonelli F, Sgorbini M, Meucci V, et al. How swimming affects plasma insulin and glucose concentration in thoroughbreds: a pilot study. Vet J 2017;226:1–3.
32. Hustace JL, Firshman AM, Mata JE. Pharmacokinetics and bioavailability of metformin in horses. Am J Vet Res 2009;70:665–8.
33. Durham AE, Rendle DI, Newton JE. The effect of metformin on measurements of insulin sensitivity and beta cell response in 18 horses and ponies with insulin resistance. Equine Vet J 2008;40:493–500.
34. Tinworth KD, Boston RC, Harris PA, et al. The effect of oral metformin on insulin sensitivity in insulin-resistant ponies. Vet J 2012;191:79–84.
35. Rendle DI, Rutledge F, Hughes KJ, et al. Effects of metformin hydrochloride on blood glucose and insulin responses to oral dextrose in horses. Equine Vet J 2013;45(6):751–4.
36. Burns TA. Effects of common equine endocrine diseases on reproduction. Vet Clin North Am Equine Pract 2016;32:435–49.
37. Hofberger S, Gauff F, Licka T. Suspensory ligament degeneration associated with pituitary pars intermedia dysfunction in horses. Vet J 2015;203:348–50.
38. Hofberger SC, Gauff F, Thaller D, et al. Assessment of tissue-specific cortisol activity with regard to degeneration of the suspensory ligaments in horses with pituitary pars intermedia dysfunction. Am J Vet Res 2018;79:199–210.
39. Goodale L, Frank N, Hermida P, et al. Evaluation of a thyrotropin-releasing hormone solution stored at room temperature for pituitary pars intermedia dysfunction testing in horses. Am J Vet Res 2015;76:437–44.
40. Beech J, Boston R, Lindborg S, et al. Adrenocorticotropin concentration following administration of thyrotropin-releasing hormone in healthy horses and those with pituitary pars intermedia dysfunction and pituitary gland hyperplasia. J Am Vet Med Assoc 2007;231:417–26.
41. Restifo MM, Frank N, Hermida P, et al. Effects of withholding feed on thyrotropin-releasing hormone stimulation test results and effects of combined testing on oral sugar test and thyrotropin-releasing hormone stimulation test results in horses. Am J Vet Res 2016;77:738–48.
42. Reeves HJ, Lees R, McGowan CM. Measurement of basal serum insulin concentration in the diagnosis of Cushing's disease in ponies. Vet Rec 2001;149:449–52.
43. Walsh DM, McGowan CM, McGowan T, et al. Correlation of plasma insulin concentration with laminitis score in a field study of equine Cushing's disease and equine metabolic syndrome. J Equine Vet Sci 2009;29:87–94.
44. McGowan CM, Frost R, Pfeiffer DU, et al. Serum insulin concentrations in horses with equine Cushing's syndrome: response to a cortisol inhibitor and prognostic value. Equine Vet J 2004;36:295–8.
45. Karikoski NP, Horn I, McGowan TW, et al. The prevalence of endocrinopathic laminitis among horses presented for laminitis at a first-opinion/referral equine hospital. Domest Anim Endocrinol 2011;41:111–7.

46. Zanettini R, Antonini A, Gatto G, et al. Valvular heart disease and the use of dopamine agonists for Parkinson's disease. N Engl J Med 2007;356:39–46.
47. Schade R, Andersohn F, Suissa S, et al. Dopamine agonists and the risk of cardiac-valve regurgitation. N Engl J Med 2007;356:29–38.
48. Davis JL, Kirk LM, Davidson GS, et al. Effects of compounding and storage conditions on stability of pergolide mesylate. J Am Vet Med Assoc 2009;234:385–9.

Borreliosis in Sport Horse Practice

Eric Lockwood Swinebroad, DVM*

KEYWORDS

- Borrelia burgdorferi • Lyme disease • Equine lyme • Neuroborreliosis
- Equine uveitis • Equine pseudolymphoma

KEY POINTS

- Given the variable clinical signs attributed to *Borrelia burgdorferi*, including infectious arthritis, neurologic disease, and behavioral changes, *B burgdorferi* is an important differential for decreased performance in sport horses.
- The primary vectors (*Ixodes* tick species in North America) are expanding their range and thus Borrelia species are located in a wider area, making exposure more likely to a naive population; however, due to regionally high seroprevalence and the vague (anecdotal) clinical signs, the diagnosis of Lyme disease (note: not exposure or infection) in the horse is believed overestimated.
- There are three confirmed clinical disease entities found in borreliosis: pseudolymphoma, neurologic disease, and uveitis.
- The definitive diagnosis of Lyme disease should be based on
  1. Exposure (reside currently, have resided, or traveled through, with a stopover, in a Lyme endemic region)
  2. Clinical signs compatible with borreliosis
  3. A careful examination, and rule out, of other differential diagnoses
  4. Positive serologic results for *B burgdorferi*
- Antibiotics are the first-line treatment of confirmed Lyme disease: tetracyclines: doxycycline, minocycline or oxytetracycline, cephalosporins, and B-lactams.
- A single positive serologic test, by itself, is not conformation of Lyme disease but is evidence of current or past infection.

Disclosure: Dr E.L. Swinebroad has no financial/funding or commercial disclosures affecting the creation or content of this article; however, he is a coauthor of the following: Divers TJ, Gardner RB, Madigan JE, Witonsky SG, Bertone JJ, Swinebroad EL, Schutzer SE, Johnson AL. Borrelia burgdorferi infection and Lyme disease in North American horses: a consensus statement. J Vet Intern Med 2018. https://doi.org/10.1111/jvim.15042.
Newmarket-Indialantic Equine, Newmarket, NH, USA
* 125 Main Street Unit # 5, Newmarket, NH 03857.
E-mail address: elsdvm@gmail.com

INTRODUCTION

The foundational work of sport horse practice is evaluating soundness and performance, defining and correcting unsoundness noted on physical examination, and returning the horse to competition. Lameness (musculoskeletal/neuromuscular unsoundness) is a factor in days lost from training and competition; it is a cause of racehorse wastage; and it is implicated in poor performance in Western equestrian sport and the seven Federation Equestre' International (FEI) disciplines, such as dressage, driving, eventing, endurance, and show-jumping.[1-5] Even though there are "no classically defined virulence factors" associated with the borrelia genome (their evolution was not one of a mammalian pathogen), these spirochetes are implicated in cases of human arthritis,[6,7] equine neurologic disease, and equine infectious synovitis (histologic evidence) and are anecdotally implicated in cases of shifting leg lameness, generalized stiffness, muscular weakness, lethargy, and behavioral abnormalities in sport horse practices across the United States.[6,8-14] As *Ixodes* tick range expands, increasing the risk of *B burgdorferi* infection and its negative effect on neuromuscular and musculoskeletal soundness, borreliosis has become a significant differential diagnosis in cases of lameness and poor performance in sport horses. With that in mind, it is counterintuitive, but imperative, to also note that care must be taken to first exclude other diseases with similar presentations, because Lyme disease is an "easy diagnosis" based on serologic prevalence and it is likely overdiagnosed in some endemic areas.[8,15-17]

Borrelia and Ixodes Biology

B garinii, *B afzelii*, *B lusitaniae*, and *B valaisiana* (and less so *B burgdorferi* sensu stricto [s.s.]) are members of the *B burgdorferi* sensu lato (s.l.) genospecies responsible for equine borreliosis in Europe and Asia.[8,12,18-22] In contrast, equine Lyme disease in North America is currently limited to the genospecies *B burgdorferi* sensu stricto (*B burgdorferi* s.s.), a distinct genotype varying in inflammatory profile and clinical disease from the European spirochete of the same name.[18] The microaerobic borrelia spirochete is an approximately 30-μm by 3-μm (length $\times$ width), unicellular, spiral microorganism. Its cell envelope is similar to gram-negative bacteria with the exception of an abundance of outer surface lipoproteins (Osps) and a lack of cell wall polysaccharides. It is motile through many tissue types, eg, connective, than most bacteria can migrate through via flagella localized in its periplasmatic space (shielding the immunogenic flagella from host immune systems).[6,13,23,24] Genospecies of borrelia are constantly being redefined or discovered, so the number of species affecting horses may be incomplete at the time of publication, for example, a new borrelia human pathogenic *B burgdorferi* s.l. genospecies, *B mayonii,* was identified in 2016 in the United States.[8,15,25,26] *B burgdorferi* s.l. are adapted to survive in different species (arachnids, mammals, reptiles, and birds) during their life span.[6,27-32] Their primary vector, the *Ixodes* tick, has a 2-year enzootic life cycle.[33,34] *B burgdorferi* DNA can also be found in the American dog tick (*Dermacentor variabilis)* and the lone star tick (*Amblyomma americanum*); however, acquired spirochetal larval infections in these tick species are short lived. *D variabilis* and *A americanum* are highly immunocompetent, using plasma borreliacidal proteins and phagocytosis by tick hemocytes to limit tissue dispersal and clear the infection so rapidly that these ticks are not vectors for Lyme disease.[35-37] *B burgdorferi* s.s. has also been identified in the midgut of the mosquitoes *Culex pipiens* and *Aedes vexans*, so transmission may be possible by vectors other than arthropods, although to date this has not been validated in North America, Europe, or Asia.[13,38-42]

In North America, *Ixodes scapularis* (eastern black-legged tick; previously classified as *I dammini*) and *I pacificus* (western black-legged tick) are the species involved with pathogen colonization, whereas in Europe and Asia the arachnid species are *I ricinus* (European sheep tick) and *I persulcatus* (taiga tick), respectively.[6,13,29,43,44] *I scapularis* may also harbor *Anaplasma* and *Piroplasmosis* organisms along with *B burgdorferi* s.s. and thus coinfections are possible from a single tick attachment.[12,17,45,46] *Ixodes* feed once at each of 3 life-cycle stages (larvae, nymph, and adult), and drop off the host in-between feedings to molt (larvae-nymph and nymph-adult) or to lay eggs (adult). Transstadial transmission occurs, but transovarial transmission is less than 2%; thus, the *Ixodes* multispecies feeding pattern is helpful for borrelia transfer to multiple hosts for overwintering. Tick survival and population expansion are also regulated by microclimate (humidity and moisture) and ticks are noted to be inactive at 45°F (7°C). In the first season, small mammals, primarily the white-footed mouse (*Peromyscus leucopus*), serve as an *Ixodes* larval food source, reservoir for Borrelia spirochete survival, and larvae to nymph maturation. In season 2, nymphs feed and molt into adult ticks (summer and fall). Adults subsequently feed and overwinter via larger mammals, for example, white-tailed deer (*Odocoileus virginianus*), horses, and humans. *Ixodes* adults complete their feeding, drop off in the final spring, and gravid female *Ixodes* deposit eggs into the environment as the cycle begins anew (**Fig. 1**). As noted, the *Ixodes* eggs do not contain *B burgdorferi*. There are select mammalian hosts, for example, Virginia opossum (*Didelphis virginiana*), that have an ability to increase *Ixodes* larval mortality at feeding. Within this tick cycle, horses and humans are considered aberrant, dead-end hosts.[8,20,22,27,32,33,35,47–49]

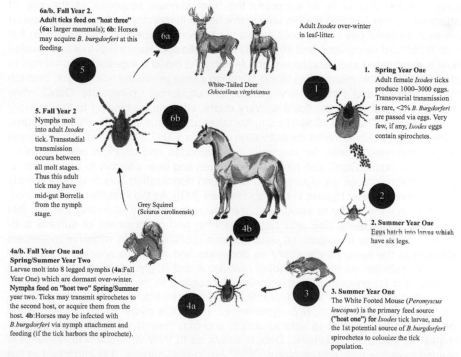

6a/b. Fall Year 2.
Adult ticks feed on "host three"
(**6a**: larger mammals); **6b**: Horses
may acquire *B. burgdorferi* at this
feeding.

6a

Adult *Ixodes* over-winter
in leaf-litter.

White-Tailed Deer
Odocoileus virginianus

1. Spring Year One
Adult female *Ixodes* ticks
produce 1000–3000 eggs.
Transovarial transmission
is rare, <2% *B. Burgdorferi*
are passed via eggs. Very
few, if any, *Ixodes* eggs
contain spirochetes.

5. Fall Year 2
Nymphs molt
into adult *Ixodes*
tick. Transstadial
transmission
occurs between
all molt stages.
Thus this adult
tick may have
mid-gut Borrelia
from the nymph
stage.

Grey Squirrel
(*Sciurus carolinensis*)

2. Summer Year One
Eggs hatch into larvae which
have six legs.

**4a/b. Fall Year One and
Spring/Summer Year Two**
Larvae molt into 8 legged nymphs (**4a**:Fall
Year One) which are dormant over-winter.
Nymphs feed on "host two" Spring/Summer
year two. Ticks may transmit spirochetes to
the second host, or acquire them from the
host. **4b**:Horses may be infected with
B.burgdorferi via nymph attachment and
feeding (if the tick harbors the spirochete).

3. Summer Year One
The White Footed Mouse (*Peromyscus
leucopus*) is the primary feed source
("host one") for *Ixodes* tick larvae, and
the 1st potential source of *B.burgdorferi*
spirochetes to colonize the tick
population.

Fig. 1. *Ixodes* tick life cycle. (*Courtesy of* Nicole Mariko Godusky, BA, BS, Coopersburg, PA; with permission.)

SPIROCHETE TRANSFER IN BORRELIOSIS

Ticks "quest" (extend and wave their forelegs and grab onto a passing host), attach, and feed via hypostome mouthparts thru an entrance wound. Horses become infected with *B burgdorferi* as the spirochete migrates from a nymph or adult tick's salivary gland to the horse's dermis at the time of attachment. The blood meal is obtained at the end of the process, because the majority of time is spent on saliva injection into the host's skin leading to immune system inhibition, for example, the uptake of immunosuppressive tick salivary proteins, such as Salp15, and the transformation of borrelia outer surface proteins (Osp), for example, OspA to OspC.[6,33,45] Evidence suggests *Borrelia burgdorferi* s.s. transmission to a host, that is, infection, may be accomplished within 16 hours or less. The time frame to infection is dependent on factors, such as the *Ixodes* species, for example, *Borrelia* spirochetes were noted to have greater systemic dissemination in *I persulcatus* versus *I scapularis;* the *Borrelia* species, for example, *B afzelii* (a European pathogen), was noted to transmit spirochetes to a mammalian host faster than *B bergdorferi* s.s.; tick surface antigen modification speed, that is, down-regulation of OspA in the tick midgut and up-regulation of OspC in tick salivary glands, and the location of *B burgdorferi* within the tick at the time of attachment to the host, that is, spirochetes residing in salivary glands, are considered more virulent and are transferred more rapidly, than those in the midgut. This time frame is shorter than noted in many evidenced-based articles, which state greater than 24 hours to 48 hours are necessary for infection to occur.[22,26,33,47,50,51] This biology of infection has become better elucidated over time, and it is detailed in several publications.[8,13,33] In summary, a mixture of bioactive chemicals (eg, anticoagulants, vasodilators, lymphocyte suppressors, cytokines, and complement inhibitors) in tick saliva work to suppress the host immune response at the site of attachment. The fact that the Borrelia spirochete's immunogenic flagella are located beneath an outer cell wall, a position unique to Borrelia species, also assists in the inability of host recognition and elimination.[6] Borrelia species survival in a mammalian host is augmented after attachment and feeding. As blood is ingested, OspA binds to plasminogen within mammalian blood, allowing passage into the tick midgut, through the hemocoel, and into salivary glands. *B burgdorferi* up-regulate OspC while migrating to and within the tick's salivary ducts, allowing for binding to tick salivary protein Salp15. The OspC/Salp15 complex takes advantage, in acute infection stages, of the saliva's ability to inhibit the activation of T cells (CD4$^+$ and natural killer cells) and antigen processing cells, for example, macrophages and dendrite cells, to infect mammalian hosts. OspC also binds plasminogen and uses plasmin to access extracellular matrix tissues via glycoprotein and fibrin degradation (this may be a means of blood-brain barrier bypass in neuroborreliosis [NB]). As the infection disseminates, Borrelia have the ability to avoid host immune responses by recruiting the variable outer surface proteins VlsE and OspF (masking and replacement of surface antigens).[13,50–54] Other *B burgdorferi* outer surface proteins include adhesive molecules assisting in the spirochete's ability to penetrate and attach to specific tissues, for example, collagen via decorin-binding proteins A and B, glycosaminoglycan-binding protein, and fibronectin-binding protein, all assisting in the pathology of Borrelia-associated synovitis.[13,47] In unfavorable host environments, or in the present of antimicrobials (eg, β-lactams), *B burgdorferi* s.l. nonmotile cystic forms appear. Such forms might be resistant to antimicrobials, and may "reconvert to vegetative spirochetes" in favorable conditions. Debate exists as to their virulence and research is needed to define their pathobiology.[45,55,56] For in-host survival, it is important to not think of bacteria in general, and *B burgdorferi* specifically, as surviving in a host as a single, free-floating cell. Bacteria most often persist attached to surfaces within a structured biofilm ecosystem. There are no research or clinical studies stating *Borrelia* species are innately antibiotic resistant; however, hydrogel biofilms, in which *B burgdorferi* colonies exist as a coordinated and functional community, are significantly more resistant to antibiotic treatment and phagocytosis than are freely floating (planktonic) cells.[57–59] Once situated in a mammalian host, *Borrelia* species cannot, as do many bacteria, biosynthesize all the nutrients necessary for survival. They rely on their arthropod and mammalian hosts to supply several needed factors, for example, nucleotides, amino acids, fatty acids, and enzyme cofactors. One unique exception to this obligate parasite life cycle is that iron is not required cofactor for *B Bergdorferi* survival.[13,52]

SEROPREVALENCE

As the geographic range of *Ixodes* expands, so does that of *B burgdorferi* (**Fig. 2**).[8] Current hypotheses are that favorable climatic change has enabled *Ixodes* expansion (along with deer and mice), notably through Canada (southern Ontario), New England (New York, Maine, Vermont, and New Hampshire) and south into Pennsylvania and Ohio. There has also been an increased expansion of ticks into the Midwest (Indiana, Illinois, and Michigan) and the Southeast (North Carolina, Virginia, and West Virginia).[8,15,60–62]

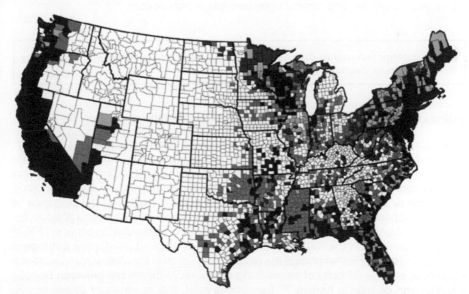

Fig. 2. Changes in county status for *I scapularis* and *I pacificus* from December 1996 to August 2015. Black color indicates that county statue was established, and gray color indicates reported sightings, for *I scapularis* or *I pacificus* and considered the same in this study. Red or orange color indicates that the status of a county changed from no records to established (*red*) or from reported to established (*orange*). Green color indicates that the status of a county changed from no records to reported. (*From* Eisen RJ, Eisen L, Beard CB. County-scale distribution of *Ixodes* scapularis and *Ixodes* pacificus (Acari: Ixodidae) in the continental United States. J Med Entomol 2016;53:383. Open access; with permission.)

Nationwide seroprevalence studies of equine borreliosis are sparse. Articles are often biased, with horses selected specifically for clinical examination findings consistent with borreliosis. Regardless of bias, as environmental changes favor *Ixodes* migration and the frequency of regional transport of sport horses increases, *Borrelia* seroprevalence in horses becomes more evident across the United States.[8,63] Positive serologic rates range from 58.7% (Michigan) and 59% (New York and Connecticut) to as high as 94% (Maryland) when sampling horses suspected of having Lyme disease.[38,61,62,64] When addressing the significance of positive serologic tests, it is critical to consider the seroprevalence of horses selected at random, that is, not based on clinical examination findings consistent with borreliosis, and these rates ranged from 0.2% (Texas), 14.8% (Oregon and Washington), and 33% in Virginia to as high as 75% in New England.[10,11,38,64,65]

DIFFERENTIATION OF LYME INFECTION VERSUS LYME DISEASE

It is imperative to emphasize, when considering equine borreliosis, that infection and disease are 2 different entities. Infection, the invasion and multiplication of microbiological agents, simply implies a foreign agent is within the body, whereas disease, the end result of infection, implies a set of defined clinical signs due to the body's response to the presence of the organism. In clinical sport horse practice, this means that serology may be the basis of diagnosing past or current Borrelia infection, but it is a poor positive predictor of current or future Lyme disease.[8,12,66] Most infected horses are asymptomatic, and case studies estimate that only 5% to 10% of horses exposed to *B burgdorferi* s.l. organisms will develop clinical signs consistent with disease.[60,67,68]

> Positive serologic tests confirm *Borrelia* infection and support a diagnosis of Lyme disease. They do not confirm, or diagnose, Lyme disease.

LABORATORY TESTS AND LYME INFECTION

Laboratory testing for *Borrelia* infection (in support of a diagnosis of disease) is, to a degree, limited to serology. The low-level spirochetemia induced by *B burgdorferi* s.s. infections make hematological polymerase chain reaction (PCR) testing insensitive and blood culture unrewarding. There are no pathognomonic changes in complete blood cell counts or biochemical profiles associated with borreliosis; and the presence of thrombocytopenia is indicative of infection, or coinfection, with *Anaplasma phagocytophilia* rather than that of *B burgdorferi*.[8,12,69] Coinfections were noted to occur in 15% of 47 horses sampled in the Netherlands, and these overlooked coinfective pathogens may be one reason that "explain[s] the biological variation in the clinical manifestations described, and the difficulty of establishing a conclusive causal link between Borrelia infection and disease in horses."[12] Exceptions exist, that is, cases of uveitis or NB, where culture and PCR should be attempted. In pseudolymphoma cases, skin biopsies (culture, PCR, and histology) may be beneficial in achieving a definitive diagnosis.[38,70,71] Serum amyloid A (SAA) values are variable and pathogen nonspecific. As in any infectious disease, a sharp rise in SAA is expected within 4 hours to 8 hours of *B burgdorferi* s.s. infection with a gradual decrease in units (μg/mL) over time. SAA was elevated (200–400 μg/mL) in joint and tendon fluid collected from a suspected case of *Borrelia*-induced synovitis in a horse (Heinrich Anhold, personal communication, 2018).[72,73] A positive serologic test for *Borrelia* antibodies is required in equine practice to define a patient as having, or having had in the past, an infection due to *B burgdorferi*. Numerous serologic tests are available to equine clinicians, using differing methodologies and antigens, with varying sensitivities, specificities, and positive or negative disease predilections. Equine practices selecting multiple testing modalities for a single case may find a lack of agreement that muddles the results. This is especially true in regions into which ticks are beginning to migrate (ie, areas of low prevalence of Lyme exposure)[29,31] In addition, an equine practice submitting serologic tests for borreliosis must expect a lag time, as in the human infection-disease complex, between the initial infection and a horses's humoral anybody response (>3 weeks). Current serologic tests cannot discern whether there was treatment failure, reinfection, or endogenous recrudescence in post-treatment testing, where the serology either remains positive, or when initially negative returns to a positive value over time.[74,75] The current consensus, within the American College of Veterinary Internal Medicine (ACVIM), is that serology not be used as a screening technique, for example, at prepurchase examinations or in horses that do not have clinical signs consistent with borreliosis, and that practitioners be aware of false-positive results due to cross-reactivity to flagellar proteins (eg, *Leptospira* spp); non–Lyme disease *Borrelia* strains, such as *Borrelia miyamotoi*; or postantibiotic, attenuated, noninfectious spirochetes.[8,25,28,31,76,77]

Commercially available serologic tests include the whole-cell lysate tests, that is, indirect fluorescent antibody (IFAT) and whole-cell ELISA; a multiple-antigen, bead-based, ELISA assay (multiplex); the Western blot (WB); and, a point-of-care canine ELISA (C_6 IDEXX SNAP, One IDEXX Drive, Westbrook, Maine) test used in horses. These tests do not consistently identify Borrelia infections at less than 3 weeks' duration, and there is not a current consensus as to a gold-standard test for *B burgdorferi* infection.[8,17,29,78–80] Whole-cell lysate testing (IFAT and ELISA), because they are more prone to false-positive results, must be confirmed by WB or multiplex testing. In addition, the whole-cell ELISA and IFAT tests do not differentiate between infection and vaccination.[8,62] The multiplex and WB serologic tests differentiate between vaccination and infection, and they can often give evidence as to infection duration (acute vs chronic). Outer surface proteins, as measured by multiplex testing, have a fixed time frame of expression by the spirochete; that is, OspC titers are noted in acute infections at 3 weeks to 5 weeks postexposure, declining into the negative range in approximately 5 months. OspF titers are noted 5 weeks to 8 weeks postexposure and may last for month to years postinfection. One reference suggests OspF half-life is short and that positive OspF serologic results correlate to the systemic presence of the organism.[7,8,66,80,81] OspA titers are noted in vaccinated horses as well as a low percentage of nonvaccinates (where they may correlate, as in human medicine, to long-term infections).[66,79] The canine C_6 snap test is validated for horses, with a high sensitivity (indicating a high negative predictive value) and a variable sensitivity (63%–96%).[78,79,82] C_6 snap test results correlate to OspF multiplex titers, but OspF titers are often produced earlier in the onset of infection, and the C_6 test has more false-positive and false-negative interpretations. As with whole-cell lysate testing, a positive SNAP C_6 test should be verified by WB or multiplex testing.[8,78,79] Severity of disease is related to an individual horse's inflammatory response, not direct damage by (or exact numbers of) spirochetes. Statements regarding correlation of serologic tests to level of infection or presence of disease are incorrect. Clinicians must realize the magnitude of serologic titers have no direct or linear correlation to spirochete numbers, severity or presence of disease, or prognosis.[8,83–85] It is important to emphasize that positive serologic tests simply "indicate the presence of antibodies against *B burgdorferi*" at the time of sampling. A disease state is not always the end outcome of infection because a horse's immune system can eliminate infections prior to the onset of recognized clinical signs (disease), or positive serology indicates vaccination (ie, OspA and/or OspC values increased via vaccination). Negative serologic tests in horses with suspected exposure greater than 3 weeks, and in the absence of immunosuppressive disorders, are a positive predictor noninfection (ie, a high negative predictive value).[66]

Serologic tests available to equine practitioners are summarized in **Table 1**.

CLINICAL SYNDROMES AND THE DIAGNOSIS OF LYME DISEASE

The pathogenesis of equine borreliosis, especially late-stage disease, is not well elucidated. Experimental infection of ponies via *B burgdorferi* s.s.–infected ticks failed to result in gross clinical signs of disease over a 9-month period. Histopathologic abnormalities were noted, for example, lymphohistiocytic dermatitis (2-mm nodules within the mid-dermis to deep dermis), nonsuppurative synovitis (1 pony), neuritis, and meningitis, all of which correlate to the clinical syndromes and anecdotal symptoms in suspected Lyme cases in the field.[8,38,86]

A diagnosis of equine Lyme disease should (minimally) be based on 4 principles[8,16,79,81]:

1. Risk: horse resides in, has stabled in, or passed through, an *Ixodes*/Borrelia endemic region

2. Clinical examination: chief complaint and presenting physical examination findings suspicious of equine borreliosis "eg, proven and anecdotal clinical signs as noted within this text", as they are so diverse and variable in clinical practice that listing all would defeat the purpose of a succinct table.

3. A complete and thorough rule out of common differentials: diseases consistent with the chief complaint and physical examination and possibly more common than borreliosis, must be ruled out.

4. Laboratory conformation of infection and in support of the clinical signs of disease
   4a. Serologic conformation of *B burgdorferi* s.l. (and/or)
   4b. Identification of organism/DNA (PCR or culture)

According to current ACVIM consensus, the documented equine diseases definitively associated with *B burgdorferi* s.s. infection are limited to 3 clinical presentations: cutaneous pseudolymphoma, uveitis, and Neuroborreliosis (NB).[8,71,84,87–89]

Pseudolymphoma is an uncommon papule-nodular dermatitis associated with a tick bite It is not as relevant to sport horse performance as are uveitis and NB. Pseudolymphoma must be differentiated, however, from cutaneous lymphoma, for example, T-cell rich, B-cell lymphoma, and cancers do affect performance and life span. Immunohistochemistry (mixed lymphoid tissue) with a positive PCR for Borrelia, the lack of subcuticular or muscular cellular infiltrations, and specialized silver staining techniques identifying argyrophilic spirochetes (poorly stained by Gram or acid-fast staining techniques) rule out neoplasia. Untreated, the skin lesions can last for months to years; treated, the prognosis for recovery is very good.[8,71,90–92]

Uveitis is the most common cause equine blindness. The most frequently isolated organisms are *Leptospiral* spirochetes. Uveitis is noted to be a sequela of *B burgdorferi* s.l. infections in rare cases. A single European study suggested there was no correlation between signs of equine recurrent uveitis and seropositivity for *B burgdorferi*; however, there are case reports of seropositivity present in cases of significant ocular disease. Ophthalmologic examination is of value in serologically positive horses, for example, neurologic horses with concurrent uveitis lead to a higher suspicion of NB.[70,71,87,93,94] *B burgdorferi* uveitis is often bilateral with significant anterior chamber inflammation and debris (a yellowish-green, fibrinous, aqueous humor) (**Fig. 3**).

Table 1
Serologic test for *Borrelia burgdorferi* exposure in horses

Test	Laboratory	Antibody Targets	Interpretation	Pros	Cons
ELISA, IFAT (Serum, CSF, joint fluid)	CVMDL Also available at other laboratories[a]	• Whole-cell lysate from cultured Bb	• Quantitative; results expressed as antibody titer • Positive results must be confirmed by WB • Cross-reactions occur with antibodies against other *Borrelia* or spirochete spp or against flagella • Does not differentiate vaccinal vs natural exposure antibodies	• Identify broad range of antibodies against Bb proteins • Quantitative • Increasing levels may indicate active infection	• Require second confirmatory test (WB) • Cross-reactivity is a concern • Provide no information regarding infection stage or vaccination status • Vaccination affects results
WB (Serum, CSF, joint fluid)	CVMDL Also available at other laboratories[a]	• Whole-cell lysate from cultured Bb • Antigens separated by molecular weight	• Qualitative; band pattern visually (subjectively) interpreted • Can give qualitative information regarding vaccination status and infection stage	• Identifies broad range of antibodies against Bb proteins • Can elucidate infection stage and vaccination status	• Labor-intensive, subjective interpretation • Nonquantitative results

(continued on next page)

Table 1
(continued)

Test	Laboratory	Antibody Targets	Interpretation	Pros	Cons
Equine multiplex assay (Serum and CSF)— not synovial fluid	AHDC, Cornell	3 recombinant antigens: OspA, OspC, and OspF	• Quantitative; results expressed as MFIs • Anti-OspA antibodies–vaccination and/or infection; correlate to antibodies detecting the 31-kDa band on WB • Anti-OspC antibodies–early infection; correlate to antibodies detecting approximate 22-kDa band on WB • Anti-OspF antibodies–chronic infection; correlate to antibodies detecting 29-kDa band on WB	• Detection of low-level antibody (pg/mL) • Potentially elucidates infection stage and vaccination status • Quantitative • Increasing levels may indicate active infection	• False-negative results might occur due to genetic variation in OspC • Experimental infection studies in horses confirming antibody kinetics have not been published • Dilutional linearity not reported
SNAP 4Dx (Serum, plasma, or anticoagulated whole blood)	IDEXX	• Synthetic peptide (C₆) that mimics specific Bb antigen (IR6, a highly conserved protein of VlsE)	• Qualitative; color development visually (subjectively) interpreted • Positive results indicate natural exposure, not vaccination • Anti-C₆ antibodies correlate to antibodies that detect the 39-kDa band on WB	• Inexpensive, easy to perform in clinic • Rapid results • Good agreement with multiplex OspF and WB • Vaccination status unlikely to affect results	• Subjective interpretation • Nonquantitative results

Abbreviations: AHDC, Cornell, Animal Health Diagnostic Center, Cornell University College of Veterinary Medicine; Bb, *Borrelia burgdorferi;* CVMDL, Connecticut Veterinary Medical Diagnostic Laboratory, University of Connecticut; ELISA, enzyme-linked immunosorbent assay; IR, immunodominant region; VlsE, Vmp-like sequence, expressed.

ᵃ Quality control may vary between differential laboratories.

From Divers TJ, Gardner RB, Madigan JE, et al. Borrelia burgdorferi infection and lyme disease in north american horses: a consensus statement. J Vet Intern Med 2018;https://doi.org/10.1111/jvim.15042; with permission.

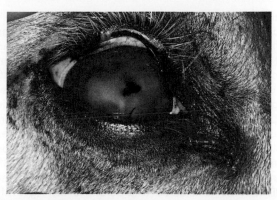

Fig. 3. Clinical photograph of the right eye of a 15-year-old Haflinger gelding with recurrent fibrinous anterior uveitis. A fibrin clot is obscures a miotic pupil with aqueous flare present. The corpora nigrans is visible through the dorsal aspect of the clot, with a linear, deep red blood clot present ventrally on the corneal endothelium. (*Courtesy of* Allison Clode, DVM, DACVO, Port City Veterinary Referral Hospital, Portsmouth, NH; with permission.)

Clinically, equine cases present as a chronic, severe, uveitis, that is, miotic pupils, aqueous flare, corpora nigra destruction, iris scarring (synechiae), neovascularization, and fibrovascular tissue on the iris' anterior surface, with glaucoma or phthisis bulbi.[95] Antibody (multiplex: OspA, OspC, and OspF) and/or PCR testing of ocular fluids is indicted when the risk of *Borrelia* uveitis is present. Vitreal tissue antibody testing and histology is indicated when enucleation is required. Spirochetes have been detected in neutrophils obtained from the vitreous humor. Wright stain or silver stains for example, Warthin–Starry and Steiner, of vitreal histologic sections can reveal spirochetes (*Leptospira* species stain poorly vs *Borrelia* species with these stains).[70,87,96] The prognosis for sight retention is poor to grave, but prognosis for survival with uncomplicated uveitis is excellent.[70,87]

Early-stage NB affects equine performance and can mimic musculoskeletal/neuromuscular disease. Albeit rare, it is of clinical importance to sport horse practitioners. The anecdotal impression that *Borrelia* induces muscle loss may be related to clinical examination findings associated with NB, that is, atrophy of spinous muscles, facial paresis, neck and back stiffness/pain, effusive joints, agitation or depression (behavioral changes), dermal hyperesthesia, laryngeal dysfunction/dysphagia with episodic respiratory distress, and cardiac arrhythmias.[8,83,88,89,93,94,97] NB may induce radiculoneuritis, spinal ataxia, and cranial nerve deficits, mimicking common equine neurologic diseases (eg, equine protozoal myeloencephalitis), so involvement of other anatomic systems such as uveitis (perhaps prior to neurologic deficits), joint effusion, and/or cardiac arrhythmias give additional support to a working diagnosis of NB, that is, "when presented with a horse displaying ataxia, cranial nerve deficits, and weight loss, with historic or current evidence of uveitis, collapse, or dysphagia...consider neuroborreliosis regardless of CSF analysis or serologic results."[83] Antemortem confirmation of *B burgdorferi* s.s. is difficult. Current literature and research do not provide sufficient data to assist the practitioner in determining a single, definitive, diagnosis. Serology determines infection, not disease, and serology can be negative if the organism is in a "immunologically privileged" site, such as the central nervous system (CNS) or anterior chamber.[70] In human cases of Lyme NB, where appropriate clinical signs are present, the antemortem diagnosis is based on cerebrospinal fluid (CSF) B-cell pleocytosis and, specifically, the intrathecal production of antibodies against Borrelia.[9,98] In NB, CSF cytology has been nonspecific as both lymphocytic (similar to human CNS borreliosis) and neutrophilic, (xanthrochromic) cellular transudates have been identified. Antemortem PCR (low sensitivity), culture, and cytologic examination of the CSF is often unrewarding because spirochetes reside in tissue (eg, dura mater and leptomeninges) and are not freely floating within CSF. Assessing intrathecal antibody production in horses is limited by the potential lack of linearity of multiplex (median fluorescent intensity [MFIs]) results, especially at low or high levels, a lack of validated cutoff values, and the physiologically and clinically unsupported assumption of a normal blood-brain barrier. Dilution (multiplex serum 1:400, multiplex CSF: undiluted) for accurate comparison of intrathecal antibody production must also be taken into consideration. NB may be considered with serum to CSF IgG ratios of less than 130:1 (ie, serum multiplex × 400/CSF multiplex), although this ratio is unvalidated in horses. The treatment of equine NB has been unrewarding, and the prognosis is currently poor to grave.[8,19,83]

Postmortem, a definitive diagnosis of equine NB may be based on its unique histologic findings on necropsy. The lesions reported are

1. Multifocal, pleocellular leptomeningitis
2. Encephalomyelitis (with perivasculitis and sclerosing vasculitis)
3. Radiculoneuritis and ganglionitis (cranial and peripheral lesions)

Lesions, and spirochetes when present, predominate in leptomeninges and dura mater with fewer lesions affecting brain or spinal cord parenchyma.[83,88,93,96,97]

Of specific interest to sport horse practices are the myriad anecdotal behavioral (lethargy or resistance to work), joint, and musculoskeletal symptoms attributed to infection with B burgdorferi s.l. These include shifting/multiple limb lameness, arthritis, and joint swelling (synovitis).[8,9,14,38,62,69-71,81,83,87,88,99] There are clinicians suggesting the most common clinical presentation of B burgdorferi–induced disease in sport horse practice is lameness.[69,72,81] Borrelia-associated synovitis is reported in the veterinary literature, and histologic evidence of joint inflammation was noted in a research pony infected with B burgdorferi s.s.[8,38] Lyme arthritis has been documented in humans (ie, knee inflammation) and dogs, which lends some, albeit poor, support for a similar condition existing in sport horses.[7,8,14,28,72,82,87] Unfortunately, for the equine sports medicine clinician, the symptoms of poor performance, that is, lameness, stiffness, agitation, and so forth, are the least well documented clinical signs of B burgdorferi s.s. infection. Case reports, that is, the synovitis cases discussed previously, are only a modest grade of evidence, and future research and/ or clinical evaluations may disprove the clinical interpretation of B burgdorferi s.l. as a cause of equine lameness. Experimental infections in dogs found lameness to be "inconsistent" and a "poorly sensitive manifestation of Lyme disease."[8,100] Still, when surveyed, equine sports medicine practices reported a wide variety of clinical signs they strongly associated with Lyme disease, and these invariably included stiffness and lameness.[8,14,22,101] In a similar thread, Internet searches for "Lyme disease in horses" reveal "facts" ad nauseam about borreliosis from equine practices, holistic practitioners, "case reports" from lay equine online journals, and advice from horse care blogs via Internet equine sites. These report a plethora of anecdotal clinical cases, with varying symptoms, for example, laminitis and head-shaking, most if not all cured in rapid fashion. The current ACVIM consensus statement includes hepatitis, nephritis, and fistulous withers into this category of cases, which are often incompletely worked up, with limited clinicopathologic data, questionable treatment regimens, and thus a nondefinitive diagnosis. There are no clinical or research data to date indicating that any of these presentations have a *B burgdorferi* s.l. etiology.[8] Diagnosis of Borrelia-associated lameness and/or synovitis must be based on the principles set forth at the beginning of this section: that is, risk of exposure, differentials ruled out, clinical signs consistent with borrelia, and positive serology and/or other confirmative laboratory tests of infection. Cytologic examination of joint fluid, synovial histopathology, and PCR may be beneficial; however, the chronic arthritis noted in humans is not generally associated with presence of *B burgdorferi*, but with the production of T-cell and macrophage cytokines (eg, interleukin [IL]-6). IL-6, and other cytokines, lead to the production of additional proinflammatory agents, for example, IL-1β and tumor necrosis factor α, creating a painful joint environment and overt lameness. Multiple tests are recommended because causation of disease is not proved by finding *B burgdorferi*, or borrelia proteins (PCR), within tissues because they are present in horses where no clinical signs of disease exist.[8,72] The most important component in the examination process, when considering *B burgdoferi* s.l. as the cause of lameness in the horse, is the complete and thorough examination for, and rule out of, the more common clinical conditions leading to the presenting lameness(es), for example, osteoarthritis, osteochondritis dissecans, recurrent exertional rhabdomyolysis, polysaccharide stage myopathy, racehorse chip fractures, and repetitive strain injuries of bone and soft tissues.[1,2,4,5,102,103] Until research and convincing clinical evidence dictate otherwise, equine borreliosis should be on a list of differential diagnoses for sport horse lameness in endemic regions, but it should not be at the top of that list. The steps suggested to come to a definitive diagnosis, if equine borreliosis is on a differential list, are included in **Fig. 4**, via the ACVIM Consensus Statement flowchart of criteria for Lyme disease diagnosis.

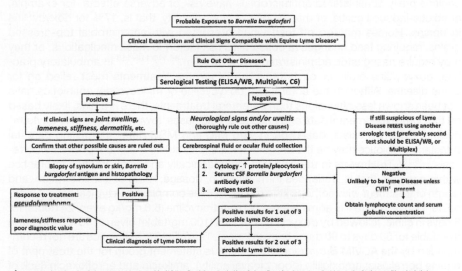

Fig. 4. ACVIM Consensus Statement proposed criteria for antemortem diagnosis of equine Lyme disease. (*From* Divers TJ, Gardner RB, Madigan JE, et al. Borrelia burgdorferi infection and Lyme disease in North American horses: a consensus statement. J Vet Intern Med 2018;https://doi.org/10.1111/ jvim.15042; with permission.)

TREATMENT OVERVIEW

Effective antimicrobials for *B burgdorferi* s.l. disease in equids are poorly refined. Antemortem diagnosis is difficult because research has yet to identify appropriate equine disease models for Borrelia; thus, in vivo drug evaluations are limited. Few articles are in agreement with standardized testing for antimicrobial sensitivity of pathogenic spirochetes, for example, Borrelia minimum inhibitory concentration (MIC) values are loosely based on dark field microscopy identifying no motile spirochetes after "x" (eg,48–72) hours of antimicrobial incubation. Experimental evidence and case reports in human and equine peer-reviewed literature identified treatment failures (persistent infections) with recommended, efficacious, in vitro–evaluated antibiotics. There is limited knowledge of Borrelia species behavior in the presence of antibiotics, and what is known has come from in vivo experiments on mice, or in vitro experiments on few *B burgdorferi* s.l. isolates.[8,104–106] Equine treatment regimens are based on human guidelines, anecdotal therapy in field cases, in vitro antibiotic susceptibility of *B burgdorferi* s.l. (using MIC and minimal bactericidal concentration [MBC]), and a single study of 16 ponies exposed to *Ixodes* ticks (with a 50%–60% Borrelia infection rate). Treatments are often empirical, generically directed against a febrile infectious (nonviral) disease. Evidence, suggesting 1 medication or dosing interval over another in horses, is subjective because experimental data is from research where few animals per treatment group make statistical power poor or from case reports containing no control groups.[8,86,104,107–112] In human *B burgdorferi* s.l. cases, the standard treatment period is 2 weeks to 4 weeks, with, argumentatively, little scientific evidence confirming benefit in administering antibiotics for longer periods.[8,9,45,112,113] Equine cases may require weeks of medication administration as well, making intravenous (IV) or intramuscular (IM) treatments, on a ranch or stable environment, difficult. Horse compliance with daily IM injections may be short lived. Long-term IV catheterization of nonhospitalized equine patients have a risk of catheter damage and complications, for example, thrombophlebitis. Available and efficacious orally administered antimicrobials have risk of adverse effects, for example, antibiotic-induced colitis, or may be of low-bioavailability, that is, 17% for doxycycline in horses. Horses may go off-feed when presented with antimicrobial top-dressed grains, requiring feed changes (a colic/colitis risk factor) to mask medications, or they may require nasogastric administration by a clinician.[86,110,114–116] In ambulatory practice, doxycycline orally or oxytetracycline IV are the treatments most relied on for Lyme disease. Although the enteral (eg, doxycycline or minocycline) antibiotics have not been shown less efficacious than parenteral treatments, there is a bias, likely based on the pony experimental data and anecdotal field cases, toward the use of IV oxytetracycline. Evidence exists, based on in vitro MIC and MBC data, suggesting parental β-lactam antibiotics may be the drugs of choice for first-line treatment of equine borreliosis.[8,38,107] Treatments in the field vary geographically and from practice to practice within a region, that is, variances in medication, dosage, route of administration, and length of treatment with perhaps little regard to case complexity. A typical case (Northeastern United States) is administered IV oxytetracycline (6.6 mg/kg every 24 hours) for 5 days in clinic, followed by doxycycline tablets (100 mg/tablet given at 10–20 mg/kg) in the stable for 30 days to 90 days, or even longer. The following antibiotics are not recommended by the ACVIM *B burgdorferi* consensus statement group for the treatment of equine borreliosis: amoxicillin (poor bioavailability): amikacin and enrofloxacin (lack of efficacy); azithromycin, ceftriaxone, and erythromycin (colitis/colic risk and anaphylaxis); tilmicosin (injection site reaction and anaphylaxis); enteral tetracycline: oral administration of a compounded or avian formulation (poor oral bioavailability, colitis risk, and compounding errors); and chloramphenicol (lack of clinical data).[8,97,104,117,118]

Table 2
Antibiotic recommendations for *Borrelia burgdorferi* sensu lato infections

Drug	Dosage	Comments	Minimum Inhibitory Concentration for *Borrelia burgdorferi* sensu stricto or (*Borrelia burgdorferi* sensu lato Isolate)(Reference 8 Has All Authors Identified)	Quick Reference Disease Indications (Subjective)
Cefotaxime	25 mg/kg IV q6h Standard 500-kg horse: 12.5 g q6h NB 500-kg horse: 25 g q6h	High dosages (eg, 50 mg/kg IV q6h) for equine NB Excellent tissue penetration so efficacious in ocular and joint infections Suitable for distal limb perfusion (synovitis and osteoarthritis) Higher doses may lead to adverse effects (eg, colitis)	≤0.125 µg/mL 0.01–1 µg/mL	CNS Joint infections, intra-articular and distal limb perfusion Ocular infections
Ceftiofur	Ceftiofur sodium (Naxcel) 2.2 mg/kg IV q12h 500-kg horse: 1.1 g q12h Ceftiofur crystalline free acid (CFA, Exceede) 6.6 mg/kg IM days 1 and 4, then q7d 500-kg horse: 3.3 g per Rx	Research (REF 3a) indicates less "relapse" (increased Osp levels) post-treatment when compared with doxycycline. Excellent tissue penetration so efficacious in ocular and joint infections Long intervals between injections may increase patient comfort and compliance (Exceede) Sodium salt (Naxcel) suitable for distal limb perfusion (synovitis and osteoarthritis) Higher doses may lead to adverse effects (eg, colitis)	<0.04–0.08 µg/mL	CNS infections Ocular infections Joint infections, intra-articular and distal limb perfusion

(continued on next page)

Table 2
(continued)

Drug	Dosage	Comments	Minimum Inhibitory Concentration for *Borrelia burgdorferi sensu stricto* or (*Borrelia burgdorferi sensu lato* Isolate)(Reference 8 Has All Authors Identified)	Quick Reference Disease Indications (Subjective)
Doxycycline	10 mg/kg PO q12h 500-kg horse, 100-mg tablets: 50 tablets q12h	The most common antibiotic used for equine borreliosis Peak synovial fluid concentrations > than serum concentrations Use in suspected *B burgdorferi* synovitis is recommended Can be used in Borrelia-induced uveitis or NB, but mocular and CNS concentrations vs doxycycline @ 10 mg/kg ([see text]), has the additional benefit of intra-articular MMP inhibition/anti-inflammation	0.125–0.25 µg/mL ≤0.125–0.25 µg/mL	Joint and musculoskeletal disease
Metronidazole	15–25 mg/kg PO q6–8h 500-kg horse at 20 mg/kg = 10 g q6–q8h	Considered ineffective against motile spirochetes and effective vs resistant, round body ("stationary" or cystic) forms in vitro Used in concert with one of the other antibiotic choices on chart, which is effective for motile spirochetes. Oral administration may lead to patient inappetence IV formulation is expensive in adult horses	0.06–32 µg/mL 0.25–0.50 µg/mL	Chronic (resistant) Lyme disease in concert with an antibiotic effective vs motile spirochetes
Minocycline	4 mg/kg PO q12h 500-kg horse/ 100-mg tablets, 20 tablets q12h	Superior aqueous humor and CSF penetration (vs doxycycline) but tissue levels in vivo are questionable (may be below MIC for target organism) ±Recommended for ophthalmic and CNS cases of borreliosis Synovial concentrations are inferior to doxycycline, therefore a secondary choice for synovitis/ osteoarthritis	0.03–1 µg/mL 0.4–0.8 µg/mL	CNS and ocular infection

Penicillin G	Na/K salts 22,000–44,000 IU/kg IV q6h procaine 22,000–44,000 IU/kg IM q12h 50-kg horse 1.1–2.2 million units per Rx	Higher dosage range recommended for NB IM penicillin may be used, but dose and duration likely lead to muscle soreness and patient noncompliance Higher doses may lead to adverse effects (eg, colitis)	0.03–8 µg/mL	CNS infection
Oxytetracycline	6.6 mg/kg IV q24h 500-kg horse 200 mg/mL (eg, LA-200) 3.3 g/16.5 mL q24h	IV oxytetracycline commonly used for Borrelia infection in horses The only treatment, in research ponies, to eliminate organism acute (3 mo) Borrelia infections without a return to positive serologic values Oral oxytetracycline not recommended (per ACVIM Borrelia Consensus Statement)	0.25 µg/mL. 0.01–20 µg/mL	Early treatment (<4 mo): All infections
Trimethoprim/sulfa	25 mg/kg PO q12h 500-kg horse 960-mg tablet 13 tablets q12h	Sulfamethoxazole is not effective against motile forms of Borrelia but has some effect against stationary forms. Trimethoprin is effective against both the motile and the stationary (eg, round body) forms in vitro Not recommended as a solo antibiotic for "active" B burgdorferi s.s. disease but may have an effect in combination therapies (similar to metronidazole comments)		Chronic (resistant) Lyme disease in concert with an antibiotic effective vs motile spirochetes

Adapted from Divers TJ, Gardner RB, Madigan JE, et al. Borrelia bergdorferi and Lyme disease in North American horses: a consensus statement. J Vet Intern Med 2018;https://doi.org/10.1111/jvim.15042; with permission.

Antibiotics that are recommended, by ACVIM, for B burgdorferi s.l. disease are summarized in **Table 2**.[8]

PROPHYLAXIS OF SUSPECTED BORRELIA EXPOSURE (IE, TICK BITE WOUND, TICK ATTACHED)

Research and case reports suggest early treatment of Lyme disease results in improved outcomes with less risk of developing long-term sequelae.[110] Although not universally accepted, prophylaxis post Ixodes tick bite has been proposed for humans, in endemic Lyme regions, via a single IV injection of oxytetracycline (200 mg) within 72 hours of (black-legged tick) removal. An exception to this recommendation is I pacificus attachment, due to the low rate of borrelia infection in I pacificus, even in endemic regions.[111,119] Conversely, a meta-analysis, examining "risk and consequences" of Lyme infection versus "cost and adverse effects" of prophylactic treatments advised against the use of antibiotics in patients suspected of tick bite and possible borrelia exposure.[110] Taking into consideration the results of the meta-analysis when questioning the use of prophylactic antibiotics in suspected equine B burgdorferi exposure, where the species of tick is rarely determined, the time attached and volume of engorgement are unknown, and the efficacy of single-dose antibiotic administration in horses is ill defined, the conclusion is identical: post-tick attachment prophylaxis in horses, without clinical signs of disease, is not recommended.[109–111,120]

ANTIMICROBIAL TREATMENT OF SUSPECT SHORT-TERM BORRELIOSIS AND CUTANEOUS PSEUDOLYMPHOMA

For uncomplicated cases of borreliosis, for example, pseudolymphoma or even the anecdotal behavioral horse case presentation, when the 4 principles of diagnosis have been satisfied, the first line of antimicrobials are the β-lactam (penicillin and cephalosporin) and tetracycline (oxytetracycline, doxycycline, and minocycline) antibiotics.[8,9,121,122] IV tetracycline was the only antibiotic to completely eliminate B burgdoreri s.s. from ponies 90 days postexposure and that may be the best drug of choice if practical and affordable to the client[38]

TREATMENT OF UVEITIS

Although treatment of Borreliosis in horses is generally accomplished with the tetracycline class of antibiotics, there is a difference in class pharmacokinetics. Minocycline (4 mg/kg every 12 hours), lipophilic and less protein bound, has improved ocular penetration versus oxytetracycline and doxycycline.[102,109,123] Doxycycline has been shown to have only 7.5% to 10% of serum values in ocular fluids, but there is evidence that minocycline tissue levels do not reach acceptable MIC values, so the choice of which medication to use is still debated and clinical decisions may be made by the attending veterinarian.[8,106,124] Cefotaxime levels in tissues are generally well within the range required for clinical efficacy, that is, 2 µg/g to 5 µg/g MIC; therefore, cephalosporins also seem a rational choice for B burdorferi–induced uveitis.[125] Treatment of infectious uveitis often occurs late in the disease process (phthisical/nonvisual eyes; enucleation is the treatment of choice) and the eye is an immune-privileged site, difficult for medications to penetrate; thus parenteral, well distributed antibiotics (see ceftiofur/cefotaxime), using higher dose/shorter intervals, are suggested as first-line treatments.[8,126–128]

For uncomplicated equine Lyme disease (ie, no cardiac, ocular, or CNS involvement), a 14-day to 28-day course of tetracyclines or β-lactam antibiotics is recommended[8]

Ophthalmic medications, for example, topical anti-inflammatories and antibiotics, specifically in regard to Borrelia uveitis, are not defined in the veterinary literature. Recommendations are based on recurrent equine uveitis guidelines, with the exception of systemic corticosteroids, which are not believed beneficial for B bergdorferi systemic disease and may be contraindicated.[8,126–128]

Ophthalmic (topical) medications for B burgdorferi uveitis

- Antimicrobial
  - Tetracycline ophthalmic ointment (Terramycin): administer approximately 4-mm strip onto corneal surface, every 2 hours to 8 hours.
- Anti-inflammatory
  - Diclofenac 0.1%: administer 1 drop q24 hours for 10 days.
  - Cyclosporin A 0.2% (Optimmune): administer a 6 mm strip onto the corneal surface q 12 hours.
- Mydriatic
  - Atropine 1%: administer approximately 4-mm strip onto corneal surface to effect and then only to maintain pupillary dilation, every 4 hours to 6 hours (do not administer at shorter duration).
    - Pupil may remain dilated for a week or more from a single dose.
    - Monitor gastrointestinal motility, because the topical application can lead to decreased motility and colic.
- Fibrin/hypopion reduction
  - Tissue plasminogen activator (Cathflo Activase) approximately 50 μg intracameral to 150 μg intracameral

TREATMENT OF NEUROBORRELIOSIS

The treatment of NB, based on case reports, is difficult with a guarded to poor prognosis.[8] Within the tetracycline group, minocycline has been reported to have improved CNS concentrations along with anti-inflammatory and neuroprotective (antiapoptotic and antioxidant) properties independent of its antimicrobial activity.[102,109,123] In the β-lactam group, as it is for uveitis, cefotaxime levels in the CNS are well within the range for efficacy.[125] Although this sounds encouraging, in horses, it is based on few cases. In human NB, where there is more research, and minocycline has a longer half-life than doxycycline, the recommendations for treating neurological cases with an antibiotic that crosses the blood-brain barrier are still based on low-quality clinical evidence, from a few small, heterogeneous, trials, with limited statistical power and varying outcomes and efficacy endpoints. Recommendations for human NB include 28-day courses of IV ceftriaxone or high doses of IM penicillin G and recommendations, in the author's opinion, until research or case-based evidence is compelling for a different regimen, are the same for equine NB.[111,129]

TREATMENT OF SUSPECTED MUSCULOSKELETAL AND JOINT INFECTIONS

Although primarily derived from anecdotal case reports in the field, B burgdorferi s.s. synovitis has been produced under experimental conditions, and lameness due to suspected borreliosis is a common concern in private practice[38]. Treatments can be targeted versus the organism and the region of interest with few modifications, for example, doxycycline, via increased joint concentration, may be a more effective choice than minocycline. Orally and parenterally administered treatments have similar outcomes, so ease of administration/patient compliance or economics may dictate the choice of medication and route of administration without likely affecting prognosis.[102,104,130] Orsini and colleagues,[131] based on pharmacokinetic data, suggests that cefotaxime (25 mg/kg IV every 6 hours) is an appropriate albeit time-intensive, choice for bacterial induced arthritis in horses. If the number and location of structures involved permit, regional limb perfusion of a joint or tendon sheath with a cephalosporin (ceftiofur sodium or cefotaxime; 2 g diluted to 60 mL of perfusate), or penicillin (25%–50% of the systemic dose of the Na^+ or K^+ salt), is an option at 24-hour intervals. The targeted injection of joint and/or tendon sheath via intrasynovial injection, for example, ceftiofur sodium, 150 mg/joint PRN, is also effective. In experimentally induced septic arthritis, white blood cell counts decrease significantly within 24 hours in perfused joints and regional therapy provides significant antimicrobial concentrations within synovial structures.[132–134] Intra-articular administration of 150 mg of ceftiofur (intrasynovial half-life: 5 hours) gives an effective MIC value within the joint for a significantly longer period than do IV injections (>24 hours vs 8 hours).[135] It is intuitive to suggest that in addition to antibiotics, anti-inflammatory drugs are indicated in Lyme synovitis/arthritis. In human cases, they reduce the symptoms of inflammation and lead to rapid case resolution.[86] Phenylbutazone, firocoxib, and flunixen at recommended dosages are considered rational adjunct therapy in cases of equine infectious arthritis. The tetracycline class of antibiotics has matrix metalloproteinase (MMP) inhibitory properties (discussed later) and may be used systemically in conjunction with regional injections/perfusions at antimicrobial or anti-inflammatory dosages.

TETRACYCLINES AS ANTI-INFLAMMATORY AGENTS

Tetracycline antibiotics have considerable anti-inflammatory properties. Doxycycline and minocycline are therapeutic agents for human osteoarthritis due to their inhibition of MMPs, such as MMP-13, which is a locally produced articular cartilage collagenase. Tetracyclines block MMPs directly, via chelating Zn^{+2} as well as inhibiting MMP synthesis. Doxycycline has the strongest affinity for zinc, making it the most effective anti-inflammatory of the antibiotic class.[46,54,102,135,136] Doxycycline reduces MMP-13 in synoviocytes with doses as low as 5 mg/kg, that is, 25 (100-mg) tablets to a 500-kg horse, because the drug is concentrated within the joint in comparison to plasma levels.[102,130] The lowest possible anti-inflammatory dose of doxycycline for use in equine osteoarthritis currently is not known. Based on in vivo data, the recommendations of 1 veterinary research group's anti-MMP doxycycline dosing for equine synovitis/osteoarthritis is week one, 5 mg/kg PO once daily; week two, 5 mg/kg PO every other day; and week three, 5 mg/kg PO every third day.[130,137] Doxycycline's efficacy as a disease-modifying osteoarthritic drug is one reason that a response to therapy, that is, improvement of suspected Borrelia-associated synovitis or lameness post–antibiotic administration, is not considered significant evidence in support of a definitive diagnosis of B burgdorferi disease.[8,46,81,102,130,137]

LONG-TERM TREATMENT, PERSISTENCE OF INFECTION (ANTIBODY) AND FORMATION OF CYSTIC OR RESISTANT STRUCTURES

Antibiotic refractory, chronic Lyme infection is a serologic based diagnosis. Antibody persistence may be from Borrelia DNA fragments, serologic memory, a new infection, or true antibiotic resistance with recrudescence of *B burgdorferi* disease. In experimentally infected ponies, 75% of doxycycline and 50% of ceftiofur-treated cases returned to positive serologic test levels within 4 months of treatment[38] In unforgiving environments, for example, bathed in antibiotics, such as doxycycline (reducing motile spirochetes), *B burgdorferi* s.l. increases cell wall blebbing and forms granular, spherical/cystic structures. In vivo, Borrelia biofilm colonies are created, of which only 30% to 50% are reduced by recommended antimicrobials. The debate whether these are biologically active bacteria that revert back to motile forms and contribute to long-term disease is on-going. Antibiotic treatment of "chronic/post lyme" disease in a majority of cases is unsuccessful.[8,23,86,112,113,122,138] Metronidazole, ineffective against motile borrelia, has efficacy against spheroid shapes that may be resistant to the first-line antimicrobials. It is considered, by some, an adjunct antibiotic and may be combined with a class of antibiotic effective versus motile spirochetes.[23,110] Tetracyclines exist, which may be superior to current therapies, for example, tigecycline (Tygacil. 50 mg/vial, Pfizer, Canada). Tigecycline is effective against both spirochetal and round body forms by approximately 80% to 90%, but it is administered slow IV (over 60 minutes) in humans, and pharmacologic data for horses are not available.[24,139]

SEROLOGIC RESPONSE TO TREATMENT

Based on pony experimental data, veterinarians have an expectation that serologic values decrease after successful antibiotic treatment of Lyme disease and such results are used as an assessment of treatment response. Serologic decreases are inconsistent in field cases; however, tests show an antibody decline within 3 months post-treatment may be considered supportive evidence of effective treatment. Regardless, treatment duration should never be based solely on a serologic test result. Improved soundness does not necessarily support a diagnosis of Lyme disease or effective treatment of the infection, if tetracyclines are used (ie, anti-inflammatory properties).[8,107]

VACCINATION AND PREVENTION

There are no Food and Drug Administration–approved equine Lyme vaccines. Five canine approved vaccines are on the market (**Table 3**) and are used in practice, with varying protocols, for horses. Clinical trials evaluating canine vaccines in horses indicated that an aluminum-adjuvanted OspA vaccine (1 mL IM) as well as the dual-antigen (OspA/C) bacterins, that is, Nobivac Lyme and Duramune Lyme (1 mL IM), and a nonadjuvanted, recombinant, OspA vaccine, that is, Recombitek Lyme (1 mL SQ), can induce *B borrelia* s.s. antibody production. Increased vaccine volume (2 mL) enhances initial antibody response (OspA and C), but the 2-mL volume did not prolong vaccine efficacy versus 1-mL IM (adjuvanted), and subcutaneous (nonadjuvanted only) routes were equally effective. The vaccines studied induced OspA antibodies inconsistently and often not to a level considered positive (>2000 MFI); thus, serologic testing prior to vaccination and 3 weeks to 4 weeks post–initial series completion is suggested. Vaccination should be done in proximity to tick feeding (eg, adult ticks in spring and fall).[23,45,100,107,129,140–142]

Whole bacterin vaccines may interfere with certain diagnostic tests because they induce OspA, OspC, and C_6 antibodies, a response amplified in horses with previous exposure to Borrelia. The Vanguard crLyme (recombinant OspA and heterogeneous OspC) effect on serologic tests are unknown, or unpublished by the manufacturer, at this time.[26,81,140] OspA and OspC are heterogeneous; therefore, monovalent OspA vaccines from the United States likely are not protective

Table 3
Canine Lyme (*Borrelia burgdorferi* s.s) vaccinations currently approved, for dogs, on the US market

Brand Name	Recombitek Lyme	Duramune Lyme	Novibac Lyme	Lyme Vax	VANGUARD crLyme
Manufacturer	Merial	Boehringer Ingelheim	Merck (Intervet, CN)	Zoetis	Zoetis
Vaccine antigen	Recombinant plasma-derived, subunit vaccine (OspA)	Killed whole-cell, bivalent bacterin (OspA, OspC)	Killed whole-cell, bivalent bacterin (OspA, OspC)	Killed whole-cell, bivalent bacterin (OspA, OspC)	Recombinant OspA and chimeric OspC
Adjuvant	None	Proprietary adjuvant	Proprietary non-Al adjuvant	Non-Al adjuvant	None
Dosing recommendations	1-mL sq vaccine; dogs should be administered 2 doses, 2–3 wk apart. Annual revaccination recommended	1-mL sq vaccine; dogs should be administered 2 doses, 2–4 wk apart. Annual revaccination recommended Do not administer sq to horses	1-mL sq vaccine; dogs should be administered 2 doses, 2–4 wk apart. Annual revaccination recommended Do not administer sq to horses	1-mL sq vaccine; dogs should be administered 2 doses, 2–3 wk apart. Annual revaccination recommended Do not administer sq to horses	1-mL sq vaccine; dogs should be administered 2 doses, 3 wk apart. Annual revaccination recommended

Dosing recommendations are for dogs. Horse dosages may vary and are off-label use only.

to horses in Europe and vice versa. Vaccination does not eliminate Borrelia from a previous infection, or protect against other vector pathogens, for example, *A phagocytophilia*.[23,45,100,129,140,141]

The optimal dose, route, and booster intervals are not yet delineated. It is reasonable to vaccinate horses in high risk (*Ixodes* tick and Lyme endemic) regions, because the vaccines have the potential to protect horses from infection. Two-vaccine initial series protocols have induced a response but, as with equine influenza vaccination, a second booster (third dose) extends the duration of response.[81,143] With no consensus (dose, route, and boosters) to lend consistency to practice protocols, a vaccination program (based on the current literature) for *B Burgdorferi*–naive horses vaccination consistency is suggested:

Initial vaccine: 2 mL subcutaneously (nonadjuvanted) or IM (adjuvanted) vaccine on day 0.
First booster vaccine administered: (1-mL dose IM or subcutaneously, as described previously) on day 28 to day 90.
Second booster administered: (1-mL dose as described previously) day 108 to day 226.
Interval (postseries): (1 mL) minimally 2× a year; targeting spring and fall, when adult tick feeding is increased.

Equine clinicians must remember that the optimum vaccination program is unknown and individual horse response varies, such that even if the suggested protocol is administered, there is no guarantee of protection from Lyme infection and disease.

In addition to vaccination, protecting a horse from infection requires a reduction of the vector population harboring the tick or *B burgdorferi*. *Ixodes* feeding may be rapid, but evidence that the longer a tick is attached the greater the risk of borreliosis is still relevant; therefore, recommendations to remove ticks as soon as they are located is sound advice.[8,32,33] Because microclimate affects tick populations, cutting grasses shorter, removing leaf litter, and keeping woods and thickets cut back from the paddocks reduce vector (ticks and small mammal) numbers and equine exposure risk.[48] Reducing mouse populations, eg, eliminating stone walls where they congregate and acorns as a food source, while selecting for less-competent intermediate hosts (eg, opossum) over competent hosts (eg, white-footed mouse, eastern chipmunk, and meadow vole) reduces exposure risk to horses.[49,144–147] Decreasing the number of deer in the area lowers the adult *Ixodes* and *B burgdorferi* concentration.[146,148] Novel approaches, mimicking fly control in barn manure piles, via introduction of a native tick predator (ie, the tick wasp *Ixodiphagus hookerl*) can decrease *Ixodes* numbers. This specific wasp uses *Ixodes* species as a food source by depositing eggs into engorged larvae or unfed nymphal ticks.[146] Lastly, the use of topical acaricides applied to mammalian vectors, the horse, and the environment, reducing *Ixodes* numbers, can be used. Pyrothrin applied to horses limbs, pyrothrin-soaked cotton balls (rodent nesting material), and rodent bait boxes containing tick repellents, for example, fipronil, are commercially available, as are Environmental Protection Agency–approved acaricides for environmental applications (online at www.caes.state.ct.us).[149–151]

REFERENCES

1. Dabareiner RM, Cohen ND, Carter GK, et al. Lameness and poor performance in horses used for team roping: 118 cases (2000-2003). J Am Vet Med Assoc 2005;226(10):1694-9.

2. Dabareiner RM, Cohen ND, Carter GK, et al. Musculoskeletal problems associated with lameness and poor performance among horses used for barrel racing: 118 cases (2000-2003). J Am Vet Med Assoc 2005;227(10):1646–50.

3. Olivier A, Nurton JP, Guthrie AJ. An epizoological study of wastage in thoroughbred racehorses in Gauteng, South Africa. J S Afr Vet Assoc 1997; 68(4):125–9 [En.].

4. Wilsher S, Allen WR, Wood JLN. Factors associated with failure of Thoroughbred horses to train and race. Equine Vet J 2006;38(2):113–8.

5. Jeffcott LB, Rossdale PD, Freestone J, et al. An assessment of wastage in thoroughbred racing from conception to 4 years ago. Equine Vet J 1982;14:185–98.

6. Tilly K, Rosa PA, Stewart PE. Biology of infection with borrelia burgdorferi. Infect Dis Clin North Am 2008;22:217–34.

7. Arvikar SL, Steere AC. Diagnosis and treatment of lyme arthritis. Infect Dis Clin North Am 2015;29:269–80.

8. Divers TJ, Gardner RB, Madigan JE, et al. Borrelia burgdorferi infection and lyme disease in North American horses: a consensus statement. J Vet Intern Med 2018. https://doi.org/10.1111/jvim.15042.

9. Sanchez JL. Clinical manifestations and treatment of Lyme disease. Clin Lab Med 2015;35:765–78.

10. Funk RA, Pleasant RS, Witonsky SG, et al. Seroprevalence of Borrelia burgdorferi in horses presented for coggins testing in southwest Virginia and change in positive test results approximately 1 year later. J Vet Intern Med 2016;30: 1300–4.

11. Metcalf KB, Lilley CS, Revenaugh MS, et al. The prevalence of antibodies against Borrelia burgdorferi found in horses residing in the northwestern United States. J Equine Vet Sci 2008;28:587–9.

12. Butler CM, Sloet van Oldruitenborgh-Oosterbaan MM, Werners AH, et al. Borrelia burgdorferi and Anaplasma phagocytophilum in ticks and their equine hosts: a prospective clinical and diagnostic study of 47 horses following removal of a feeding tick. Pferdeheilkunde 2016;32:335–45.

13. Krupka M, Raskaa M, Belakovaa J, et al. Biological aspects of Lyme disease spirochetes: UniqueBacteria of the Borrelia burgdorferi species group. Biomed Pap Med Fac Univ Palacky Olomouc Czech Repub 2007;151(2):175–86.

14. DeVilbiss BA, Mohammed HO, Divers TJ. Perception of equine practitioners regarding the occurrence of selected equine neurologic diseases in the northeast over a 10-year period. J Equine Vet Sci 2009;29:237–46.

15. Burtis JC, Sullivan P, Levi T, et al. The impact of temperature and precipitation on blacklegged tick activity and Lyme disease incidence in endemic and emerging regions. Parasit Vectors 2016;9:606–16.

16. Bartol J. Is Lyme disease over-diagnosed in horses? Equine Vet J 2013;45: 529–30.

17. Cutler SJ, Rudenko N, Golovchenko M, et al. Diagnosing borreliosis. Vector-Borne Zoonot 2017;17:2–11.

18. Cerar T, Strle F, Stupica D, et al. Differences in genotype, clinical features, and inflammatory potential of Borrelia burgdorferi sensu stricto strains from Europe and the United States. Emerg Infect Dis 2016;22:818–27.

19. Pietikäinen A, Maksimow M, Kauko T, et al. Cerebrospinal fluid cytokines in Lyme neuroborreliosis. J Neuroinflamm 2016;13(1):273–83.

20. Hovius J, van Dam A, Fikrig E. Tick-host-pathogen interactions in Lyme borreliosis. Trends Parasitol 2007;23:434–8.

21. Veronesi F, Laus F, Passamonti F, et al. Occurrence of B. lusitaniae infection in horses. Vet Microbiol 2012;160:535–8.

22. Butler CM, Houwers DJ, Jongejan F, et al. Borrelia burgdorferi infections with special reference to horses. A review. Vet Q 2005;27:146–56.

23. Brorson O, Brorson SH. An in vitro study of the susceptibility of mobile and cystic forms of Borrelia burgdorferi to metronidazole. APMIS 1999;107:566–76.

24. Boroson O, Boroson S-H, Scythe J, et al. Destruction of spirochete Borrelia burgdorferi round-body propagules (RBs) by the antibiotic tigecycline. Proc of the Natl Acad Sci U S A 2009;106(44):18565–661.

25. Pritt BS, Mead PS, Hoang-Johnson DK, et al. Identification of a novel pathogenic Borrelia species causing Lyme borreliosis with unusually high spirochaetaemia: a descriptive study. Lancet Infect Dis 2016;165:556–64.

26. Slaughter KM, Halland SK, Schur LA, et al. Humoral response of Borrelia burg-dorferi outer surface protein A (OspA) vaccination in equids. Equine Vet Educ 2017;29(10):572–6.

27. Barbour AG, Bunikis J, Fish D, et al. Association between body size and reser-voir competence of mammals bearing Borrelia burgdorferi at an endemic site in the northeastern United States. Parasit Vectors 2015;30:299.

28. Shin SJ, Chang YF, Jacobson RH, et al. Cross-reactivity between B. burgdorferi and other spirochetes affects specificity of serotests for detection of antibodies to the Lyme disease agent in dogs. Vet Microbiol 1993;36:161–74.

29. Schvartz G, Epp T, Burgess HJ, et al. Comparison between available serologic tests for detecting antibodies against Anaplasma phagocytophilum and Borrelia burgdorferi in horses in Canada. J Vet Diagn Invest 2015;27:540–6.

30. Levine JF, Apperson CS, Howard P, et al. Lizards as hosts for immature Ixo-des scapularis (Acari: Ixodidae) in North Carolina. J Med Entomol 1997;34(6):594–8.

31. Durden LA, Oliver JH Jr, Banks CW, et al. Parasitism of lizards by immature stages of the blacklegged tick, Ixodes scapularis (Acari, Ixodidae). Exp Appl Acarol 2002;26(3–4):257–66.

32. Kazimírová M, Štibrániová I. Tick salivary compounds: their role in modulation of host defenses and pathogen transmission. Front Cell Infect Microbiol 2013;3:43, 1–19.

33. Cook MJ. Lyme borreliosis: a review of data on transmission time after tick attachment. Int J Gen Med 2014;19(8):1–8.

34. Parola P, Raoult D. Tick-borne diseases emerging in Europe. Clin Microbiol Infect 2001;7:80–3.

35. Piesman J, Sinsky RJ. Ability of ixodes scapularis, Dermacentor variabilis, and Amblyomma americanum (Acari: Ixodidae) to acquire, maintain, and transmit Lyme disease spirochetes (Borrelia burgdorferi). J Med Entomol 1988;25(5):336–9.

36. Johns R, Ohnishi J, Broadwater A, et al. Contrasts in tick innate immune re-sponses to Borrelia burgdorferi challenge: immunotolerance in ixodes scapula-ris versus immunocompetence in Dermacentor variabilis (Acari: Ixodidae). J Med Entomol 2001;38(1):99–107.

37. ej Hajdušek O, Šíma R, Ayllón N, et al. Interaction of the tick immune system with transmitted pathogens. Front Cell Infect Microbiol 2013;3(26):1–15.

38. Chang YF, Novosol V, McDonough SP, et al. Experimental infection of ponies with Borrelia burgdorferi by exposure to Ixodid ticks. Vet Pathol 2000;37:68–76.

39. Halouzka J, Wilske B, Stunzner D, et al. Isolation of Borrelia afzelii from overwin-tering Culex pipiens biotype molestus mosquitoes. Infection 1999;27:275–7.

40. Žakovská A, Nejedlá P, Holíková A, et al. Positive findings of Borrelia burgdorferi in Culex (Culex) pipiens pipiens larvae in the surrounding of Brno city determined by the PCR method. Ann Agric Environ Med 2002;9:257–9.
41. Halouzka J, Postic D, Hubálek Z. Isolation of the spirochaete Borrelia afzelii from the mosquito Aedes vexans in the Czech Republic. Med Vet Entomol 1998;12:103–5.
42. Krupka I, Straubinger RK. Background, diagnosis, treatment and prevention of infections with Borrelia burgdorferi sensu stricto. Vet Clin Small Anim 2010;40:1103–19.
43. Marcus LC, Patterson MM, Gilfillan RE, et al. Antibodies to Borrelia burgdorferi in New England horses: serologic survey. Am J Vet Res 1985;46:2570–1.
44. Steere AC. Lyme disease. N Engl J Med 2001;345(2):115–25.
45. Stricker RB. Counterpoint: long-term antibiotic therapy improves persistent symptoms associated with lyme disease. Clin Infect Dis 2007;45:149–57.
46. Griffin MO, Fricovsky E, Ceballos G, et al. Tetracyclines: a pleitropic family of compounds with promising therapeutic properties. Review of the literature. Am J Physiol Cell Physiol 2010;299(3):C539–48.
47. Pal U, Yang X, Chen M. OspC facilitates Borrelia burgdorferi invasion of Ixodes scapularis salivary glands. J Clin Invest 2004;113:220–30.
48. Greenfield BPJ. Environmental parameters affecting tick (Ixodes ricinus) distribution during the summer season in Richmond Park, London. Bioscience Horizons 2011;4(2):140–8.
49. Fish D, Daniels TJ. The role of medium sized mammals as reservoirs of Borrelia burgdorferi in Southern New York. J Wildl Dis 1990;26(3):339–45.
50. Caine JA, Coburn J. Multifunctional and redundant roles of Borrelia burgdorferi outer surface proteins in tissue adhesion, colonization, and complement evasion. Front Immunol 2016;7:442–53.
51. Templeton TJ. Borrelia outer membrane surface proteins and transmission through the tick. J Exp Med 2004;199:603–6.
52. Berndtson K. Review of evidence for immune evasion and persistent infection in Lyme disease. Int J Gen Med 2013;6:291–306.
53. Grab DJ, Perides G, Dumler JS, et al. Borrelia burgdorferi, host- derived proteases, and the blood-brain barrier. Infect Immun 2005;73(2):1014–22.
54. Plane JM, Shen Y, Pleasure DE, et al. Prospects for minocycline neuroprotection. Arch Neurol 2010;67:1442–8.
55. Miklossy J, Kasas S, Zurn AD, et al. Persisting atypical and cystic forms of Borrelia burgdorferi and local inflammation in Lyme neuroborreliosis. J Neuroinflammation 2008;5(40):1–18.
56. Murgia R, Piazzetta C, Cinco M. Cystic forms of Borrelia burgdorferi sensu lato: induction, development, and the role of RpoS. Wien Klin Wochenschr 2002; 114(13–14):574–9.
57. Davey ME, O'Toole GA. Microbial biofilms: from ecology to molecular genetics. Microbiol Mol Biol Rev 2000;64(4):847–67.
58. Gilbert P, Das J, Foley I. Biofilms susceptibility to antimicrobials. Adv Dent Res 1997;11:160–7.
59. Costerton J, Lewandowski Z, Caldwell DE, et al. Microbial biofilms. Ann Rev Microbiol 1995;5(49):711–45.
60. Wagner B, Erb H. Dogs and horse with antibodies to outer surface protein C as on time sentinels for ticks infected with B. burgdorferi in 2011. Prev Vet Med 2012;107:275–9.
61. Durrani AZ, Goyal SM, Kamal N. Retrospective study on seroprevalence of Borrelia burgdorferi antibodies in horses in Minnesota. J Equine Vet Sci 2011;31(8): 427–9.

62. Magnarelli E, Fikrig E. Detection of antibodies to B. burgdorferi in naturally infected horses in the USA by enzyme linked immunosorbent assay using whole cell recombinant antigens. Res Vet Sci 2005;79:99–103.

63. Eisen R, Eisen L, Beard CB. County scale distribution of Ixodes scapularis and Ixodes pacificus (Acari: Ixodidae) in the continental United States. J Med Entomol 2016;53:349–86.

64. Cohen ND, Heck FC, Heim B, et al. Seroprevalence of antibodies to Borrelia burgdorferi in a population of horses in central Texas. J Am Vet Med Assoc 1992;201:1030–4.

65. Lindenmayer J, Weber M, Onderdonk A, et al. Borrelia burgdorferi infection in horses. J Am Vet Med Assoc 1989;186:1384.

66. Johnson A, Wagner B. Borrelia bergdorferi. In: Pusterla N, Higgins J, editors. Interpretation of laboratory diagnostics. 1st edition. Hoboken (NJ): John Wiley & Sons; 2018. p. 191–6.

67. Burbelo P, Bren KE, Ching KH, et al. Antibody profiling of Borrelia burgdorferi infection in horses. Clin Vaccine Immunol 2011;18:1562–7.

68. Levy SA, Magnarelli LA. Relationship between development of antibodies to Borrelia burgdorferi in dogs and the subsequent development of limb/joint borreliosis. J Am Vet Med Assoc 1992;200:344–7.

69. Manion TB, Bushmich S, Khan MI, et al. Suspected clinical lyme disease in horses: serological and antigen testing differences between clinically Ill and clinically normal horses from an endemic region. J Equine Vet Sci 2001;21(5):229–34.

70. Priest HL, Irby NL, Schlafer DH, et al. Diagnosis of Borrelia-associated uveitis in two horses. Vet Ophthalmol 2012;15:398–405.

71. Sears KP, Divers TJ, Neff RT, et al. A case of Borrelia-associated cutaneous pseudolymphoma in a horse. Vet Dermatol 2012;23:153–6.

72. Passamonti F, Veronesi F, Cappelli K, et al. Polysynovitis in a horse due to Borrelia burgdorferi sensu lato infection: case study. Ann Agric Environ Med 2015; 22:247–50.

73. Jacobsen S, Thomsen H, Nanni S. Concentrations of serum amyloid A in serum and synovial fluid from healthy horses and horses with joint disease. Am J Vet Res 2006;67(10):1738–42.

74. Halperin JJ, Baker P, Wormser GP. Common misconceptions about Lyme disease. Am J Med 2013;126(3):264.e1-7.

75. Hunfeld KP, Ruzic-Sabljic E, Norris DE, et al. Vitro susceptibility testing of Borrelia burgdorferi sensu lato isolates cultured from patients with erythema migrans before and after antimicrobial chemotherapy. Antimicrob Agents Chemother 2005;49(4):1294–301.

76. Krause PJ, Narasimhan S, Wormser GP, et al. Borrelia miyamotoi sensu lato seroreactivity and seroprevalence in the northeastern United States. Emerg Infect Dis 2014;20:1183–90.

77. Brockenstodt LK, Mao J, Hodzic E, et al. Detection of attenuated, noninfectious spirochetes in Borrelia burgdorferi infected mice. J Infect Dis 2002;186:1430–7.

78. Wagner B, Goodman LB, Rollins A, et al. Antibodies to OspC, OspF and C6 antigens as indicators for infection with Borrelia burgdorferi in horses. Equine Vet J 2013;45:533–7.

79. Johnson AL, Divers TJ, Chang YF. Validation of an in-clinic enzyme-linked immunosorbent assay kit for diagnosis of Borrelia burgdorferi infection in horses. J Vet Diagn Invest 2008;20:321–4.

80. Wagner B, Freer H, Rollins A, et al. Development of a multiplex assay for the detection of antibodies to Borrelia burgdorferi in horses and its validation using

Bayesian and conventional statistical methods. Vet Immunol Immunopathol 2011;144:374–81.

81. Guarino C, Asbie S, Rohde J, et al. Vaccination of horses with Lyme vaccines for dogs induces short-lasting antibody responses. Vaccine 2017;35:4140–7.

82. Hansen MG, Christoffersen M, Thuesen LR, et al. Seroprevalence of Borrelia burgdorferi sensu lato and Anaplasma phagocytophilum in Danish horses. Acta Vet Scand 2010;52(3):1–6.

83. Johnstone LK, Engiles JB, Aceto H, et al. Retrospective evaluation of horses diagnosed with neuroborreliosis on postmortem examination: 16 cases (2004-2015). J Vet Intern Med 2016;30:1305–12.

84. Divers TJ, Grice AL, Mohammed HO, et al. Changes in Borrelia burgdorferi ELISA antibody over time in both antibiotic treated and untreated horses. Acta Vet Hung 2012;60:421–9.

85. Magnarelli LA, Flavell RA, Padula SJ, et al. Serologic diagnosis of canine and equine borreliosis: use of recombinant antigens in enzyme-linked immunosorbent assays. J Clin Microbiol 1997;35:169–73.

86. Girschick HJ, Morbach H, Tappe D. Treatment of Lyme borreliosis. Arthritis Res Ther 2009;11:258–68.

87. Burgess EC, Gillette D, Pickett JP. Arthritis and panuveitis as manifestations of Borrelia burgdorferi infection in a Wisconsin pony. J Am Vet Med Assoc 1986; 189:1340–2.

88. Imai DM, Barr BC, Daft B, et al. Lyme neuroborreliosis in 2 horses. Vet Pathol 2011;48:1151–7.

89. Burgess EC, Mattison M. Encephalitis associated with Borrelia burgdorferi infection in a horse. J Am Vet Med Assoc 1987;191:1457–8.

90. Mullegger RR. Dermatological manifestations of Lyme borreliosis. Eur J Dermatol 2004;14:296–309.

91. Boudova L, Kazakov DV, Hes O, et al. Pseudolymphoma of the breast nipple. The problem overview. Rozhl Chir 2005;84:66–9.

92. Zanconati F, Cattonar P, Grandi G. Histochemical and immunohistochemical methods for demonstration of spirochetes in skin biopsies. Acta Dermatovenerol Alp Pannonica Adriat 1994;3:99–104.

93. Hahn CN, Mayhew IG, Whitwell KE, et al. A possible case of Lyme borreliosis in a horse in the UK. Equine Vet J 1996;28:84–8.

94. Mikkila HO, Seppala IJ, Viljanen MK, et al. The expanding clinical spectrum of ocular lyme borreliosis. Ophthalmology 2000;107:581–7.

95. Ostfeld RS, Canham CD, Oggenfuss K, et al. Climate, deer, rodents, and acorns as determinants of variation in Lyme-disease risk. PLoS Biol 2006;4(6):e145.

96. Elias JM, Greene C. Modified Steiner method for the demonstration of spirochetes in tissue. Am J Clin Pathol 1979;71:109–11.

97. James FM, Engiles JB, Beech J. Meningitis, cranial neuritis, and radiculoneuritis associated with Borrelia burgdorferi infection in a horse. J Am Vet Med Assoc 2010;237:1180–5.

98. Djukic M, Schmidt-Samoa C, Lange P, et al. Cerebrospinal fluid findings in adults with acute Lyme neuroborreliosis. J Neurol 2012;259:630–6.

99. Aguero-Rosenfeld ME, Wormser GP. Lyme disease: diagnostic issues and controversies. Expert Rev Mol Diagn 2015;15:1–4.

100. Grosenbaugh DA, Rissi DR, Krimer PM. Demonstration of the ability of a canine Lyme vaccine to reduce the incidence of histological synovial lesions following experimentally-induced canine Lyme borreliosis. Vet Immunol Immunopathol 2016;180:29–33.

101. Bosler EM, Cohen DP, Schulze TL, et al. Host responses to Borrelia burgdorferi in dogs and horses. Ann N Y Acad Sci 1988;539:221–34.
102. Maher MC, Schnabel LV, Cross JA, et al. Plasma and synovial fluid concentration of doxycycline following low-dose, low-frequency administration, and resultant inhibition of matrix metalloproteinase-13 from interleukin-stimulated equine synoviocytes. Equine Vet J 2014;46:198–202.
103. Dyson SJ. Lesions of the equine neck resulting in lameness or poor performance. Vet Clin North Am Equine Pract 2011;27(3):417–37.
104. Kim D, Kordick D, Divers T, et al. In vitro susceptibilities of Leptospira spp. and Borrelia burgdorferi isolates to amoxicillin, tilmicosin, and enrofloxacin. J Vet Sci 2006;7:355–9.
105. Sicklinger M, Wienecke R, Neuber U. In vitro susceptibility testing of four antibiotics against Borrelia burgdorferi: a comparison of results for the three genospecies: Borrelia afzelii, Borrelia garinii, and Borrelia burgdorferi sensu stricto. J Clin Microbiol 2003;41(4):1791–3.
106. Hunfeld KP, Brade V. Antimicrobial susceptibility of Borrelia burgdorferi sensu lato: what we know, what we don't know, and what we need to know. Wien Klin Wochenschr 2006;118:659–68.
107. Chang YF, Ku YW, Chang CF, et al. Antibiotic treatment of experimentally Borrelia burgdorferi-infected ponies. Vet Microbiol 2005;107:285–94.
108. Ates L, Hanssen-Hubner C, Norris DE, et al. Comparison of in vitro activities of tigecycline, doxycycline, and tetracycline against the spirochete Borrelia burgdorferi. Ticks Tick Borne Dis 2010;1:30–4.
109. Schnabel LV, Papich MG, Divers TJ, et al. Pharmacokinetics and distribution of minocycline in mature horses after oral administration of multiple doses and comparison with minimum inhibitory concentrations. Equine Vet J 2012;44:453–8.
110. Caol S, Divers T, Crisman M, et al. In vitro susceptiblility of Borrelia burgdorferi isolates to three antibiotics commonly used for treating equine Lyme disease. BMC Vet Res 2017;13(1):293.
111. Wormser GP, Nadelman RB, Dattwyler RJ, et al. Practice guidelines for the treatment of Lyme disease. Clin Infect Dis 2006;43:1089–134.
112. Berende A, ter Hofstede HJM, Voset FJ, et al. Randomized trial of longer-term therapy for symptoms attributed to Lyme disease. N Engl J Med 2016;374:1209–20.
113. Klempner MA, Hu LT, Evans J, et al. Two controlled trials of antibiotic treatment in patients with persistent symptoms and a history of Lyme disease. N Engl J Med 2001;345(2):85–92.
114. Agwuh KN, MacGowan A. Pharmacokinetics and pharmacodynamics of the tetracyclines including glycylcyclines. J Antimicrob Chemother 2006;58(2):256–65.
115. Zozaya H, Gutierrez L, Bernad MJ, et al. Pharmacokinetics of a peroral single dose of two long-acting formulations and an aqueous formulation of doxycycline hyclate in horses. Acta Vet Scand 2013;55(21):1–7.
116. Reeves MJ, Salman MD, Smith G. Risk factors for equine acute abdominal disease (colic): results from a multi-center case-control study. Prev Vet Med 1996;26(3):285–301.
117. Basile RC, Rivera GG, Del Rio LA, et al. Anaphylactoid reaction caused by sodium ceftriaxone in two horses experimentally infected by Borrelia burgdorferi. BMC Vet Res 2015;11:197.

118. Ringger NC, Pearson EG, Gronwall R, et al. Pharmacokinetics of ceftriaxone in healthy horses. Equine Vet J 1996;28:476–9.
119. Wormser GP, Dattwyler RJ, Shapiro ED. The Clinical assessment, treatment, and prevention of Lyme disease, human granulocytic anaplasmosis, and babesiosis: clinical practice guidelines by the infectious diseases society of America. Clin Infect Dis 2006;43(9):1089–134.
120. Clark RP, Hu LT. Prevention of Lyme disease (and other tick borne infections). Infect Dis Clin North Am 2008;22(3):381–96.
121. Barthold SW, Hodzic E, Imai DM, et al. Ineffectiveness of tigecycline against persistent Borrelia burgdorferi. Antimicrob Agents Chemother 2010;54(2):643–51.
122. Kersten A, Poitschek C, Rauch S, et al. Effects of penicillin, ceftriaxone, and doxycycline on morphology of Borrelia burgdorferi. Antimicrob Agents Chemother 1995;39(5):1127–33.
123. Bernardino ALF, Kaushal D, Philipp MT. The antibiotics doxycycline and minocycline inhibit inflammatory responses to the Lyme disease spirochete Borrelia burgdorferi. J Infect Dis 2009;199:1379–88.
124. Davis JL, Salmon JH, Papich MG. Pharmacokinetics and tissue distribution of doxycycline after oral administration of single and multiple doses in horses. Am J Vet Res 2006;67(2):310–6.
125. Novick WJ Jr. Levels of cefotaxime in body fluids and tissues: a review. Rev Infect Dis 1982;4(2):S346–53.
126. Brooks D. Equine ophthalmology. In: Proceed of the AAEP, vol. 48. 2002. p. 300–13.
127. Prabhu SS, Shtein RM, Michelotti MM, et al. Topical cyclosporine A 0.05% for recurrent anterior uveitis. Br J Ophthalmol 2016;100(3):345–7.
128. Gilger BC. Equine recurrent uveitis: the viewpoint from the USA. Equine Vet J Suppl 2010;37:57–61.
129. Cadavid D, Auwaerter PG, Rumbaugh J, et al. Antibiotics for the neurological complications of Lyme disease. Cochrane Database Syst Rev 2016;(12):CD006978.
130. Schnabel LV, Papich MG, Watts AE, et al. Orally administered doxycycline accumulates in synovial fluid compared to plasma. Equine Vet J 2010;42(3):208–12.
131. Orsini JA, Moate PJ, Engiles J, et al. Cefotaxime kinetics in plasma and synovial fluid following intravenous administration in horses. J Vet Pharmacol Ther 2004; 27(5):293–8.
132. Pille F, De Baere S, Ceelen L, et al. Synovial fluid and plasma concentrations of ceftiofur after regional intravenous perfusion in the horse. Vet Surg 2005;34(6): 610–7.
133. Whitehair KJ, Bowersock TL, Blevins WE, et al. Regional limb perfusion for antibiotic treatment of experimentally induced septic arthritis. Vet Surg 1992;21(5): 367–73.
134. Rubio-Martínez LM, Cruz AM. Antimicrobial regional limb perfusion in horses. J Am Vet Med Assoc 2006;228(5):706–12, 655.
135. Mills ML, Rush BR, Jean GS, et al. Determination of synovial fluid and serum concentrations, and morphologic effects of intra-articular ceftiofur sodium in horses. Vet Surg 2000;29:398–406.
136. Feng J, Zhang S, Shi W, et al. Activity of sulfa drugs and their combinations against stationary phase B. burgdorferi in vitro. Antibiotics (Basel) 2017;6(1):10.
137. Fortier L. Current Concepts in Joint Therapy. In: Proceedings of the 11th International Congress of World Equine Veterinary Association, 2009.
138. Sapi E, Kaur N, Ananwu S, et al. Evaluation of in-vitro antibiotic susceptibility of different morphological forms of Borrelia burgdoferi. Infect Drug Resist 2011;4: 97–113.

139. Yang X, Nguyen A, Qiu D, et al. In-vitro susceptibility of tigecycline against multiple strains of Borrelia burgdorferi. J Antimicrob Chemother 2009;63:709–12.
140. Chang Y, Novosol V, McDonough SP, et al. Vaccination against lyme disease with recombinant Borrelia burgdorferi outer-surface protein A (rOspA) in horses. Vaccine 1999;18:540–8.
141. Wikle RE, Fretwell B, Jarecki M, et al. Canine Lyme disease: one-year duration of immunity elicited with a canine OspA monovalent Lyme vaccine. Intern J Appl Res Vet Med 2006;4(1):23–8.
142. Polanda GA, Jacobsonb RM. The prevention of Lyme with a vaccine. Vaccine 2001;19(17–19):2303–8.
143. Töpfera KH, Straubinger KH. Characterization of the humoral immune response in dogs after vaccination against the Lyme borreliosis agent: a study with five commercial vaccines using two different vaccination schedules. Vaccine 2007;25(2):314–26.
144. Hanincová K, Kurtenbach K, Diuk-Wasser M, et al. Epidemic spread of Lyme borreliosis, northeastern United States. Emerg Infect Dis 2006;12:605–11.
145. Keesing F, Brunner J, Duerr S, et al. Hosts as ecological traps for the vector of Lyme disease. Proc Biol Sci 2009;276:3911–9.
146. Stafford KC III, Denicola AJ, Kilpatrick HJ. Reduced abundance of ixodes scapularis (Acari: Ixodidae) and the tick parasitoid ixodiphagus hookeri (Hymenoptera: Encyrtidae) with reduction of white-tailed deer. J Med Entomol 2003;40(5):642–52.
147. Shaw MT, Keesing F, McGrail R. Factors influencing the distribution of larval blacklegged ticks on rodent hosts. Am J Trop Med Hyg 2003;68(4):447–52.
148. Deblinger RD, Wilson ML, Rimmer DW, et al. Reduced abundance of immature Ixodes dammini (Acari: Ixodidae) following incremental removal of deer. J Med Entomol 1993;30:144–50.
149. Stafford III, KC. Managing ticks on your property. Connecticut Agricultural Experiment Station Brochure. Available at: http//:www.caes.state.ct.us. Accessed February 17, 2018.
150. Georgilis KM, Peacocke M, Klempner MS. Fibroblasts protect the Lyme disease spirochete, Borrelia burgdorferi, from ceftriaxone in vitro. J Infect Dis 1992;166:440–4.
151. Brouqui P, Badiaga S, Raoult D. Eucaryotic cells protect Borrelia burgdorferi from the action of penicillin and ceftriaxone but not from the action of doxycycline and erythromycin. Antimicrob Agents Chemother 1996;40:1552–4.

Management and Rehabilitation of Joint Disease in Sport Horses

Erin K. Contino, MS, DVM

KEYWORDS

- Sport horse • Joint disease • Osteoarthritis • Joint therapy • Physical therapy
- Rehabilitation

KEY POINTS

- Successful management of joint disease often requires a multimodal approach consisting of systemic medications and supplements, traditional or biologic intra-articular therapies, physical therapy, and management considerations.
- An accurate diagnosis is critical in the successful management of joint disease because it allows for the most appropriate targeted treatments to be selected.
- There are multiple nonmusculoskeletal factors that influence treatment selection, including endocrine status, history of gastrointestinal ulceration or kidney dysfunction, rules of the sports governing body, and various owner factors, such as expectations and finances.

INTRODUCTION

The successful treatment of joint disease in sport horses requires an accurate diagnosis, an honest evaluation of the treatment goals, and a clear understanding of an owner's expectations. Joint disease is a broad statement and attempts should be made to deduce which of the joint components are contributing to the joint disease so that the most appropriate treatment(s) can be pursued. Additionally, the entire horse should be evaluated, not only from a musculoskeletal standpoint but also to detect systemic disorders or concerns that may influence treatment choices.

MANAGEMENT CONSIDERATIONS

It is well understood in humans and dogs the negative effects of body weight on osteoarthritis (OA). In humans, every pound of body weight lost results in a 4-lb decrease in

Disclosure Statement: Minor financial interest in a commercial stem cell company (Advanced Regenerative Therapies, Fort Collins, CO).
Department of Clinical Sciences, Colorado State University, 300 West Drake, Fort Collins, CO 80523, USA
E-mail address: erin.contino@colostate.edu

Vet Clin Equine 34 (2018) 345–358
https://doi.org/10.1016/j.cveq.2018.04.007
0749-0739/18/© 2018 Elsevier Inc. All rights reserved.

forces on the knee.[1] Dogs with hip OA have less lameness after an 11% to 18% decrease in weight,[2] and a landmark study demonstrated longer life spans and delayed onset of chronic disease in dogs fed a restricted diet.[3] Similar benefits would be expected in horses so it is interesting that the role of weight is so commonly overlooked. Recommending weight loss in a clearly overweight horse seems appropriate.

Housing and environment also play a role in managing joint disease. Like humans, horses with OA, particularly of the axial skeleton or multiple limbs, tend to be stiff and to warm up slowly, particularly in cold weather and/or after stall confinement. Therefore, providing adequate shelter from the elements and means to stay warm and allowing regular access to turnout are beneficial. In particular, older horses do better with regular, consistent exercise compared with infrequent intense exercise. Fortunately, most sport horses are kept in routine work, which may be an effective, although unintentional, management strategy.

SYSTEMIC TREATMENTS
Nonsteroidal Anti-inflammatory Drugs

Nonsteroidal anti-inflammatory drugs (NSAIDs) are a mainstay of pain management for horses with joint disease due to their efficacy, availability, and ease of administration. The most commonly used NSAIDs include phenylbutazone, flunixin meglumine, and firocoxib; a topical NSAID is also available (**Table 1**). Nonspecific cyclooxygenase (COX) inhibitors, such as phenylbutazone, can cause gastrointestinal (GI) ulceration and kidney disease in a dose-dependent fashion. In an otherwise healthy horse, without history of GI or kidney disease, phenylbutazone is still a reasonable first line of defense.

Firocoxib is a newer COX-2 selective NSAID that spares the protective effects of the COX-1 pathway. At the labeled dose, firocoxib is fairly safe, even for long-term administration, but adverse effects can be seen when administered in excess and/or when combined with another NSAID.[4] Multiple studies have shown firocoxib to be effective in reducing naturally occurring lameness,[5,6] with similar efficacy to phenylbutazone for decreasing lameness.[7] Clinically, phenylbutazone seems more potent, so in cases of acute and/or moderate to severe lameness, the author prefers phenylbutazone for short-term and firocoxib for long-term administration. Because firocoxib takes several days to reach steady state, a loading dose should be given on the first day followed by the label dose each day thereafter.

Injectable Joint Products

The use of injectable products, such as Legend (sodium hyaluronate [HA], Bayer Healthcare LLC, Shawnee Mission, KS, USA), Adequan (polysulfated glycosaminoglycan [PSGAG], Luitpold Animal Health, Shirley, NY, USA), and Pentosan EQ (pentosan polysulfate sodium [PPS], Ceva Animal Health, Glenorie, New South Wales, Australia) are widespread. In a survey of 831 equine practitioners, 63% reported using Legend and 57% reported using Adequan.[8] These products, and many others, have been tested in the equine carpal chip model at Colorado State University Orthopaedic Research Center. Briefly, this model entails surgical creation of an osteochondral fragment off the distal aspect of the radiocarpal bone. Two weeks later, treatment is initiated and horses begin treadmill exercise to induce OA of the middle carpal joint. At the end of the study (day 70) various clinical, gross, and histopathologic outcomes are measured.

Using this model, intravenous (IV) HA (40 mg once weekly for 3 weeks) resulted in significantly less lameness (grade 1 vs grade 1.75 of 5), less synovial fluid inflammation, and improved synovial membrane scores.[9] These results indicate that injectable HA is both a symptom-modifying and disease-modifying OA drug, making it a

Table 1
Commonly used medications in the management and treatment of joint disease in sport horses

	Dosing/Frequency	Benefits/Uses/Pros	Contraindications/Cautions/Cons
NSAIDs			
Phenylbutazone	• IV, PO • 2.2 mg/kg BID or • 4.4 mg/kg q 24 h	• Effective, fast acting anti-inflammatory • Readily available	• Can cause GI ulceration/kidney disease • Do not combine with other systemic NSAIDs
Firocoxib	• IV, PO • 0.3 mg/kg day 1 (loading) • 0.1 mg/kg daily (maintenance)	• Useful for long-term administration • Less risk of GI/kidney disease	• Do not combine with other systemic NSAIDs • Use loading dose on day 1
Flunixin meglumine	• IV, PO • 500 mg once daily	• Effective, fast acting anti-inflammatory	• Can cause GI ulceration/kidney disease • Do not combine with other systemic NSAIDs
Diclofenac cream	• Topical • 1–2× daily	• Safe for long-term administration • Minimal systemic side effects	• Wear gloves when handling • Can cause skin irritation/dermatitis
Systemic therapy			
IV HA	• Loading: 40 mg q 7 d × 4 treatments • Maintenance: once monthly	• Used for general joint support • Low-grade multilimb lameness	
IM PSGAG	• 500 mg IM q 4 d × 7 treatments • Repeat 1–2× year	• Used for general joint support • Cases of synovitis	
IM PPS	• Loading: 3 mg/kg q 7 d × 4 treatments • Maintenance: once monthly	• Used for general joint support • Low-grade multilimb lameness	• FDA-approved product not currently available • Can cause discoloration of hair at injection site

(continued on next page)

Table 1
(continued)

	Dosing/Frequency	Benefits/Uses/Pros	Contraindications/Cautions/Cons
IA			
Corticosteroids		• Relatively inexpensive • Potent anti-inflammatory effect	• Avoid in horses with metabolic disease • Avoid frequent repeat injection (>2× year)
Betamethasone	• 4–14 mg/joint • ≤18–40 mg/horse	• Fast onset of action	• Shorter acting
Methylprednisolone	• 20–80 mg/joint • ≤200 mg/horse	• May be less likely to cause corticosteroid-induced laminitis	• Can be harmful to articular cartilage • Can cause dystrophic soft tissue mineralization • Avoid in high-motion joints
Triamcinolone	• 3–10 mg/joint • ≤18–40 mg/horse	• Chondroprotective • High-motion joints	• May be more likely to cause steroid-induced laminitis
Other		• IA treatment of metabolic horses • No drug withdrawal times	
HA	• 11–22 mg/joint once or every 7 d × 3 treatments	• Chondroprotective effects • Cases of synovitis	• Can cause postinjection flare (≤12%)
IRAP	• 2–10 mL (based on joint volume) • Every 3–10 d × 3 treatments	• Good alternative to corticosteroids • May aid in soft tissue healing	• Do not administer with IA antibiotics • Requires 1 d to process • Can cause postinjection flare
MSCs	• 10–20 million/joint • ≤50 million/horse • Administer with HA	• Regenerative properties • Can aid in surfacing joints and repair of soft tissue injuries	• Can cause postinjection flare • Do not administer with IA antibiotics • Expensive
PRP	• 2–6 mL/joint	• Available stallside	• Can cause postinjection flare • IA use not substantiated scientifically in horses
PSGAG	• 1–2 mL/joint	• Good for treating synovitis	• Administer with IA antibiotics • Not steadily available from manufacturer

Other therapies		
Shockwave	• 1500–2000 pulses/joint • Single treatment, as needed • Or q 7–10 d × 3 treatments	• Noninvasive • Well-tolerated, safe	• Fairly expensive • Not within 4 d of competition

Bisphosphonates		• Licensed for navicular syndrome
		• Useful in managing back OA/back pain
		• Cases of bone pain/edema
			• Contraindicated in young/pregnant horses
			• Can cause kidney dysfunction
			  ○ Check kidney values first
			  ○ Do not administer with NSAIDs

Tiludronate disodium	• 1 mg/kg administered in 10 L IV fluids over 90 minutes • 1 mg/kg administered in 10 L IV fluids over 90 minutes		• Can causes colic-like symptoms • Time consuming to administer
Clodronate disodium	• 1.8 mg/kg IM (≤900 mg total) • Divide into 3 IM injection sites	• Ease of administration	• Can cause irritation, nervousness, mild colic-like symptoms

justifiable addition to the sport horse maintenance regime. Clinically, horses are administered a loading dose of 40 mg once weekly for 4 weeks, followed by 40 mg monthly for maintenance. Adverse effects are rare and there is little risk with more frequent administration; thus, many upper-level performance horses and/or horses competing under strict drug rules are commonly treated at shorter intervals leading up to and during competition.

Scientific results are less favorable for intramuscular (IM) PSGAG (500 mg every 3 days for 7 treatments), with 2 experimental studies showing minimal differences between treated and control joints.[10,11] In a model of chemically induced carpitis, however, horses treated with IM PSGAG (500 mg every 4 days for 7 treatments) showed more improvement in lameness, stride length, and carpal joint flexion compared with horses treated with IV HA (40 mg every 7 days for 3 treatments).[12] This model produced a marked degree of synovitis and may indicate that IM PSGAG is most beneficial in cases of synovitis. Given the widespread use of IM PSGAG among sport horse practitioners, there is likely a positive clinical effect beyond a placebo effect and lackluster experimental results. Clinically, some horses respond well to IV HA but not to IM PSGAG and vice versa. In the author's experience, there is no way to predict which product will yield a superior result in a given horse so it is often trial and error, based on subjective analysis. Other than cost, there is no reason that horses cannot be treated with both IV HA and IM PSGAG, and many sport horses are. Administration of PSGAG has drifted away from the manufacturer recommended dosing of 7 treatments every 4 days for 28 days, with many practitioners recommending a loading dose (500 mg IM weekly for 4 weeks) followed by monthly administration. There is no evidence to support the latter dosing regime, so the author prefers the 28-day course, given as needed or twice yearly for routine maintenance.

In the carpal chip model, treatment with IM PPS (3 mg/kg once weekly for 4 weeks) performed well.[13] PPS is currently licensed in Australia; a Food and Drug Administration (FDA)-approved product (Pentosan EQ) was briefly available in the United States but has since been removed from the market with no indication of resurfacing. This is unfortunate because initial use of PPS suggested it was popular and clinical results seemed promising, with a majority of horses showing improvement in lameness and general way of going. The most common side effect was permanent discoloration (darkening) of the hair at the injection site, which was reported with both the FDA-approved and compounded versions. There have been anecdotal reports of sudden fatality after IV injection; thus, PPS must only be given IM. The author does not advocate the use of compounded products so cannot recommend its use clinically at this time.

Nutraceuticals

The companion animal, including equine, nutraceutical market has been reported to be in excess of $1 billion annually. Unfortunately, oral supplements and nutraceuticals are not FDA regulated so efficacy does not have to be proved. Additionally, independent laboratory analyses reveal the majority of these products fall short of the labeled amounts. This creates a buyer beware market and many veterinarians are left making recommendations based on limited research from the company and/or based on a company's reputation.

Equithrive (Equithrive, Biological Prospects, LLC, Lexington, KY, USA) is an oral supplement containing resveratrol, a plant extract found in red wine. In a double-blinded study of horses treated (intra-articular [IA] corticosteroid) for naturally occurring distal hock joint OA, those supplemented with resveratrol (n = 21) were more likely improved (per rider feedback) at 2 months (95% vs 70%) and at 4 months (86% vs 50%) compared with placebo-treated horses. Although subjective lameness scores did not differ between groups, objectively, lameness was decreased at 4 months in the resveratrol group.[14] This study supports the use of oral resveratrol as an adjunct therapy in horses that suffer from OA. It may be particularly useful for horses that cannot tolerate NSAID administration and/or in horses subject to NSAID regulations by their sports governing body. As with many other supplements, clinical results vary. It seems that a greater effect is realized when administered at the twice-daily dose (loading dose), which was the dose tested in the study. Other than cost, there do not seem to be any disadvantages to the twice-daily dosing.

An avocado and soybean unsaponifiable (ASU) oral supplement (fed days 0–70) was tested in the carpal chip model. Compared with the placebo group, treated horses showed disease-modifying effects (decreased articular cartilage erosion and synovial hemorrhage and increased articular cartilage glycosaminoglycan synthesis)[15] but no differences in clinical presentation. Although the formulation is not identical to the ASU tested in the study, there is a commercially available product available in the United States (Cosequin ASU, Nutramaxx Laboratories Inc., Lancaster, SC, USA).

INTRA-ARTICULAR THERAPIES

Typically, the more specific the diagnosis and the more pinpointed the therapy, the greater the treatment effect. Therefore, IA therapy often provides the most bang for the buck. IA medications most commonly consists of corticosteroids, HA, biologics (interleukin-1 receptor antagonist protein [IRAP], platelet-rich plasma [PRP], and mesenchymal stem cells [MSCs]), and PSGAG.

Corticosteroids

Despite the advances of regenerative and biologic therapies, IA corticosteroids are a cornerstone for managing joint disease and for good reason. Corticosteroids are potent, effective, and inexpensive. Betamethasone, methylprednisolone acetate (MPA), and triamcinolone acetate (TCA) are the most commonly used IA corticosteroids. Betamethasone was temporarily unavailable, which may have given TCA a market edge, although clinically these 2 corticosteroids yield similar results and are sometimes used interchangeably. Experimentally, TCA seems to outperform betamethasone—whereas betamethasone did not show any detrimental effects on treated joints,[16] TCA was shown to be chondroprotective.[17] The same study demonstrated that TCA is both disease modifying and symptom modifying and, interestingly, disease-modifying effects were realized even when administered remotely, in the contralateral carpal joint.

Conversely, there is evidence that MPA is harmful to articular cartilage in a dose-dependent fashion. In the carpal chip model, horses treated with IA MPA (100 mg, days 14 and 28) had significantly worse articular cartilage grades not only when the OA joint was treated but also when administered remotely (ie, in the contralateral limb).[18] Additionally, MPA retarded cartilage healing[19] and repeated IA injections resulted in decreased mechanical properties of articular cartilage.[20] These results give reason to question IA MPA use, particularly when TCA was shown to be chondroprotective. The use of TCA in high-motion joints and MPA in low-motion joints is fairly widespread[8] but considering MPA caused cartilage degradation when administered remotely, treating low-motion joints with MPA may not be entirely harmless. There is widespread belief that MPA is more potent and/or longer acting than TCA but this is not substantiated clinically or by the literature. In the author's opinion, the negative effects of MPA do not manifest clinically to the degree the scientific research would suggest and may have a limited a place in treating joint disease. For example, in horses that require IA treatment of multiple joints, using MPA in low-motion joints and/or the sacroiliac region and TCA in other joints allows a lower total body dose of each corticosteroid. MPA has a longer detection time compared with TCA, which may limit its use in competition horses, in particular those competing under Federation Equestre Internationale (FEI) regulations.

Although IA corticosteroids are heavily used, there are many contraindications. When administered in the acute phase of injury, corticosteroids delay soft tissue healing so should not be used to treat joint disease that involves an acute soft tissue injury. Because corticosteroids can diffuse from synovial cavities to surrounding soft tissues, even if the soft tissue injury is extracapsular (eg, collateral ligament or patellar ligament), corticosteroid treatment of the underlying joint may be contraindicated. There are anecdotal reports of horses developing severe collateral ligament desmopathy within 2 weeks of IA coffin joint corticosteroid treatment; it is highly likely these horses had preexisting, subclinical desmopathy that was exacerbated after corticosteroid injection. For this reason, it is advisable to evaluate the soft tissues of the joint to the fullest extent possible prior to treating with IA corticosteroids, which are too often administered flippantly.

In general, the sport horse population is much older than the race horse or western performance horse population. With this comes a greater proportion of horses with endocrine disorders that are at an increased risk of developing laminitis secondary to corticosteroid administration. The author is of the opinion that horses with equine metabolic syndrome are more likely to develop steroid-induced laminitis compared with horses with Cushing disease although this has not yet been substantiated by the literature. Nonetheless, the risk of laminitis is almost always going to outweigh the potential benefits of IA corticosteroids in metabolic horses. There is a common belief that the total body dose of TCA should not exceed 18 mg; this is based on data from 1200 horses treated with less than or equal to 18 mg TCA, none of whom foundered.[21] More recently, of 2000 cases, most of which were treated with 20 mg to 45 mg TCA, only 3 (0.15%) developed laminitis, of which 2 were ponies that had previously foundered.[22] This study has led many practitioners to increase the total TCA dose to less than or equal to 45 mg; however, the majority of the 2000 cases were young Thoroughbred racehorses—a population presumably much less likely to suffer from endocrine-related steroid-induced laminitis compared with middle-aged to older sport horses.

Sodium Hyaluronate

The use of serial IA HA injections in humans with knee OA is common and is considered more efficacious than systemic NSAIDs or IA corticosteroids.[23] Clinically in horses, IA HA is used to treat mild to moderate synovitis although its greatest benefit may be its long-term disease-modifying effects, including evidence that it is chondroprotective.[24] When used alone, IA HA is often not enough to decrease lameness substantially and it has a flare rate of 12%. For these reasons, HA is commonly administered with corticosteroids. A recent study demonstrated that treatment outcomes were no better with HA and TCA injections compared with TCA injections alone.[25] It has yet to be seen if this study will cause a major shift in practitioners foregoing traditional combination HA and corticosteroid therapy in favor of corticosteroids only.

Polysulfated Glycosaminoglycans

PSGAG is most commonly used IM but from a scientific standpoint, it may be more effective IA, particularly in cases of synovitis.[26] IA Adequan is associated with an increased incidence of joint sepsis but this risk is alleviated with the addition of amikacin IA, 125 mg.[27] In the author's experience, IA PSGAG is effective at decreasing clinical lameness in some cases and, therefore, may be useful IA alternative to corticosteroids in horses with metabolic disease.

Polyacrylamide Hydrogel

Polyacrylamide hydrogel is used in Europe with promising results but is currently only available in the United States experimentally. In a prospective study of 43 horses with naturally occurring OA, treatment with 2 mL polyacrylamide gel resulted in significant decreases in lameness and effusion, with treatment effects apparent to 24-months, at which time 82% of horses were considered sound.[28] The author has treated only a handful of joints with polyacrylamide gel with mixed results. This treatment warrants further investigation.

Biologics

Biologic therapies are used with increasing frequency. They are often a good substitute for IA corticosteroids and, therefore, are important in managing joint disease in horses with metabolic issues. Biologics are useful in the face of acute soft tissue injuries and are used for their various anti-inflammatory, growth factor, and/or regenerative properties.

Interleukin-1 receptor antagonist

IRAP is increasingly becoming a cornerstone of managing joint disease, particularly in sport horses.[9] Experimentally, IRAP (6 mL IA every 7 days for 4 treatments) not only produces disease-modifying effects but also decreases lameness,[29] as is the case clinically. IRAP is typically administered every 7 days to 10 days for 3 treatments, especially in acute cases of joint disease. For long-term maintenance of chronic joint disease, a single injection, as needed, seems effective.

IRAP takes 1 day to process, and, although logistically inconvenient, the efficacy of IRAP and its use as an alternative to corticosteroids outweigh this minor drawback. IRAP is not subject to any drug regulations (other than United States Equestrian Federation [USEF] prohibiting any intrasynovial injection within 4 days of competition), thus can be administered closer to competition than corticosteroids. IRAP is also superior to corticosteroids in treating joint disease with a concurrent soft tissue injury. Not only is IRAP less detrimental to soft tissue healing than corticosteroids but also recent studies have shown that it may be beneficial. Finally IRAP may have an advantage over corticosteroids in very young horses when many practitioners feel more comfortable treating a joint with a biologic versus a corticosteroid.

Platelet-rich plasma and autologous protein solution

The majority of research on PRP, particularly in horses, surrounds its use in soft tissue injuries and there is minimal evidence to support its use in treating joint disease. Clinically, however, many sport horses practitioners report positive results with IA use. Recently, a stallside autologous protein solution (APS) (Pro-Stride, Owl Manor Veterinary, Warsaw, IN, USA) has gained quick and widespread traction among sport horse practitioners. Compared with blood, APS contains significantly higher concentrations of anti-inflammatory proteins (>3×) and white blood cells (12.1×) but not platelets (1.6×). A quasi-clinical trial reported improved lameness and joint range of motion in treated horses at 2 weeks with positive client feedback (nonblinded) at 3 months and 12 months.[30] The study used 2 kits per joint, double what typically is used clinically. Commercially, APS is marketed as a combination PRP/IRAP product, which may not be entirely accurate, but this is semantics because anecdotally the clinical results have been favorable.

Mesenchymal stem cells

The use of MSCs in treating OA in humans and horses is a relatively new frontier. Impressive results were seen in a severe model of goat OA, in which the medial meniscus and cranial cruciate ligament were excised.[31] Treated goats (10 million IA MSCs injected 6 weeks postsurgery) showed marked regeneration of the medial meniscus and significantly less progression of OA compared with controls. Although the first experimental study in horses produced underwhelming results,[32] the clinical results have been more positive. MSCs are a good choice for joints with cartilage damage and/or soft tissue injury because MSCs can resurface the joint and aid in soft tissue healing. Anecdotally, MSC therapy seems particularly beneficial for stifle injuries, especially those with meniscal damage.

As with other biologics, IA MSCs can result in postinjection joint flare in approximately 10% of patients. MSCs are often administered with HA due to evidence that HA extends the viability of MSCs. This is problematic from a postinjection flare standpoint because it is nearly impossible to determine which caused the flare. Current recommendations are for 10 million to 20 million MSCs per joint, up to 50 million MSCs total body dose, but the specifics of optimizing timing and dosing are not fully established. It seems that waiting until the acute inflammatory phase subsides may produce superior results compared with immediate administration. Clinically, this timing works well because culture expansion of bone marrow–derived MSCs takes several weeks.

OTHER THERAPIES
Shockwave

Focused extracorporeal shockwave therapy was compared with IM PSGAG (500 mg every 4 days for 7 treatments) in the carpal chip model. Shockwave horses received 2000 pulses with a 12-mm focal head followed 2 weeks later by 1500 pulses. Shockwave-treated horses had significantly less lameness compared with controls (grade 1.3 vs grade 2.1 of 5) and this persisted 1 month after treatment. Shockwave therapy is noninvasive and well tolerated and has minimal side effects.[10] It is expensive and cannot be performed within 4 days of competition under USEF guidelines. Clinically, it seems particularly useful for low-motion joints (eg, pasterns and hocks) and in treating enthesopathy, which can occur at the joint capsule insertion.

Bisphosphonates

Bisphosphonates alter bone metabolism by irreversibly binding to osteoclasts, which in turn decreases osteoblast activity and bone turnover, thus the rationale for use in cases with overactive osseous activity. In the United States, the 2 FDA-approved bisphosphonates (tiludronate [Tildren, Ceva Animal Health, LLC, Lenexa, KS, USA] and clodronate [OsPhos, Dechra Veterinary Products, Overland Park, KS, USA]) are licensed only for the treatment of navicular syndrome. A few, albeit weak, clinical studies have shown efficacy in treating hock and back OA[33,34] which is in line with clinical bisphosphonate use as adjunct therapy in managing cases of back pain due to thoracolumbar OA and/or kissing spine, navicular syndrome particularly in cases of flexor cortex erosion, and OA of low-motion joints. Additionally, bisphosphonates may be a reasonable choice when bone pain is suspected or diagnosed (eg, bone marrow–like lesion, bone bruising, or enthesopathy).

The clinical effects of bisphosphonate therapy are not immediately evident and usually take approximately 2 months. Horses that respond well to treatment can be treated once to twice yearly; however, excessive and/or prolonged use can cause bone fragility so bisphosphonates should only be used for specific indications, as needed, and not prophylactically. Because bisphosphonates can cause kidney disease, it is advisable to evaluate kidney serum biomarkers prior to administration. Concurrent NSAID administration is contraindicated due to the increased risk to the kidneys; this is problematic because many practitioners pre-emptively administer

NSAIDs to limit the colic-like symptoms that are not uncommon secondary to bisphosphonate administration.

PHYSICAL THERAPY

Considering the numerous ways that joint disease can alter proprioception, muscle timing, and balance, it is logical to incorporate physical therapy into the management plan. Unfortunately, many of the modalities that are used in physical therapy lack rigorous scientific support, leaving equine practitioners to evaluate limited human literature and extrapolate when appropriate. In regard to the plethora of physical therapy modalities available, an open mind and healthy skepticism should be used.

Underwater Treadmill Therapy

In one of the few controlled physical therapy studies in horses, underwater treadmill therapy (UWT) showed impressive results. Compared to matched controls exercised on a land treadmill, horses that underwent UWT treadmill therapy had more even weight distribution between the forelimbs, increased symmetry of muscle firing, better postural control, increased range of motion, among other positive results.[35] Although UWT did not improve the lameness compared with controls, there were clearly positive outcomes that would benefit horses with joint disease long term. When using UWT, it is important to establish a specific treatment goal because various factors influence the therapeutic effects. For example, if the goal is to decrease weight-bearing forces on the limb(s) during a period of rehabilitation, a higher water level is appropriate to increase buoyancy. Alternatively, many horses with chronic OA suffer from decreased range of motion, in which case having the water level just above the joint of interest may be most appropriate because this yields the greatest range of motion of that joint. At the author's institution, UWT is used frequently in the rehabilitation of joint injuries. Once acclimated to the UWT, horses are exercised 5 times per week, up to 20 minutes once or twice daily at a walk.

Other Physical Therapy Techniques

The ways in which physical therapy techniques can be applied to horses to improve balance, postural control, proprioception, neuromuscular timing, coordination, and so forth are limited only by the imagination. Various examples are provided (**Box 1**) but the critical concept is that a practitioner must have a specific problem and/or

---

Box 1
Examples of various physical therapy exercises that could be used to target specific problems in horses suffering from joint disease

- Standing a horse on postural pads (spongy foam blocks) to increase balance and encourage equal loading of the fore or hind limb pairs.
- Utilizing varied terrain and/or ground poles and cavalettis set at various distances, heights, and angles to improve coordination and proprioception.
- Targeting muscle atrophy of a specific muscle(s) with neuromuscular stimulation to increase muscle strength.
- Applying tactile stimulators to produce exaggerated flexion of the target limb.
- Increasing joint stability through physical conditioning aimed at strengthening surrounding musculature.
- Passive range-of-motion exercises to decrease joint effusion and increase joint flexion.

treatment goal in mind to curtail the exercise as specifically as possible. Thus successful physical therapy programs are customized to the individual horse.

SUMMARY

Joint disease in sport horses is prevalent and successful management often requires a multimodal approach. There are a plethora of systemic and IA medications as well as various other modalities, such as shockwave therapy, physical therapy exercises, and management techniques from which to choose. Thoroughly assessing a patient, understanding the expectations and goals, and understanding the advantages and disadvantage the various treatments allows making the best decisions regarding treatment and management for that patient.

REFERENCES

1. Messier SP, Gutekunst DJ, Davis C, et al. Weight loss reduces knee-joint loads in overweight and obese older adults with knee osteoarthritis. Arthritis Rheum 2005; 52(7):2026–32.
2. Impellizeri JA, Tetrick MA, Muir P. Effect of weight reduction on clinical signs of lameness in dogs with hip osteoarthritis. J Am Vet Med Assoc 2000;216(7): 1089–91.
3. Kealy RD, Lawler DF, Ballam JM, et al. Effects of diet restriction on life span and age-related changes in dogs. J Am Vet Med Assoc 2002;220(9):1315–20.
4. Kivett L, Taintor J, Wright J. Evaluation of the safety of a combination of oral administration of phenylbutazone and firocoxib in horses. J Vet Pharmacol Ther 2014;37(4):413–6.
5. Orsini JA, Ryan WG, Carithers DS, et al. Evaluation of oral administration of firocoxib for the management of musculoskeletal pain and lameness associated with osteoarthritis in horses. Am J Vet Res 2012;73(5):664–71.
6. Back W, MacAllister CG, van Heel MC, et al. The use of force plate measurements to titrate the dosage of a new COX-2 inhibitor in lame horses. Equine Vet J 2009; 41(3):309–12.
7. Doucet MY, Bertone AL, Hendrickson D, et al. Comparison of efficacy and safety of paste formulations of firocoxib and phenylbutazone in horses with naturally occurring osteoarthritis. J Am Vet Med Assoc 2008;232(1):91–7.
8. Ferris DJ, Frisbie DD, McIlwraith CW, et al. Current joint therapy usage in equine practice: a survey of veterinarians 2009. Equine Vet J 2011;43(5):530–5.
9. Kawcak CE, Frisbie DD, Trotter GW, et al. Effects of intravenous administration of sodium hyaluronate on carpal joints in exercising horses after arthroscopic surgery and osteochondral fragmentation. Am J Vet Res 1997;58(10):1132–40.
10. Yovich JV, Trotter GW, McIlwraith CW, et al. Effects of polysulfated glycosaminoglycan on chemical and physical defects in equine articular cartilage. Am J Vet Res 1987;48(9):1407–14.
11. Frisbie DD, Kawcak CE, McIlwraith CW. Evaluation of the effect of extracorporeal shock wave treatment on experimentally induced osteoarthritis in middle carpal joints of horses. Am J Vet Res 2009;70(4):449–54.
12. White GW, Jones EW, Stites T, et al. The efficacy of systemically administered anti-arthritic drugs in an induced equine carpitis model. J Equine Vet Sci 1996; 16(4):139–45.
13. McIlwraith CW, Frisbie DD, Kawcak CE. Evaluation of intramuscularly administered sodium pentosan polysulfate for treatment of experimentally induced osteoarthritis in horses. Am J Vet Res 2012;73(5):628–33.

14. Watts AE, Dabareiner R, Marsh C, et al. A randomized, controlled trial of the effects of resveratrol administration in performance horses with lameness localized to the distal tarsal joints. J Am Vet Med Assoc 2016;249(6):650–9.
15. Kawcak CE, Frisbie DD, McIlwraith CW, et al. Evaluation of avocado and soybean unsaponifiable extracts for treatment of horses with experimentally induced osteoarthritis. Am J Vet Res 2007;68(6):598–604.
16. Foland JW, McIlwraith CW, Trotter GW, et al. Effect of betamethasone and exercise on equine carpal joints with osteochondral fragments. Vet Surg 1994; 23(5):369–76.
17. Frisbie DD, Kawcak CE, Trotter GW, et al. Effects of triamcinolone acetonide on an in vivo equine osteochondral fragment exercise model. Equine Vet J 1997; 29(5):349–59.
18. Frisbie DD, Kawcak CE, Baxter GM, et al. Effects of 6alpha-methylprednisolone acetate on an equine osteochondral fragment exercise model. Am J Vet Res 1998;59(12):1619–28.
19. Shoemaker RS, Bertone AL, Martin GS, et al. Effects of intra-articular administration of methylprednisolone acetate on normal articular cartilage and on healing of experimentally induced osteochondral defects in horses. Am J Vet Res 1992; 53(8):1446–53.
20. Murray RC, DeBowes RM, Gaughan EM, et al. The effects of intra-articular methylprednisolone and exercise on the mechanical properties of articular cartilage in the horse. Osteoarthritis Cartilage 1998;6(2):106–14.
21. Genovese RL. The use of corticosteroids in racetrack practice. In: Proc. Effective Use of Corticosteroids in Veterinary Practice. Veterinary Learning Systems. Princeton, 1983.
22. Bathe AP. The corticosteroid laminitis story: 3. The clinician's viewpoint. Equine Vet J 2007;39(1):12–3.
23. Bannuru RR, Schmid CH, Kent DM, et al. Comparative effectiveness of pharmacologic interventions for knee osteoarthritis: a systematic review and network meta-analysis. Ann Intern Med 2015;162(1):46–54.
24. McIlwraith CW. Use of sodium hyaluronate (Hyaluronan) in equine joint disease. Equine Vet Educ 1997;9(6):296–304.
25. de Grauw JC, Visser-Meijer MC, Lashley F, et al. Intra-articular treatment with triamcinolone compared with triamcinolone with hyaluronate: a randomised open-label multicentre clinical trial in 80 lame horses. Equine Vet J 2016;48(2):152–8.
26. McIlwraith CW. Management of joint disease in the sport horse. In: 17th Proc. of the 2010 Kentucky Research Nutrition Conference. Lexington, April 26–27, 2010. p. 61–81.
27. Gustafson SB, McIlwraith CW, Jones RL, et al. Further investigations into the potentiation of infection by intra-articular injection of polysulfated glycosaminoglycan and the effect of filtration and intra-articular injection of amikacin. Am J Vet Res 1980;50(12):2018–22.
28. Tnibar A, Schougaard H, Camitz L, et al. An international multi-centre prospective study on the efficacy of intraarticular polyacrylamide hydrogel in horses with osteoarthritis: a 24 months follow-up. Acta Vet Scand 2015;57(1):20.
29. Frisbie DD, Kawcak CE, Werpy NM, et al. Clinical, biochemical, and histologic effects of intra-articular administration of autologous conditioned serum in horses with experimentally induced osteoarthritis. Am J Vet Res 2007;68(3):290–6.
30. Bertone AL, Ishihara A, Zekas LJ, et al. Evaluation of a single intra-articular injection of autologous protein solution for treatment of osteoarthritis in horses. Am J Vet Res 2014;75(2):141–51.

31. Murphy JM, Fink DJ, Hunziker EB, et al. Stem cell therapy in a caprine model of osteoarthritis. Arthritis Rheum 2003;48(12):3464–74.
32. Frisbie DD, Kisiday JD, Kawcak CE, et al. Evaluation of adipose-derived stromal vascular fraction or bone marrow-derived mesenchymal stem cells for treatment of osteoarthritis. J Orthop Res 2009;27(12):1675–80.
33. Gough MR, Thibaud D, Smith RKW. Tiludronate infusion in the treatment of bone spavin: a double blind placebo-controlled trial. Equine Vet J 2010;42(5):381–7.
34. Coudry V, Thibaud D, Riccio B, et al. Efficacy of tildronate in the treatment of horses with signs of pain associated with osteoarthritic lesions of the thoracolumbar vertebral column. Am J Vet Res 2007;68(3):329–37.
35. King MR, Haussler KK, Kawcak CE, et al. Biomechanical and histologic evaluation of the effects of underwater treadmill exercise on horses with experimentally induced osteoarthritis of the middle carpal joint. Am J Vet Res 2017;78(5):558–69.

Regenerative Medicine and Rehabilitation for Tendinous and Ligamentous Injuries in Sport Horses

Kyla F. Ortved, DVM, PhD

KEYWORDS

- Tendonitis • Desmitis • Regenerative medicine • Rehabilitation • Stem cell
- Platelet-rich plasma

KEY POINTS

- Tendon and ligament injuries are common in athletic horses.
- Spontaneous healing of tendon and ligaments occurs; however, repair tissue is usually biomechanically inferior leading to high reinjury rates.
- Regenerative medicine therapies have been used with increasing frequency to improve the quality of repair tissue.
- Regenerative medicine therapies including stem cell therapy, platelet-rich plasma, and autologous conditioned serum lead to improved repair of tendon and ligament lesions.
- A tailored rehabilitation program, including controlled exercise and adjunctive treatments, is also key to success in cases of tendonitis and desmitis.

INTRODUCTION

Tendon and ligament injuries are common in all sports horses, with specific injuries being overrepresented in certain disciplines. Most tendon and ligament injuries are categorized as overstrain injuries, especially in racehorses where tendons are operating close to their functional limits.[1] Tendons and ligaments are highly organized tissues that depend on the strength and structure of the extracellular matrix (ECM) to function. Overloading can lead to physical damage and degeneration. If peak loads on a tendon or ligament are greater than the structural strength, fibrillar slippage, breakage of cross-linking, fibrillary rupture, and tendon tearing can occur.[2,3] Although tendons and ligaments have the ability to spontaneously heal with time, the scar tissue that

Disclosure Statement: The author declares no conflict of interest related to this report.
Department of Clinical Studies, New Bolton Center, University of Pennsylvania, 382 West Street Road, Kennett Square, PA 19348, USA
E-mail address: kortved@vet.upenn.edu

fills lesions is biomechanically inferior leading to high reinjury rates and recurrent lameness.

The therapeutic objective for horses with tendonitis and/or desmitis is to return the horse to its previous athletic level and prevent reinjury. Rehabilitation has been a mainstay of therapy following tendon and ligament injuries. More recently, regenerative medicine has been used to "promote self-healing through endogenous recruitment or exogenous delivery of appropriate cells, biomolecules and supporting structures,"[4] such that the healed product more closely resembles native tissue. Restoration of normal biomechanical function and structure would allow horses to perform at previous athletic levels with reduced risk of reinjury.[5,6]

The goal of regenerative medicine is to restore normal structure and function of injured tissues, with the three main components of regenerative medicine including scaffolds, cells, and bioactive signals. Stem cell therapy, platelet-rich plasma (PRP), and autologous conditioned serum or plasma are the main orthobiologic products currently used in equine musculoskeletal injuries, although growth factor therapy and amnion are occasionally used. All of these injectable orthobiologic therapies can be used in the treatment of superficial digital flexor (SDF) tendonitis, proximal suspensory desmitis, suspensory branch desmitis, and various other tendon and ligament injuries. Acute, subacute, or chronic tendinitis/desmitis with hypoechoic areas noted on ultrasonographic examination are amenable to intralesional injection. Through slightly different mechanisms, the previously mentioned therapies work to modulate the inflammatory process and regulate tissue repair. Combined with controlled rehabilitation, regenerative medicine has become an important treatment option for horses with tendon and ligament lesions.

REGENERATIVE MEDICINE
Growth Factor Therapy

Treatment of tendon and ligament lesions with several different growth factors has been reported. Growth factors are used to stimulate cellular differentiation, angiogenesis, and ECM synthesis. The beneficial effects of insulin-like growth factor (IGF)-I[7,8] and platelet-derived growth factor[9] have been demonstrated in equine tendons. IGF was shown to improve the ultrasonographic appearance of SDF tendon (SDFT) and decrease swelling following intralesional injection in an equine collagenase-induced tendonitis model.[7] When used in horses with naturally occurring SDF tendonitis, IGF-I was associated with improved ultrasonographic appearance of lesions; however, treatment carried only a moderate prognosis for return to racing (62%) with a moderate rate of reinjury (46%).[8] Conversely, intramuscular injection of recombinant equine growth factor was found to have significant negative effects on healing in a collagenase-induced SDF tendonitis model.[10] One major downfall of the growth factor approach, is the limited number of growth factors that can be injected at one time. More recently, the concentrated milieu of growth factors in PRP has been exploited as high concentrations of numerous growth factors are simultaneously administered.

Platelet-Rich Plasma Therapy

PRP is defined as a volume of plasma with a platelet count greater than that of whole blood, although the fold increase in platelet count is highly variable between different products.[11] The therapeutic effect of PRP is in large part caused by degranulation of platelet α-granules.[12] Degranulation leads to release of a milieu of growth factors including PDGT, transforming growth factor-β, fibroblast growth factor, vascular endothelial growth factor, and epidermal growth factor that modulate the healing response in damaged tissue.[13–15]

PRP can be prepared patient side following centrifugation or gravity filtration of autologous blood because platelets are smaller and less dense than erythrocytes and leukocytes (**Fig. 1**). Several commercial systems are available including Arthrex autologous protein solution (Arthrex, Naples, FL), GPS III (Zimmer Biomet, Warsaw, IN), Magellan (Arteriocyte, Hopkinton, MA), Harvest SmartPrep (Terumo BCT, Lakewood, CO), Restigen PRP (Owl Manor Veterinary, Warsaw, IN), V-PET (Pall Medical, Port Washington, NY). There is great variability in final platelet and leukocyte concentration in the PRP produced by different systems.[16] PRP is classified by its leukocyte concentration with leukocyte-reduced preparations considered to be pure-PRP and leukocyte-rich preparations referred to as leukocyte-PRP. The effect of leukocytes on tendon and ligament healing has been questioned because *in vitro* studies by McCarrel and colleagues[17] found that expression of catabolic cytokines (interleukin [IL]-1β, tumor necrosis factor-α) and degradative enzymes (matrix metalloproteinase-13) were higher in tendon explants treated with leukocyte-rich PRP; however, a definitive conclusion has not been reached.

PRP promotes healing by enhancing cell migration, proliferation, and differentiation; improving matrix synthesis; and stimulating angiogenesis.[18,19] Several equine experimental and clinical studies have found that PRP-treated tendon and ligament lesions have improved strength and elasticity compared with control, and that reinjury rates are decreased.[20–23] Early *in vitro* studies by Schnabel and colleagues[24] demonstrated that SDFT explants cultured in PRP had enhanced expression of tendon-specific genes including cartilage oligomeric matrix protein, a much desired increased collagen I/collagen III ratio, and no increase in matrix metalloproteinase expression. A similar study showed comparable responses of suspensory ligament explants to PRP.[25] Several *in vivo* experiments have also demonstrated the benefit of PRP in healing of experimentally created lesions in the SDFT.[20,21,26] After surgical induction of SDF tendonitis, lesions were injected with PRP under ultrasound guidance. Tendons treated with PRP, when compared with saline-treated tendons, had improved quality of repair tissue histologically, significantly more collagen and glycosaminoglycan content, and superior neovascularization. Perhaps most importantly, improved

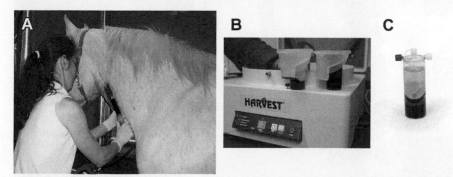

Fig. 1. Platelet-rich plasma (PRP) can be prepared patient-side using many different commercial products. (*A*) Blood is drawn sterilely from the jugular vein. (*B*) In the Harvest SmartPrep (Terumo BCT) system, blood is placed into the blood chamber of the process disposable (right) and then centrifuged such that PRP is concentrated in the bottom of the side chamber (left). (*C*) Restigen PRP (Owl Manor Veterinary) is prepared using a specialized processing tube and centrifugation. (*Courtesy of* [A] and [B] Terumo BCT, Lakewood, CO; with permission; and [C] Owl Manor Veterinary, Warsaw, IN; with permission.)

biomechanical properties including higher strength at failure and elastic modulus were demonstrated in PRP-treated tendons. Superior biomechanical properties indicates improved functionality and may translate to decreased reinjury rates in clinically treated horses.[20,21] Several reports have also described successful clinical outcomes following treatment of horses with SDF tendonitis and desmitis of the suspensory ligament, including lesions in the origin, midbody, and branches.[22,23,27–30] Despite seemingly positive clinical outcomes, the lack of a large randomized controlled trial must be considered when interpreting the results of PRP treatments.

One of the greatest benefits of PRP is that it can be prepared patient-side within 15 to 20 minutes; therefore, PRP can be used during the initial diagnostic ultrasonographic examination. If injection of PRP is planned, blood should be collected sterilely from the jugular vein and the limb should be clipped and sterilely prepared. It is recommended to block the site of injection with a local anesthetic administered locally or perineural to limit movement during the treatment injection. Following preparation of the limb, the lesion is reidentified with the ultrasound probe that has been covered with a sterile glove. Introduction of a needle into the lesion is confirmed with the ultrasound image (**Fig. 2**). Tendon and ligament lesions are best treated in the acute phase when a hypoechoic lesion is present on ultrasound. Chronic lesions with increased echogenicity are difficult to inject and likely too fibrotic to remodel effectively. The filling of hypoechogenic lesions with PRP is seen on the ultrasound image. Although no consensus has been reached regarding timing of the first injection, it seems reasonable to use PRP in the acute phase because of the inherent anti-inflammatory properties of the solution. Repeat injections are performed at 3- to 4-week intervals.

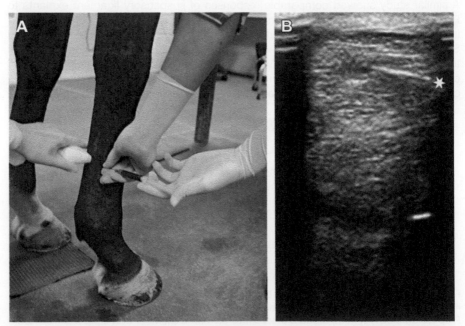

Fig. 2. Regenerative medicine therapies are injected into tendon and ligament lesions under ultrasound guidance. (*A*) Using sterile technique, the needle is inserted into the lesion parallel to the ultrasound beam. (*B*) The needle can easily be seen as a hyperechoic line in the SDFT on the ultrasound image (*yellow star*).

Stem Cell Therapy

Stem cells, or progenitor cells, are undifferentiated cells that are capable of self-renewal and are able to differentiate into different cell types (potency). The potency of stem cells varies from totipotent (able to give rise to all cells types [eg, early embryonic cell]), pluripotent (able to differentiate into any of the three germ layers [eg, embryonic- and early fetal-derived stem cells]), multipotent (able to differentiate into several closely related cells [eg, adult-derived stem cell]), to unipotent (able to give rise to only one cell type [eg, progenitor cell]).[31,32] Mesenchymal stem cells (MSCs) are used most commonly in the treatment of tendon and ligament injuries in the horse. They are multipotent cells derived from mesoderm that are capable of differentiating into bone, cartilage, adipose, tendon, and various other types of connective tissue.[33,34]

Originally, the principle mechanism of action of stem cells was thought to be differentiation of cells into the predominant cell type of the injured tissue. Although complete differentiation and engraftment do not seem to be the principal feature, stem cells are now known to exert their effect by modulating the host's inflammatory, healing, and repair phases following injury. Through potent paracrine activity, stem cells exert immunomodulatory, angiogenic, trophic, and antiapoptotic effects,[35] while also inducing migration and differentiation of resident progenitor cell populations.[36] The combination of these activities promotes natural regeneration of injured tissues, such that the healed product more closely resembles native tissue than it would otherwise.[37–39]

Adult-derived MSCs is obtained from a variety of sources including bone marrow, fat, synovium, dental pulp, tendon, muscle, and periosteum.[40–44] Fetal MSCs have been derived from amnion, umbilical cord blood, and umbilical cord tissue.[45–47] Like adult-derived cells, fetal cells are multipotent, not pluripotent, but may have slightly increased differentiation potential.[48] Bone marrow and adipose are the most common source of MSCs used in clinical cases, although several studies have suggested that bone marrow–derived MSCs (BM-MSCs) are superior for differentiation into musculoskeletal tissue.[41,49,50] Bone marrow is easily obtained from the sedated, standing horse from the sternum or tuber coxae,[51,52] whereas fat is usually collected from either side of the tail head (**Fig. 3**). Following collection of bone marrow or fat, MSCs are immediately concentrated for subsequent use or they are culture-expanded in the laboratory. Bone marrow aspirate concentrate refers to bone marrow that undergoes immediate centrifugation following collection. The centrifugation process concentrates progenitor cells and allows for patient-side application, although the density of MSCs is significantly lower than culture-expanded products.[53] Adipose-derived stromal vascular fraction refers to adipose that is collagenase-digested before concentration of progenitor cells. This product can also be used patient-side; however, it should be noted that only approximately 2% to 4% of cells in this product are progenitor cells.[54] In many injuries, a larger population of progenitor cells is desired; therefore, BM-MSCs or adipose-derived MSCs are culture expanded over a 2- to 4-week period, depending on isolation protocol and the individual horse. Culture expansion typically yields 1 to 2 × 10⁶ MSCs, which can be cryopreserved for future use.

Dental pulp has been described as a noninvasive source of stem cells in humans and the horse, with ECM and cells being isolated from the pulp chamber of extracted teeth,[55,56] although few studies have evaluated the regenerative potential of equine dental pulp. Recently, Bertone and colleagues[57] investigated the effect of injection of an off-the-shelf product, Pulpcyte (VetGraft, Columbus, OH), in horses with osteoarthritis and tendonitis or desmitis. This commercially available product, described as

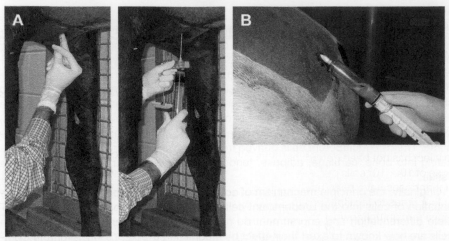

Fig. 3. Bone marrow and adipose are commonly used as a source of mesenchymal stem cells. (*A*) Bone marrow is collected from the sternum in a standing, sedated horse. The Jamshidi biopsy needle is inserted into the sternebrae by rotating the hand back and forth. The stylet is removed and bone marrow is aspirated using a 60-mL syringe. (*B*) Adipose is collected from beside the tail head in a standing, sedated horse using a 60-mL syringe with a slightly curved, large-bore, fenestrated needle. Alternatively, a skin incision is made to collect adipose. (*Courtesy of* Dr Ashlee Watts, Texas A&M University, College Station, TX; with permission.)

dental pulp connective tissue particles by the authors because of the scarcity of cells and relative abundance of ECM, was associated with improved lameness scores following intralesional injection. Despite the reported benefit of dental pulp products, further research is required before they are fully recommended.

Embryonic stem cells and induced pluripotent stem cells are also being investigated for use in musculoskeletal injuries because these cells may have greater differentiation capabilities and are available patient-side, negating the 2- to 4-week lag time. Watts and colleagues[58] evaluated healing in collagenase-induced SDF tendonitis using commercial fetal-derived embryonic-like stem cells with treated tendons showing improved tissue architecture, decreased lesion size, and superior fiber alignment. To date, embryonic stem cells for tendon and ligament healing have mainly been investigated *in vitro*.[59] Equine induced pluripotent stem cells have been described, although these cells have also not yet been used clinically.[60,61] Additionally, much interest lies in using allogeneic adult- or fetal-derived MSCs because these cells would also be available patient-side. At this time, it is uncertain whether allogeneic cells are effective or safe because of demonstrated recognition by the host immune system.[62]

Several experimental and clinical studies support the use of MSCs for SDFT and suspensory ligament injuries, with most studies showing improved tissue architecture, biomechanical function, and resistance to reinjury.[63–66] Adipose-derived stem cells in PRP,[67] adipose-derived stem cells,[68] and BM-MSCs[69] have been used in experimentally created SDFT lesions leading to improved tendon architecture and organization. In a recent clinical report, Godwin and colleagues[63] found that Thoroughbred racehorses with SDF tendonitis treated with BM-MSCs had significantly reduced reinjury rates compared with those treated conservatively. More specifically, the authors found that 111 of 113 (98%) horses raced at least once following injury with a reported reinjury rate of 27%, compared with a previously reported reinjury rate of 56%.[5]

Similarly, in a case controlled study by Pacini and colleagues[70] horses with SDFT lesions treated with BM-MSCs were less likely to reinjure (0 of 11; 0% reinjury after 2 years) compared with control horses (15 of 15; 100% reinjury within 1 year). BM-MSCs have also been associated with improved healing in other species including a rabbit Achilles tendonitis model.[71,72] Tenocyte-derived MSCs and tenogenically differentiated MSCs may be superior in tendon healing, although more research is needed.[40]

Stem cell treatment of tendon and ligament lesions can be performed under ultrasound guidance, as described previously. A 20- to 23-gauge needle is recommended to avoid shearing cells and damaging tendon/ligament.[73] The optimal number of cells to inject has not been determined with significant variability reported in the literature. A dose of 10×10^6 cells per lesion seems to be the most common[74]; however, lower and higher doses have been used. Stem cell injections are repeated every 4 weeks, three to four times to facilitate healing (**Fig. 4**). At this time, the optimal dose and dosing interval remain unknown.

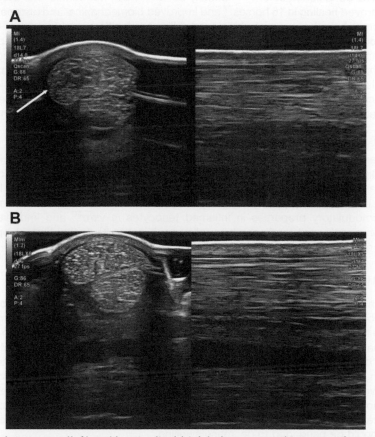

Fig. 4. (A) Transverse (*left*) and longitudinal (*right*) ultrasonographic image of an SDFT core lesion (*arrow*) in an 8-year-old Warmblood mare. (B) The same lesion 3 months after injury following three injections of bone marrow–derived MSCs under ultrasound guidance. The transverse (*left*) ultrasonographic image shows good filling of the lesion with increased echogenicity. The longitudinal (*right*) ultrasonographic image shows short fibers filling the lesion.

Extensive lesions in the SDFT or suspensory ligament can also be treated with regional limb perfusion of MSCs, instead of direct injection because of the difficulty of adequately injecting the entire lesion. Several studies have evaluated the localization of stem cells following regional perfusion[70,75]; however, the possible benefit of this technique in horses with pathology has not been published.

Autologous Conditioned Serum and Autologous Protein Solution

Autologous conditioned serum (eg, IRAP-II, Arthrex; Orthokine, Dechra Veterinary Products, Overland Park, KS) is prepared from autologous whole blood collected sterilely. The blood is injected into a tube containing borosilicate glass beads and incubated overnight at 37°C. The incubation process stimulates production of IL-1Ra, mainly by monocytes, and other growth factors including IL-10, fibroblast growth factor, vascular endothelial growth factor, IGF-1, platelet-derived growth factor, and transforming growth factor-β.[76] Limited studies have investigated the effects of autologous conditioned serum in tendonitis and desmitis; however, a single injection of autologous conditioned serum in naturally occurring SDF tendonitis was associated with improved healing in 15 horses[77] and improved biomechanical and histopathologic outcomes have been reported in a rat Achilles tendonitis model.[78]

Autologous protein solution or Pro-Stride (Owl Manor Veterinary) is a newer product that combines the benefits of IL-1Ra with those of PRP.[79] Differences in product technology have allowed Pro-Stride to be produced without overnight incubation; therefore, it is available patient-side. Although this product has been used clinically in SDF tendonitis and proximal suspensory desmitis with anecdotal success, no controlled studies on tendon and ligament healing have been performed at this time.

Amnion

Equine amnion-based products are available for treatment of wounds, ocular lesions, tendon/ligament injuries, and joints (AniCell Biotech, Chandler, AZ). Amniotic membranes are collected and decellularized such that an off-the-shelf bioscaffold is available. Limited studies have shown that human amniotic membrane has immunomodulatory properties in inflamed tenocytes *in vitro*[80] and improves pain scores in people with tendinopathies following injection.[81] At this time, support for the use of amniotic membrane is horses is mainly anecdotal.

REHABILITATION

Although orthobiologics may aid in tendon and ligament healing, proper rehabilitation and a convalescent exercise program remain paramount to success with any treatment. In the acute phase of tendon and ligament injuries, the goal should be to reduce inflammation and limit the action of proteolytic enzymes on remaining ECM. Cryotherapy is effective at decreasing swelling, secondary cellular necrosis, inflammation, and pain. The tissue temperature should be maintained at 10°C to 19°C for 15 to 20 minutes two to four times daily to optimize therapeutic effects. Temperatures less than 10°C should be avoided because this can cause further damage.[82] Nonsteroidal anti-inflammatory drugs are administered to decrease inflammation and pain, and affected limbs should be bandaged to decrease swelling.

Restricted exercise is absolutely necessary in the acute and subacute phases of tendon and ligament healing. General recommendations for exercise restriction are discussed next; however, there are many acceptable variations and severity of the injury should dictate the rehabilitation plan. Horses should be confined to a stall without purposeful hand walking or turnout until initial inflammation subsides, often up to 14 days. Hand walking is instituted once inflammation has subsided, often beginning with 5 to 10 minutes twice daily. The amount of hand walking is increased by 5 minutes per week up to 30 minutes twice daily. Mild tendonitis and desmitis cases can often begin tack walking after 30 days of hand walking, whereas moderate and severe cases usually require at least 60 days of hand walking. Repeat ultrasonographic examination should be performed 30 to 60 days after injury and every 2 to 3 months thereafter. Sonograms should be compared with previous studies to accurately monitor healing. Many horses with moderate injuries can begin tack walking after 60 to 90 days of hand walking. Trotting is introduced after 1 to 3 months of tack walking, depending on the severity of the lesion.

Small paddock turnout should not be introduced until 3 to 6 months after the initial injury, depending on lesion severity. Pasture rest has been shown to be detrimental in a study by Gillis and colleagues[83] in which the authors found that 71% (20 of 28) of Thoroughbred racehorses with SDF tendinitis returned to racing after rehabilitation with a controlled exercise program compared with only 25% (two of eight) of horses returned to racing after rehabilitation with pasture rest. Ideally, poor or deep footing and small circles should be avoided during rehabilitation. Race or jump training should not be initiated until at least 6 to 9 months following initial injury.

Other modalities that are often incorporated into tendon/ligament rehabilitation include extracorporeal shockwave therapy (ESWT), therapeutic ultrasound, cold laser therapy, and pulsed electromagnetic therapy. ESWT involves application of electromagnetic energy that is converted to high-energy shockwaves by an acoustic converter. ESWT can cause disorganization of collagen in normal tendon and microcracks in bone; therefore, exercise restriction after treatment is recommended.[84,85] Treatment protocols vary but a common protocol may entail one treatment every 1 to 3 weeks for three to five treatments. There is a paucity of literature regarding the effectiveness of ESWT in tendon and ligament injuries in horses. Shock wave was not found to improve healing in a collagenase model of SDF tendinitis but did increase vascularity; however, it was found to slightly improve the ultrasonographic appearance of collagenase-induced proximal suspensory desmitis.[86,87]

Therapeutic ultrasound,[88] laser therapy,[89] and pulsed electromagnetic therapy[90] are also used in rehabilitation of tendon and ligament injuries. However, little research currently exists supporting their use.

SUMMARY

Regenerative medicine for tendon and ligament injuries has been extensively investigated in the past 10 years, with experimental and controlled clinical studies finally catching up with clinical use. Currently, there is good evidence to support the use of PRP and stem cells in cases of tendonitis and desmitis with healed tissue that is likely to be stronger and more resistant to reinjury. Although tendon and ligament lesions demonstrate spontaneous healing, reinjury is a major problem in equine athletes. Regenerative medicine seems to significantly decrease the likelihood of reinjury, allowing more horses to continue their athletic pursuits.

REFERENCES

1. Stephens PR, Nunamaker DM, Butterweck DM. Application of a Hall-effect transducer for measurement of tendon strains in horses. Am J Vet Res 1989;50(7): 1089–95.
2. Goodship AE, Birch HL, Wilson AM. The pathobiology and repair of tendon and ligament injury. Vet Clin North Am Equine Pract 1994;10(2):323–49.

3. Avella CS, Smith RKW. Diagnosis and management of tendon and ligament disorders. In: Auer JA, Stick JA, editors. Equine surgery. St Louis (MO): Elsevier; 2012. p. 1157–79.

4. Advancing tissue science and engineering: a foundation for the future. A multi-agency strategic plan. Tissue Eng 2007;13(12):2825–6.

5. Dyson SJ. Medical management of superficial digital flexor tendonitis: a comparative study in 219 horses (1992-2000). Equine Vet J 2004;36(5):415–9.

6. Dyson S. Proximal suspensory desmitis in the hindlimb: 42 cases. Br Vet J 1994; 150(3):279–91.

7. Dahlgren LA, Nixon AJ, Bertram JEA, et al. Insulin-like growth factor-I improves cellular and molecular aspects of healing in a collagenase-induced model of flexor tendinitis. J Orthop Res 2002;20(5):1089.

8. Witte TH, Yeager AE, Nixon AJ. Intralesional injection of insulin-like growth factor-I for treatment of superficial digital flexor tendonitis in Thoroughbred racehorses: 40 cases (2000-2004). J Am Vet Med Assoc 2011;239(7):992–7.

9. Haupt JL, Donnelly BP, Nixon AJ. Effects of platelet-derived growth factor-BB on the metabolic function and morphologic features of equine tendon in explant culture. Am J Vet Res 2006;67(9):1595–600.

10. Dowling BA, Dart AJ, Hodgson DR, et al. The effect of recombinant equine growth hormone on the biomechanical properties of healing superficial digital flexor tendons in horses. Vet Surg 2002;31(4):320–4.

11. Boswell SG, Cole BJ, Sundman EA, et al. Platelet-rich plasma: a milieu of bioactive factors. Arthroscopy 2012;28(3):429–39.

12. Maynard DM, Heijnen HF, Horne MK, et al. Proteomic analysis of platelet α-granules using mass spectrometry. J Thromb Haemost 2007;5(9):1945–55.

13. Thomopoulos S, Zaegel M, Das R, et al. PDGF-BB released in tendon repair using a novel delivery system promotes cell proliferation and collagen remodeling. J Orthop Res 2007;25(10):1358–68.

14. Anitua E, Andia I, Sanchez M, et al. Autologous preparations rich in growth factors promote proliferation and induce VEGF and HGF production by human tendon cells in culture. J Orthop Res 2005;23(2):281–6.

15. Kajikawa Y, Morihara T, Sakamoto H, et al. Platelet-rich plasma enhances the initial mobilization of circulation-derived cells for tendon healing. J Cell Physiol 2008;215(3):837–45.

16. Sampson S, Gerhardt M, Mandelbaum B. Platelet rich plasma injection grafts for musculoskeletal injuries: a review. Curr Rev Musculoskelet Med 2008;1(3–4): 165–74.

17. McCarrel TM, Minas T, Fortier LA. Optimization of leukocyte concentration in platelet-rich plasma for the treatment of tendinopathy. J Bone Joint Surg Am 2012;94(19):e143.

18. Textor J. Autologous biologic treatment for equine musculoskeletal injuries: platelet-rich plasma and il-1 receptor antagonist protein. Vet Clin North Am Equine Pract 2011;27(2):275–98.

19. Molloy T, Wang Y, Murrell G. The roles of growth factors in tendon and ligament healing. Sports Med 2003;33(5):381–94.

20. Bosch G, van Schie HTM, de Groot MW, et al. Effects of platelet-rich plasma on the quality of repair of mechanically induced core lesions in equine superficial digital flexor tendons: a placebo-controlled experimental study. J Orthop Res 2010;28(2):211–7.

21. Bosch G, Moleman M, Barneveld A, et al. The effect of platelet-rich plasma on the neovascularization of surgically created equine superficial digital flexor tendon lesions. Scand J Med Sci Sports 2011;21(4):554–61.
22. Waselau M, Sutter WW, Genovese RL, et al. Intralesional injection of platelet-rich plasma followed by controlled exercise for treatment of midbody suspensory ligament desmitis in Standardbred racehorses. J Am Vet Med Assoc 2008;232(10): 1515–20.
23. Georg R, Maria C, Gisela A, et al. Autologous conditioned plasma as therapy of tendon and ligament lesions in seven horses. J Vet Sci 2010;11(2):173–5.
24. Schnabel LV, Mohammed HO, Miller BJ, et al. Platelet rich plasma (PRP) enhances anabolic gene expression patterns in flexor digitorum superficialis tendons. J Orthop Res 2007;25(2):230–40.
25. Schnabel LV, Sonea HO, Jacobson MS, et al. Effects of platelet rich plasma and acellular bone marrow on gene expression patterns and DNA content of equine suspensory ligament explant cultures. Equine Vet J 2008;40(3):260–5.
26. Romero A, Barrachina L, Ranera B, et al. Comparison of autologous bone marrow and adipose tissue derived mesenchymal stem cells, and platelet rich plasma, for treating surgically induced lesions of the equine superficial digital flexor tendon. Vet J 2017;224:76–84.
27. Zuffova K, Krisova S, Zert Z. Platelet rich plasma treatment of superficial digital flexor tendon lesions in racing thoroughbreds. Orig Pap Vet Med 2013;58(4): 230–9.
28. Torricelli P, Fini M, Filardo G, et al. Regenerative medicine for the treatment of musculoskeletal overuse injuries in competition horses. Int Orthop 2011;35(10): 1569–76.
29. Castelijns G, Crawford A, Schaffer J, et al. Evaluation of a filter-prepared platelet concentrate for the treatment of suspensory branch injuries in horses. Vet Comp Orthop Traumatol 2011;24(5):363–9.
30. Argüelles D, Carmona JU, Climent F, et al. Autologous platelet concentrates as a treatment for musculoskeletal lesions in five horses. Vet Rec 2008;162(7): 208–11.
31. Spencer ND, Gimble JM, Lopez MJ. Mesenchymal stromal cells: past, present, and future. Vet Surg 2011;40(2):129–39.
32. Corradetti B, Lange-Consiglio A, Barucca M, et al. Size-sieved subpopulations of mesenchymal stem cells from intervascular and perivascular equine umbilical cord matrix. Cell Prolif 2011;44(4):330–42.
33. Pittenger MF, Mackay AM, Beck SC, et al. Multilineage potential of adult human mesenchymal stem cells. Science 1999;284(5411):143–7.
34. Youngstrom DW, LaDow JE, Barrett JG. Tenogenesis of bone marrow-, adipose-, and tendon-derived stem cells in a dynamic bioreactor. Connect Tissue Res 2016;57(6):454–65.
35. Spees JL, Lee RH, Grogory CA. Mechanisms of mesenchymal stem/stromal cell function. Stem Cell Res Ther 2016;7(1):125.
36. Fu Y, Karbaat L, Wu L, et al. Trophic effects of mesenchymal stem cells in tissue regeneration. Tissue Eng Part B Rev 2017;23(6):515–28.
37. da Silva ML, Caplan AI, Nardi NB. In search of the in vivo identity of mesenchymal stem cells. Stem Cells 2008;26:2287–99.
38. Caplan AI, Correa D. The MSC: an injury drugstore. Cell Stem Cell 2011;9(1):11–5.
39. Ménard C, Tarte K. Immunoregulatory properties of clinical grade mesenchymal stromal cells: evidence, uncertainties, and clinical application. Stem Cell Res Ther 2013;4(3):64.

40. Durgam SS, Stewart AA, Sivaguru M, et al. Tendon-derived progenitor cells improve healing of collagenase-induced flexor tendinitis. J Orthop Res 2016; 34(12):2162–71.

41. Frisbie DD, Kisiday JD, Kawcak CE, et al. Evaluation of adipose-derived stromal vascular fraction or bone marrow-derived mesenchymal stem cells for treatment of osteoarthritis. J Orthop Res 2009;27(12):1675–80.

42. Bi Y, Ehirchiou D, Kilts TM, et al. Identification of tendon stem/progenitor cells and the role of the extracellular matrix in their niche. Nat Med 2007;13: 1219–27.

43. Radtke CL, Nino-Fong R, Esparza Gonzalez BP, et al. Characterization and osteogenic potential of equine muscle tissue- and periosteal tissue–derived mesenchymal stem cells in comparison with bone marrow– and adipose tissue–derived mesenchymal stem cells. Am J Vet Res 2013;74(5):790–800.

44. Chen Y, Caporali E, Stewart M. Bone morphogenetic protein 2 stimulates chondrogenesis of equine synovial membrane-derived progenitor cells. Vet Comp Orthop Traumatol 2016;29(5):378–85.

45. Corradetti B, Correani A, Romaldini A, et al. Amniotic membrane-derived mesenchymal cells and their conditioned media: potential candidates for uterine regenerative therapy in the horse. PLoS One 2014;9(10):e111324.

46. Desancé M, Contentin R, Bertoni L, et al. Chondrogenic differentiation of defined equine mesenchymal stem cells derived from umbilical cord blood for use in cartilage repair therapy. Int J Mol Sci 2018;19(2):537.

47. Nazari-Shafti TZ, Bruno IG, Martinez RF, et al. High yield recovery of equine mesenchymal stem cells from umbilical cord matrix/Wharton's jelly using a semi-automated process. Methods Mol Biol 2015;1235:131–46.

48. Kern S, Eichler H, Stoeve J, et al. Comparative analysis of mesenchymal stem cells from bone marrow, umbilical cord blood, or adipose tissue. Stem Cells 2006;24(5):1294–301.

49. Vidal MA, Robinson SO, Lopez MJ, et al. Comparison of chondrogenic potential in equine mesenchymal stromal cells derived from adipose tissue and bone marrow. Vet Surg 2008;37(8):713–24.

50. Guest DJ, Smith MRW, Allen WR. Monitoring the fate of autologous and allogeneic mesenchymal progenitor cells injected into the superficial digital flexor tendon of horses: preliminary study. Equine Vet J 2008;40(2):178–81.

51. Kasashima Y, Ueno T, Tomita A, et al. Optimisation of bone marrow aspiration from the equine sternum for the safe recovery of mesenchymal stem cells. Equine Vet J 2011;43(3):288–94.

52. Adams MK, Goodrich LR, Rao S, et al. Equine bone marrow-derived mesenchymal stromal cells (BMDMSCs) from the ilium and sternum: are there differences? Equine Vet J 2013;45(3):372–5.

53. Cuomo AV, Virk M, Petrigliano F, et al. Mesenchymal stem cell concentration and bone repair: potential pitfalls from bench to bedside. J Bone Joint Surg Am 2009; 91(5):1073–83.

54. Vidal MA, Kilroy GE, Lopez MJ, et al. Characterization of equine adipose tissue-derived stromal cells: adipogenic and osteogenic capacity and comparison with bone marrow-derived mesenchymal stromal cells. Vet Surg 2007; 36(7):613–22.

55. Gronthos S, Brahim J, Li W, et al. Stem cell properties of human dental pulp stem cells. J Dent Res 2002;81(8):531–5.

56. Ishikawa S, Horinouchi C, Murata D, et al. Isolation and characterization of equine dental pulp stem cells derived from Thoroughbred wolf teeth. J Vet Med Sci 2017; 79(1):47–51.
57. Bertone AL, Reisbig NA, Kilborne AH, et al. Equine dental pulp connective tissue particles reduced lameness in horses in a controlled clinical trial. Front Vet Sci 2017;4:31.
58. Watts AE, Yeager AE, Kopyov OV, et al. Fetal derived embryonic-like stem cells improve healing in a large animal flexor tendonitis model. Stem Cell Res Ther 2011;2(1):4.
59. Bavin EP, Smith O, Baird AEG, et al. Equine induced pluripotent stem cells have a reduced tendon differentiation capacity compared to embryonic stem cells. Front Vet Sci 2015;2:55.
60. Breton A, Sharma R, Diaz AC, et al. Derivation and characterization of induced pluripotent stem cells from equine fibroblasts. Stem Cells Dev 2013;22(4): 611–21.
61. Nagy K, Sung H-K, Zhang P, et al. Induced pluripotent stem cell lines derived from equine fibroblasts. Stem Cell Rev 2011;7(3):693–702.
62. Pezzanite LM, Fortier LA, Antczak DF, et al. Equine allogeneic bone marrow-derived mesenchymal stromal cells elicit antibody responses in vivo. Stem Cell Res Ther 2015;6(1):54.
63. Godwin EE, Young NJ, Dudhia J, et al. Implantation of bone marrow-derived mesenchymal stem cells demonstrates improved outcome in horses with over-strain injury of the superficial digital flexor tendon. Equine Vet J 2012;44(1):25–32.
64. Van Loon VJF, Scheffer CJW, Genn HJ, et al. Clinical follow-up of horses treated with allogeneic equine mesenchymal stem cells derived from umbilical cord blood for different tendon and ligament disorders. Vet Q 2014;34(2):92–7.
65. Smith RKW, Werling NJ, Dakin SG, et al. Beneficial effects of autologous bone marrow-derived mesenchymal stem cells in naturally occurring tendinopathy. PLoS One 2013;8(9);e75697.
66. Burk J, Berner D, Brehm W, et al. Long-term cell tracking following local injection of mesenchymal stromal cells in the equine model of induced tendon disease. Cell Transplant 2016;25(12):2199–211.
67. Ricco S, Renzi S, Del Bue M, et al. Allogeneic adipose tissue-derived mesen-chymal stem cells in combination with platelet rich plasma are safe and effective in the therapy of superficial digital flexor tendonitis in the horse. Int J Immunopa-thol Pharmacol 2013;26(1 Suppl):61–8.
68. Nixon AJ, Dahlgren LA, Haupt JL, et al. Effect of adipose-derived nucleated cell fractions on tendon repair in horses with collagenase-induced tendinitis. Am J Vet Res 2008;69(7):928–37.
69. Caniglia CJ, Schramme MC, Smith RK. The effect of intralesional injection of bone marrow derived mesenchymal stem cells and bone marrow supernatant on collagen fibril size in a surgical model of equine superficial digital flexor tendon-itis. Equine Vet J 2012;44(5):587–93.
70. Sole A, Spriet M, Galuppo LD, et al. Scintigraphic evaluation of intra-arterial and intravenous regional limb perfusion of allogeneic bone marrow-derived mesen-chymal stem cells in the normal equine distal limb using (99m) Tc-HMPAO. Equine Vet J 2012;44(5):594–9.
71. Crovace A, Lacitignola L, Rossi G, et al. Histological and immunohistochemical evaluation of autologous cultured bone marrow mesenchymal stem cells and bone marrow mononucleated cells in collagenase-induced tendinitis of equine superficial digital flexor tendon. Vet Med Int 2010;2010:250978.

72. Chong AK, Ang AD, Goh JC, et al. Bone marrow-derived mesenchymal stem cells influence early tendon-healing in a rabbit Achilles tendon model. J Bone Joint Surg Am 2007;89(1):74–81.

73. Lang HM, Schnabel LV, Cassano JM, et al. Effect of needle diameter on the viability of equine bone marrow derived mesenchymal stem cells. Vet Surg 2017;46(5):731–7.

74. Pacini S, Spinabella S, Trombi L, et al. Suspension of bone marrow-derived undifferentiated mesenchymal stromal cells for repair of superficial digital flexor tendon in race horses. Tissue Eng 2007;13(12):2949–55.

75. Spriet M, Buerchler S, Trela JM, et al. Scintigraphic tracking of mesenchymal stem cells after intravenous regional limb perfusion and subcutaneous administration in the standing horse. Vet Surg 2015;44(3):273–80.

76. Wehling P, Moser C, Frisbie D, et al. Autologous conditioned serum in the treatment of orthopedic diseases: the orthokine therapy. BioDrugs 2007;21(5):323–32.

77. Geburek F, Lietzau M, Beineke A, et al. Effect of a single injection of autologous conditioned serum (ACS) on tendon healing in equine naturally occurring tendinopathies. Stem Cell Res Ther 2015;6(1):126.

78. Genç E, Beytemur O, Yuksel S, et al. Investigation of the biomechanical and histopathological effects of autologous conditioned serum on healing of Achilles tendon. Acta Orthop Traumatol Turc 2018;26:126–40.

79. Bertone AL, Ishihara A, Zekas LJ, et al. Evaluation of a single intra-articular injection of autologous protein solution for treatment of osteoarthritis in horses. Am J Vet Res 2014;75(2):141–51.

80. Hortensius RA, Ebens JH, Harley BAC. Immunomodulatory effects of amniotic membrane matrix incorporated into collagen scaffolds. J Biomed Mater Res A 2016;104(6):1332–42.

81. Gellhorn AC, Han A. The use of dehydrated human amnion/chorion membrane allograft injection for the treatment of tendinopathy or arthritis: a case series involving 40 patients. PM R 2017;9(12):1236–43.

82. Petrov R, MacDonald MH, Tesch AM, et al. Influence of topically applied cold treatment on core temperature and cell viability in equine superficial digital flexor tendons. Am J Vet Res 2003;64(7):835–44.

83. Gillis CL. Rehabilitation of Tendon and Ligament Injuries. Proc Am Assoc Equine Pract 1997;43:306–9.

84. Bosch G, Lin YL, van Schie HTM, et al. Effect of extracorporeal shock wave therapy on the biochemical composition and metabolic activity of tenocytes in normal tendinous structures in ponies. Equine Vet J 2007;39(3):226–31.

85. Da Costa Gómez TM, Radtke CL, Kalscheur VL, et al. Effect of focused and radial extracorporeal shock wave therapy on equine bone microdamage. Vet Surg 2004;33(1):49–55.

86. McClure S, VanSickle D, Evans R, et al. The effects of extracorporeal shock-wave therapy on the ultrasonographic and histologic appearance of collagenase-induced equine forelimb suspensory ligament desmitis. Ultrasound Med Biol 2004;30(4):461–7.

87. Kersh KD, McClure SR, Van Sickle D, et al. The evaluation of extracorporeal shock wave therapy on collagenase induced superficial digital flexor tendonitis. Vet Comp Orthop Traumatol 2006;19(2):99–105.

88. Morcos MB, Aswad A. Histological studies of the effects of ultrasonic therapy on surgically split flexor tendons. Equine Vet J 1978;10(4):267–8.

89. Marr CM, Love S, Boyd JS, et al. Factors affecting the clinical outcome of injuries to the superficial digital flexor tendon in National Hunt and point-to-point race-horses. Vet Rec 1993;132(19):476–9.

90. Ramey DW, Steyn PF, Kirschvink JL. Effect of therapeutic magnetic wraps on circulation in the third metacarpal region. Proc Am Assoc Equine Pract 1998;44: 272–4.

Equine Manual Therapies in Sport Horse Practice

Kevin K. Haussler, DVM, DC, PhD

KEYWORDS

- Manual therapy • Proprioception • Neuromuscular control • Massage therapy
- Stretching exercises • Joint mobilization • Chiropractic care • Osteopathy

KEY POINTS

- Manual therapies can provide detailed diagnostic and therapeutic approaches to assess and manage neuromuscular coordination and strength in sport horses.
- Active stretching involves using the patient's own movements to induce a stretch; whereas, passive stretches are applied to relaxed muscles or connective tissues.
- Soft tissue or joint mobilization is indicated to help limit the effects of joint immobilization and to restore proprioceptive mechanisms.
- Equine chiropractic research has shown positive effects for pain relief, improving flexibility, reducing muscle hypertonicity, and restoring spinal motion symmetry.

INTRODUCTION

Manual therapies involve the application of the hands to the body, with a diagnostic or therapeutic intent. In horses, a diverse array of manual techniques, such as touch therapies, massage, joint mobilization, and manipulation (ie, chiropractic), have been applied with a primary therapeutic intent (eg, reduce pain or stiffness).[1–3] However, all of these therapies also have important diagnostic value in assessing musculoskeletal pain and dysfunction that is not possible with other more traditional physical examination approaches or imaging modalities. In sport horse practice, the primary issues that limit performance are chronic repetitive use injuries associated with long active athletic careers of pushing physical and psychological limits of horse and rider. Chronic, poorly localized pain and stiffness combined with slower reflexes or altered muscle timing contribute to poor performance issues and increase the risk of acute injury and inflammation. Manual therapies can provide detailed soft tissue, osseous, and articular evaluation techniques and unique methods to assess neuromuscular

Disclosures: The author has no commercial or financial conflicts of interest and there was not any funding source for this work.
Department of Clinical Sciences, College of Veterinary Medicine and Biomedical Sciences, Gail Holmes Equine Orthopaedic Research Center, Colorado State University, 300 West Drake Road, Fort Collins, CO 80523, USA
E-mail address: Kevin.Haussler@ColoState.edu

coordination and strength in sport horses that are not possible with routine lameness evaluation or neurologic tests.

Touch therapies and massage techniques focus on myofascial tone and the role of connective tissue (ie, fascia) in supporting optimal muscle, joint, ligament, and tendon function. Joint mobilization techniques involve assessing the quantity (eg, range of motion) and quality (ease of movement) in static and dynamic settings. Joint mobilization is used to provide subjective assessments of joint stability, passive and active joint movements patterns, and type of palpable resistance created as a joint is brought toward its end range of motion (ie, end-feel), which all provide critical insights into the biomechanical and neurologic features of an articulation. The ability to localize pain or stiffness to a specific vertebral level or defined spinal motion pattern (eg, restricted right lateral bending at C3-C4) provides a level of specificity that is required to diagnose subtle performance issues and to address vague or poorly localized sources of pain or upper limb lameness. The objectives of soft tissue and joint mobilization are typically to reduce pain, restore tissue compliance, and improve overall tissue mobility and joint range or motion.[4] Manipulation is more often used to address localized pain and joint stiffness, with less focus on the surrounding soft tissues.[5] Manual therapy techniques can also provide an adjunct to therapeutic exercises and rehabilitation of neuromotor control, where applied forces are used to induce passive stretching, weight-shifting, and activation of spinal reflexes, which help to increase flexibility, stimulate proprioception, and strengthen core musculature.[6]

IDENTIFICATION OF REHABILITATION ISSUES

Any medical, surgical, or rehabilitation plan is only as good as the diagnosis on which it is based. Veterinarians typically are good at establishing or defining diagnoses based on a known pathology or on anatomic localization (ie, pathoanatomic diagnosis). At times, they may even slide into the misguided approach of "treating the diagnostic image" without giving full consideration to determining the clinical relevance of the diagnostic imaging findings relative to the presenting or continued clinical signs of the patient. At the other end of the diagnostic-treatment spectrum are those owners and practitioners that are solely focused on the function of the horse (ie, is the horse able to do its job) despite the accumulation of known musculoskeletal injuries and chronic, multilimb lameness over a long active athletic career. Striving to find a balance between applying structural and functional approaches is ideal for managing the athletic demands and injuries in sport horses.

From the functional perspective, general rehabilitation issues to be addressed in equine athletes include, in progressing order, (1) pain management, (2) proprioceptive deficits, (3) stiffness, (4) weakness or fatigue, and (5) neuromuscular control. Pain management is always the first step in rehabilitation because it is not possible or ethical to ask a patient to exercise or do stretching when they are in pain. The body's normal protective mechanisms do not allow one to fully contract a muscle attached to an acutely stained tendon or to freely move a joint with acute synovitis. Nociceptive input by itself induces many other neurologic reflexes (eg, withdrawal reflex, crossed-extensor reflex) that function acutely to protect the body from further injury. However, chronic nociceptive input leads to peripheral and central sensitization (ie, wind-up) that has widespread neurologic and musculoskeletal effects that make clear distinctions between pain or lameness, altered proprioception or body awareness (ie, somatoesthesia), and altered gait patterns difficult to interpret.

As horses move into the proprioceptive and flexibility phases of rehabilitation, more focus is placed on how the horse is perceiving its environment through its sensory system and able to navigate through that environment with its motor system. This integration is often referred to as neuromuscular or neuromotor control and relies heavily on afferent signaling from proprioceptors, which include muscle spindle fibers in muscles, Golgi tendon organs, and many other soft tissue mechanoreceptors located in joint capsules and fascial planes. The motor component includes active and passive structures. The active structures that are addressed with rehabilitation include all motor pathways from the motor cortex in the cerebrum for control of movement, the cerebellum for balance and coordination, down to the timing and strength of muscle contractions. Passive structures include the joint capsules, ligaments, and the superficial and deep fascial layers that cover and envelop muscles and neurovascular bundles. All of the sensory and motor components and active and passive structures must function optimally for the horse to be able to progress in a defined rehabilitation or training program to build endurance and strength required for sport-specific demands.

PAIN MANAGEMENT

The goal of most rehabilitation programs is the early initiation of movement to begin the process of restoring normal joint motion, strength, and coordination. Acute pain and inflammation are typically managed with nonsteroidal anti-inflammatory drugs; cold therapies (ie, ice); restricted exercise; and compression wraps, if indicated, to protect local tissues and to limit excessive joint movement. Once the initial acute inflammatory phased has begun to subside in 3 to 5 days, then gentle, slow passive soft tissue or joint mobilization is indicated to help limit the effects of joint immobilization and to restore proprioceptive mechanisms.[7,8] Joint mobilization is usually applied in a graded manner, with each grade increasing the range of joint movement. Grades 1 to 2 joint mobilization involve inducing small degrees of joint motion around the neutral joint axis (ie, resting joint position) and then beginning to move the joint up to 50% of normal joint range of motion for a specified articulation. If passive joint motion is too painful, then applying light pressure and inducing motion of the overlying skin and subcutaneous tissues may help to improve lymphatic flow and increase mechanoreceptor stimulation in an effort to inhibit nociceptive signaling via local and spinal cord mechanisms.[9] Manual lymph drainage has been described for use in the management of lymphedema in horses; however, no controlled studies exist evaluating its effectiveness.[10] The reparative process of tissue healing includes collagen synthesis and fibrous tissue proliferation. Significant fascial restrictions or adhesions can limit injury recovery if proper mechanical stimulation and restoration of fascial glide of superficial and deep tissues is not achieved. Skin rolling techniques and deep tissue massage provide increased level of mechanical stimulation of connective tissues, which may be required in patients with extensive fibrosis or soft tissue adhesions.[2] Prolonged joint immobilization or forced stall rest are often counterproductive to maintaining musculoskeletal health.

Chronic pain often induces sensitization or wind-up, which produces generalized pain that is poorly localized and is often disassociatod from the initial inciting injury. In humans, massage therapy, joint mobilization, and manipulation are often used to address chronic pain syndromes and compensatory gait mechanisms (ie, antalgic gait). In horses, massage therapy has been shown to be effective for reducing stress-related behavior[11] and lowering mechanical nociceptive thresholds within the thoracolumbar region.[12] The use of acupuncture evaluation techniques to localize reactive loci within superficial soft tissues is useful for assessing overall nociceptive thresholds and diagnosing myofascial pain. Acupressure or ischemic compression techniques are used to treat local muscle pain or hypertonic bands (ie, trigger points).[13] Two randomized, controlled clinical trials using pressure algometry to assess mechanical nociceptive thresholds in the thoracolumbar region of horses have demonstrated that manual and instrument-assisted spinal manipulation can reduce back pain (or increase mechanical nociceptive thresholds).[12,14]

STIFFNESS

Neck or back stiffness is a common cause of poor performance in sport horses. Stiffness localized to a specific limb articulation is typically caused by joint capsule fibrosis or periarticular adhesions. Stiffness can also be produced by pain and muscle guarding associated with osteoarthritis or dorsal spinous process impingement. Muscle spasms or hypertonicity are common clinical findings in horses with neck or back pain or stiffness.[2] Detailed palpation techniques provided by manual therapy techniques can help to localize the source of stiffness to the various tissue types and possible pathophysiology of the clinical complaint.

All of the individual articulations of the proximal and distal limbs are mobilized to assess the quality and quantity of joint motion. As isolated joints are moved through full flexion and extension and accessory motions of internal and external rotation or translation, the ease of joint movement and any restrictions or painful responses are noted. A full description of the techniques for joint mobilization are beyond the scope of this article, but a simple example of assessing internal and external rotation of the coffin joint demonstrates asymmetries in the end range of motion. Gentle rotation of the hoof internally and externally helps to determine the quality and quantity of passive axial rotation of the coffin joint as the pastern region is stabilized proximally (**Fig. 1**).

Active stretching involves using the patient's own movements to induce a stretch, whereas passive stretches are applied to relaxed muscles or connective tissues during passive soft tissue or joint mobilization.[3,15] In horses, active stretches of the neck and trunk are often induced with baited (ie, carrot) stretches with the goal in increasing flexion, extension, or lateral bending of the axial skeleton.[6] Asking horses to produce active stretching of the limbs is often difficult; therefore, passive stretches are most commonly prescribed in horses.[15] In horses, passive stretching exercises of the limbs and axial skeleton have anecdotal effects of increasing stride length and joint range of motion and improving overall comfort.[15] In a noncontrolled study, passive thoracic limb stretching lowered wither height caused by possible relaxation of the fibromuscular thoracic girdle.[16] However, a randomized controlled trial in riding school

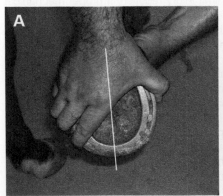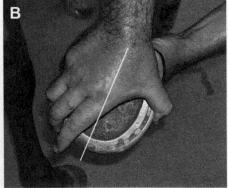

Fig. 1. Joint mobilization of the coffin joint in internal (*A*) and external (*B*) rotation. Note the reduced or asymmetric end range of motion induced during external rotation, compared with internal rotation (*white lines*).

horses evaluating the effect of two different 8-week passive stretching programs reported no significant changes in stride length at the trot but had a detrimental effect of decreasing joint range of motion within the shoulder, stifle, and hock articulations.[17]

The focus of recent equine chiropractic research has been on assessing the clinical effects of spinal mobilization and manipulation on pain relief, improving flexibility, reducing muscle hypertonicity, and restoring spinal motion symmetry. Spinal mobilization has been shown to be effective at increasing spinal flexibility in ridden horses without clinical signs of back pain.[12] Manipulation may preferentially stimulate receptors within deep intervertebral muscles, whereas mobilization techniques most likely affect more superficial axial muscles. Only one study has compared mobilization with manipulation in horses and spinal manipulation induced a 15% increase in displacement and a 20% increase in applied force, compared with mobilization.[18] At most vertebral sites studied, manipulation increased the amplitudes of dorsoventral displacement and applied force, indicative of increased spinal flexibility and increased tolerance to pressure in the thoracolumbar region of the equine vertebral column.

Manually applied forces associated with chiropractic techniques are able to produce substantial segmental spinal motion.[19] Additional studies have assessed the effects of equine chiropractic techniques on increasing passive spinal mobility (ie, flexibility)[12,18] and reducing longissimus muscle tone.[20] The effect of manipulation on asymmetrical spinal movement patterns in horses with documented back pain suggest that chiropractic treatment elicits slight but significant changes in thoracolumbar and pelvic kinematics and that some of these changes are likely to be beneficial.[21,22]

Equine osteopathic evaluation and treatment procedures have been described in textbooks and case reports, but no formal hypothesis-driven research exists.[23,24] A case series of 51 horses with chronic lameness or gait abnormalities that were poorly localized were treated with osteopathic techniques under sedation and had reported positive results in most cases from 6 to 12 months after treatment.[25]

WEAKNESS

Weakness (ie, lack of muscular strength) is a common but poorly recognized or easily localized disorder. The cause of weakness is often neurologic-based but clinically weakness is often attributed to muscular disorders because of the lack of epaxial muscle development, inability to perform advanced training techniques, asymmetrical movement patterns (eg, not bend to the left), or difficulty in clearing a jump. The most common cause of weakness is reflex inhibition caused by soft tissue or orthopedic pain. A lame horse is that is unable or unwilling to place full weight bearing on a limb also has distinct changes in muscle activation (ie, timing and amplitude of contractions). Muscles that have altered timing can include individual muscles that turn on too early or stay active too long or do not turn on at all. Muscles also have changes in the number of motor units activated, which directly correlates to the amplitude or strength of muscle contraction. A horse with a painful back often has accompanying muscle hypertonicity of varying degrees, which alters the resting muscle tone and threshold for muscle activation. A common misconception is that a hypertonic or muscle spasm is a "strong" muscle; however, because of chronic activation it is often a weak muscle with altered on-and-off timing that increases the risk of injury. Chronic pain often induces recruitment of peripheral or proximal limb muscles, which is interpreted clinically as altered gait patterns. Neurogenic atrophy is noted locally within a segmentally innervated myotome and varying degrees of disuse atrophy may be noticed more regionally over the lateral neck or dorsal trunk in horses with chronic neck or back pain.

MOTOR CONTROL

Manual forces are used to induce passive stretching, weight-shifting, or activation of spinal reflexes, which help to increase flexibility, stimulate proprioception, and strengthen core musculature.[6,26] Soft tissue mobilization has the additional effect of stimulating regional or systemic changes in neurologic signaling related to pain processing and motor control. Joint mobilization and manipulation can provide effective management of pain and neuromuscular deficits associated with musculoskeletal injuries, alterations in postural control, and locomotor issues related to antalgic or compensatory gait. In response to chronic pain or stiffness, new movement patterns are developed by the nervous system and adopted to reduce pain or discomfort. Long after the initial injury has healed, adaptive or secondary movement patterns may continue to persist, which predispose adjacent articulations or muscles to injury. Activation of proprioceptors, nociceptors, and components of the muscle spindles provide afferent stimuli that have direct and widespread influences on components of the peripheral and central nervous systems that directly regulate muscle tone and movement patterns. The various forms of manual therapy are thought to affect different aspects of joint function via diverse mechanical and neurologic mechanisms.

The goals of neuromuscular rehabilitation are to (1) identify the individual muscle or muscle groups involved; (2) diagnose the underlying cause of muscular dysfunction (or neurologic or muscular disease); (3) define the rehabilitation issue relevant for that horse on that day (ie, timing or amplitude); (4) develop and implement a focused rehabilitation plan to address the specific needs of the individual patient; and (5) provide objective outcome measures to assess accomplishment of goals and eventual return to optimal function. Manual therapy is a useful diagnostic and therapeutic tool in this process and is often combined with therapeutic exercises to help support rehabilitation process of neuromotor control.

Three-Legged Stance

The ability to stand comfortably on three limbs while one limb is elevated off of the ground is a measure of the musculoskeletal and nervous systems. If a sport horse is not able to stand quietly on one limb for a short period of time, then concerns may be raised about the strength and nociceptive and mechanoreceptive requirements to run at full speed, navigate turns or jumps, or to maintain collected movements for any period of time. The contralateral limb is required to double its weight-bearing load, which increases musculotendinous and ligamentous strain and may precipitate osteoarthritic pain. Because of the increased weight bearing and change in center of mass, the proximal musculature (ie, thoracic sling or pelvic girdle muscles) of the contralateral limb is also activated to maintain balance and stability. Sequential limb elevation is used to assess the ease of limb elevation and the quality of proprioceptive capabilities and neuromuscular strength (ie, core stability) within individual limbs.

Limb Circumduction

Static assessment is done with simple limb elevation and evaluation of the horse's ability to stand comfortably on three limbs for up to 20 to 30 seconds. Dynamic assessment includes the addition of induced distal limb circumduction in small repetitive circles about the size of a dinner plate. The circles are repeated in several locations, which include directly under the elevated forelimb, 12 inches cranial and caudal, and 12 inches lateral to the site of normal foot placement. The circumduction circles are done in either clockwise or counterclockwise directions. The horse is observed for the ability to let their distal limb be moved freely at the four different locations, which requires activation of different proximal muscle stabilization patterns and the ability to maintain balance on three limbs with mild perturbations in the center of mass. Horses without pain or neuromuscular dysfunction can easily stand while their distal limb is mobilized in these different positions. Horses with perceived weakness, pain, or poor core stability of the proximal limb musculature are not able to stand on three limbs, do not allow limb elevation or circumduction in one or all positions, or place excessive weight into the hands of the evaluator as they resist standing with their limb elevated. Limb circumduction exercises are used diagnostically and therapeutically to improve strength and proprioceptive awareness because of painful or diseased tissues within the limb.

Passive and Active-Assisted Limb Retraction

The quality and quantity of limb protraction and retraction also assesses the functional status of the musculoskeletal and nervous systems. If a sport horse is not able to readily extend its fore and hind limbs without pain or resistance or while maintaining proper balance, then concerns may be raised about flexibility issues and the nociceptive or neuromuscular status. Passive limb range of motion helps to assess the passive supporting structures of the limb and proximal attachments to the trunk, which include joint capsule, ligaments, and fascial components. Active engagement of the limb musculature during assisted limb retraction helps to assess over strength, coordination, and ability to perform these limb movements in a standing or static position and at end-ranges of overall limb motion. If horses are not able or willing to perform this type of limb movements in a low-impact setting, then questions or concerns could be raised about their optimal performance under active or ridden exercise with the high demands placed on the neuromuscular systems during athletic competition.

Active-assisted limb retraction is used diagnostically and therapeutically. While gently guiding a horse's forelimb backward (ie, retraction) to induce a slow and steady stretch, the handler asks for an "active stretch," which occurs when the horse leans into your supporting hands and actively stretches its forelimb backward (**Fig. 2**). Normally, horses should be able to retract their forelimb so that the forearm (radius and ulna) are moved caudally behind vertical with ease and comfort, which is a measure of forelimb flexibility. With active engagement and the willingness to extend the limb fully into retraction, proprioceptive signaling and motor control are assessed. In horses that do not actively retract their fore or hind limbs, lowering the hoof closer to the ground (ie, 3–6 inches off the ground) and asking for an "active stretch" again may be successful.

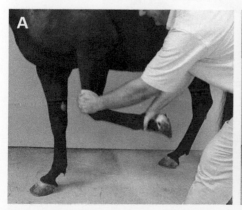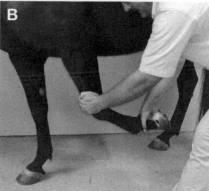

Fig. 2. Passive (*A*) and active-assisted (*B*) thoracic limb retraction stretches.

Passive and active-assisted hind limb retraction provides similar insights into hind limb range or motion and neuromuscular status. Normally, horses should be able to retract their hind limb so that the metatarsus is moved caudally behind vertical with ease and comfort. Active-assisted hind limb retraction asks for active engagement and assesses the ability and willingness to extend the limb fully into retraction (**Fig. 3**). Treatment involves using this same technique in a series of repetitions to help develop strength and coordination in the limb or direction of impairment.

Passive and Assisted Limb Protraction

Passive limb protraction induces a stretch in the supporting structures located along the caudal aspect of the limb. With the lower forelimb held in a flexed position, the stretch is localized to the upper forelimb and scapulothoracic junction (**Fig. 4**). As the forelimb is supported in full extension, then a passive stretch of the entire fore or hind limb is produced (**Fig. 5**). Hind limb flexibility in protraction is assessed by the measured distance between the forward reach of the hind hoof and the ipsilateral front hoof (**Fig. 6**). Assisted limb protraction seeks an "active stretch," which occurs when the horse leans into your support and actively stretches its forelimb forward into your supporting hands. In horses that do not actively protract their fore or hind limbs, lowering the hoof closer to the ground (ie, 3 inches off the ground) and asking for an "active stretch" again may be successful. Normally, horses should readily bring their hind foot to the level of or past the position of the front foot. This is especially true with assisted hind limb protraction, as the footfall of the hind limb is near the footfall of the forelimb during trotting exercise. In horses that readily produce active engagement at lower levels of foot placement, the hoof is raised slightly in 3-inch increments and repeated until the fore or hind limb is near horizontal position to maximize flexibility and core stability of the proximal limb attachments (**Fig. 7**).

Sternal Elevation Reflex

Horses with poor saddle fit and pain in the wither region or impinged dorsal spinous processes may benefit from trunk elevation or flexion exercises because of the induced stretching and separation of the soft tissues and bony structures along the

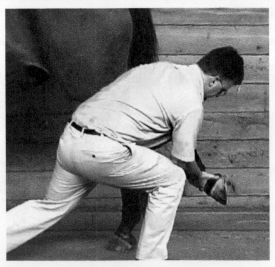

Fig. 3. Active-assisted pelvic limb retraction stretch.

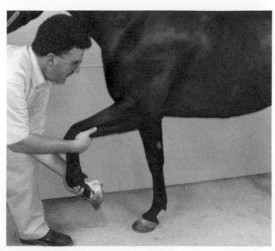

Fig. 4. Passive upper thoracic limb protraction stretch.

dorsal midline. Using spinal reflexes to diagnose and treat core stability issues is an important tool in managing sport horses. A spinal reflex that induces sternal elevation is done by applying upward fingertip pressure or scratching in a craniocaudal direction along the ventral midline of the sternum to induce active elevation of the cranial thoracic region (**Fig. 8**). As a natural response, most horses also lower their head and neck during active elevation of the withers. Initially, one may need to use strong upward pressure or fingernail pressure to induce elevation of the withers. If the horse does not respond, then the pressure may be applied with the fingernails of both hands or the pressure may be applied more caudally, at the xyphoid or along the midline of the cranial portion of the abdomen. Both the quality and quantity of movement are assessed during the spinal reflex response and the ability to hold or maintain the induced posture. The induced motion should be smooth and easy with the base of the withers elevating about 2 cm in normal horses. The goal is to help to develop core stabilization and movement of the scapulothoracic junction that forms the fibro-muscular sling between the thoracic limb and rib cage.

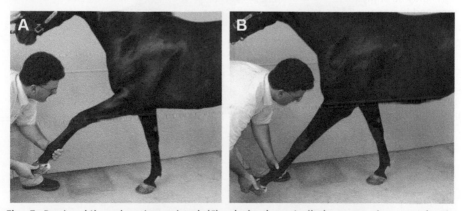

Fig. 5. Passive (*A*) and active-assisted (*B*) whole thoracic limb protraction stretch. The thoracic limb is fully extended and held at the end range of motion to promote elongation of soft tissues and increase neuromuscular activation.

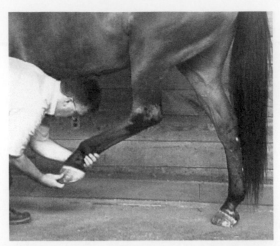

Fig. 6. Passive pelvic limb protraction stretch. The pelvic limb is brought into full extension to assess overall limb range of motion in protraction.

Horses with girth pain may react strongly to the applied pressure and often kick out, step away from the applied pressure, or maintain an elevated head and neck posture. Saddle fit and proper girth positioning, use, and fit should be evaluated in these affected horses. Some horses do not respond to any applied pressure along the ventral sternum. Asking the handler to lower the head below the height of the withers may help to assist or initiate active elevation of the withers. Rapid and repeated stimulation along the ventral midline or off to one side of the ventral midline along the edge of the deep pectoral muscle may also help to initiate the desired reflex.

Pelvic Flexion Reflex

Horses with lordosis, obvious epaxial muscle pain or hypertonicity, or trunk stiffness may benefit from induced pelvic and trunk flexion exercises. Active trunk flexion is

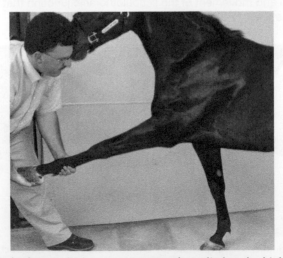

Fig. 7. Passive whole thoracic limb protraction stretch applied at the highest level possible above the ground while still remaining comfortable for this horse.

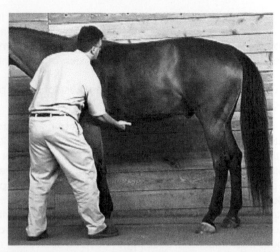

Fig. 8. Sternal elevation reflex with digital pressure applied along the ventral midline of the sternum while assessing the quality and quantity of elevation of the region caudal to the withers.

required in collective movements and horses with poor hind limb coupling or lack of impulsion may also benefit from this exercise. By applying firm digital pressure bilaterally along the intermuscular groove between the biceps femoris and semitendinosus muscles at a level lateral to the base of the tail, the natural response is induced pelvic (lumbosacral joint) flexion and elevation or induced kyphosis of the entire thoracolumbar region (**Fig. 9**). Moving the digital stimulation ventrally along the muscular groove is often required to identify the site that produces the most effective spinal reflex response. Once the horse produces active elevation of the back and flexion of the pelvis, then hold the finger contact to maintain the abdominal muscle contraction and stretch for up to 20 seconds. Again, the quality and quantity

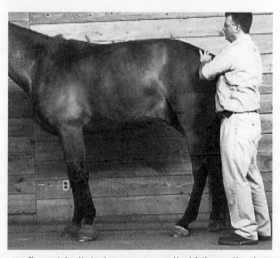

Fig. 9. Pelvic flexion reflex with digital pressure applied bilaterally along the intermuscular groove between the biceps femoris and semitendinosus muscles. Note the degree of pelvic flexion and trunk elevation (kyphosis) induced in this horse.

of movement are assessed during the induced movement. The induced motion should be smooth and fluent with clear pelvic flexion noted and elevation of the thoracolumbar junction by 2 to 4 cm. The goal is to strengthen and stimulate coordination of the muscles that lift the back and produce flexion of the trunk and pelvis (ie, collection).

Diagnostically, one of several responses occurs because of digital pressure applied over the croup region:

1. Normally, a horse without back or lumbosacral pain and with strong coupling or collection abilities strongly contracts the rectus abdominis muscle and the horse actively flexes the lumbosacral junction (ie, coupling) and elevates or flexes the trunk. Muscles responsible for producing lumbosacral flexion include the rectus abdominis, iliopsoas, and psoas minor muscles. The amount of trunk flexion produced by this exercise should at least produce flattening of the thoracolumbar spine. Optimally, a prolonged, steady kyphotic posture of the caudal thoracic and lumbar spine should be produced to induce maximal stretching of the dorsal epaxial musculature.
2. A horse with poor neuromuscular coupling or obvious back pain, muscle hypertonicity, or stiffness does not respond to any amount of applied pressure. Because this is an unusual aid, many normal horses may not respond initially to the applied pressure until they learn the desired response to the applied stimulus.
3. A horse with notable lumbosacral or gluteal pain may have an exaggerated response and buck or kick out on the hind limbs. It is always best to begin with light digital pressure and gradually increase the digital or fingernail pressure until an avoidance response or active spinal movement is noted.
4. Other horses produce active lumbosacral flexion without any elevation of the trunk or elevation of the trunk but no active flexion of the lumbosacral junction.

Therapeutically, if the horse has a weak, slow, or minimal response to the applied pressure, then repeated application of this exercise is indicated. If, after several repeated attempts, an exaggerated or painful response is consistently noted, then referral for evaluation of underlying back, lumbosacral, or pelvic pain or lameness is indicated.

Axial Tail Traction

The lateral tail pull tests or exercises are often used to assess hind limb weakness and proprioceptive status. Caudal or axial tail traction can also provide diagnostic and therapeutic insights into the horse's capabilities for lumbosacral coupling, canter movements, and pelvic stabilization. Horses with pain in the lumbosacral or sacroiliac regions and horses with poor hindquarter coupling and lack of impulsion benefit from this exercise. This exercise is best done in a quiet open space with horses that one is familiar with and if there are limited distractions in the immediate area. Cautiously move from the side and stand behind the horse while grasping the horse's tail firmly with both hands, about 6 inches below the tail head. Lean back slightly and gently apply slow and gradual caudal or axial traction to the tail. The tail and your line of pull should be parallel to the croup of the individual horse. Pull firmly for 5 seconds and monitor the contraction of both middle gluteal muscles along the top line of the pelvis (**Fig. 10**).

Diagnostically, one of several responses typically occurs during the application of tail traction:

1. Normally in a horse without back or tail pain and good coupling or collection abilities, you see a strong contraction of both croup (gluteal) muscles and the horse actively pull against you.

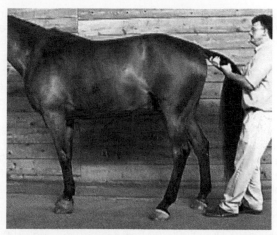

Fig. 10. Axial tail traction with firm, constant pressure applied caudally to induce a counter-resistive response and activation of bilateral middle gluteal muscles.

2. A horse with poor coupling or who is disunited allows you to pull on their tail but there is no visible gluteal muscle contraction or attempt to lean forward to resist your traction on the tail.
3. A horse with potential lumbosacral or tail pain dances from side-to-side and does not allow you to apply any pressure to the tail. If this response is seen, immediately discontinue the applied traction and reassess the horse's back, pelvic, and tail regions with your veterinarian.
4. Some horses contract only one gluteal muscle or consistently stand on one pelvic limb. If a horse consistently unweights one hind limb or refuses to stand on one limb, then applying traction slightly to the affected or unweighted limb helps the horse to redistribute its weight evenly on both hind limbs and begin equal contraction of both gluteal muscles.

Therapeutically, if the horse has a weak, slow, or minimal response, then slowly release the traction for 2 seconds and apply again for 2 seconds. Rhythmically repeat the applied traction and release procedures for up to 30 to 40 repetitions. When finished with the exercise, slowly release the applied traction on the tail. Do not let go of the horse's tail too fast because some horses resent this and kick out.

SUMMARY

Touch therapies, massage, joint mobilization, and manipulation are all critical components in the management of muscular, articular, and neurologic components of select injuries in performance horses. Musculoskeletal conditions that are chronic or recurring, not readily diagnosed, or are not responding to conventional veterinary care may be indicators that manual therapy evaluation and treatment is needed.

REFERENCES

1. Tellington-Jones L, Lieberman B. The ultimate horse behavior and training book. North Pomfret (VT): Trafalgar Square Books; 2006.
2. Scott M. The basic principles of equine massage/muscle therapy. Camden (SC): Massage/Muscle Therapy Productions; 2003.

3. Blignault K. Stretch exercises for your horse. London: J. A. Allen; 2003.
4. Bromiley MW. Massage techniques for horse and rider. Wiltshire (England): The Crowood Press Ltd; 2002.
5. Haussler KK. Chiropractic evaluation and management. Vet Clin North Am Equine Pract 1999;15:195–209.
6. Stubbs NC, Clayton HM. Activate your horse's core: unmounted exercises for dynamic mobility, strength and balance. Mason (MI): Sport Horse Publications; 2008.
7. Plaza-Manzano G, Vergara-Vila M, Val-Otero S, et al. Manual therapy in joint and nerve structures combined with exercises in the treatment of recurrent ankle sprains: a randomized, controlled trial. Man Ther 2016;26:141–9.
8. Weerasekara I, Osmotherly P, Snodgrass S, et al. Clinical benefits of joint mobilization on ankle sprains: a systematic review and meta-analysis. Arch Phys Med Rehabil 2017. [Epub ahead of print].
9. Jones LE, O'Shaughnessy DF. The pain and movement reasoning model: introduction to a simple tool for integrated pain assessment. Man Ther 2014;19:270–6.
10. Fedele C, Berens von Rautenfeld D. Manual lymph drainage for equine lymphoedema-treatment strategy and therapist training. Equine Vet Educ 2007; 19:26–31.
11. McBride SD, Hemmings A, Robinson K. A preliminary study on the effect of massage to reduce stress in the horse. J Equine Vet Sci 2004;24:76–82.
12. Sullivan KA, Hill AE, Haussler KK. The effects of chiropractic, massage and phenylbutazone on spinal mechanical nociceptive thresholds in horses without clinical signs. Equine Vet J 2008;40:14–20.
13. Zidonis NA, Snow A, Soderberg MK. Equine acupressure: a working manual. Larkspur (CO): Tallgrass Publishers, LLC; 2001.
14. Haussler KK, Erb HN. Pressure algometry: objective assessment of back pain and effects of chiropractic treatment. Proceedings of the 49th Annual Convention of the American Association of Equine Practitioners. New Orleans, Louisiana, November 21–25, 2003. pp. 66–70.
15. Frick A. Fitness in motion: keeping your equine's zone at peak performance. Guilford (CT): The Lyons Press; 2007.
16. Giovagnoli G, Plebani G, Daubon JC. Withers height variations after muscle stretching. Proceedings of the Conference on Equine Sports Medicine and Science (CESMAS). Oslo, Norway, September 24–26, 2004. p. 172–6.
17. Rose NS, Northrop AJ, Brigden CV, et al. Effects of a stretching regime on stride length and range of motion in equine trot. Vet J 2009;181:53–5.
18. Haussler KK, Hill AE, Puttlitz CM, et al. Effects of vertebral mobilization and manipulation on kinematics of the thoracolumbar region. Am J Vet Res 2007; 68:508–16.
19. Haussler KK, Bertram JEA, Gellman K. In-vivo segmental kinematics of the thoracolumbar spinal region in horses and effects of chiropractic manipulations. Proc Amer Assoc Equine Practitioners 1999;45:327–9.
20. Wakeling JM, Barnett K, Price S, et al. Effects of manipulative therapy on the longissimus dorsi in the equine back. Equine Comp Exerc Physiol 2006;3:153–60.
21. Faber MJ, van Weeren PR, Schepers M, et al. Long-term follow-up of manipulative treatment in a horse with back problems. J Vet Med A Physiol Pathol Clin Med 2003;50:241–5.
22. Gomez Alvarez CB, L'Ami JJ, Moffat D, et al. Effect of chiropractic manipulations on the kinematics of back and limbs in horses with clinically diagnosed back problems. Equine Vet J 2008;40:153–9.

23. Verschooten F. Osteopathy in locomotion problems of the horse: a critical evaluation. Vlaams Diergeneeskd Tijdschr 1992;61:116–20.
24. Pusey A, Colles C, Brooks J. Osteopathic treatment of horses: a retrospective study. Br Osteopathic J 1995;16:30–2.
25. Colles CM, Nevin A, Brooks J. The osteopathic treatment of somatic dysfunction causing gait abnormality in 51 horses. Equine Vet Educ 2014;26:148–55.
26. Goff LM. Manual therapy of the horse-a contemporary perspective. J Equine Vet Sci 2009;29:799–808.

Understanding the Basic Principles of Podiatry

Raul J. Bras, DVM, CJF, APF[a],*, Ric Redden, DVM[b]

KEYWORDS

- Podiatry • Therapeutic shoeing • Foot-related lameness • Mechanics

KEY POINTS

- Principles of therapeutic shoeing are based on the mechanical thought process of altering the internal forces as a means to aid preventing and/or treating the ill effects of foot-related lameness that frequently occur with the performance horse.
- Equine podiatry can be defined as a professional field of service that requires the efforts and dedicated responsibility of foot-focused veterinarians and pathologic focused farriers.
- The primary goal for therapeutic applications is to offset the mechanical limitations and enhance the healing environment.

Foot-related lameness is one of the most frequently encountered problems in the equine industry. Therapeutic shoeing is a frequently used preventative discipline for the treatment of many causes of lameness.[1-3] The primary goal for therapeutic applications is to offset the mechanical limitations and enhance the healing environment. The mechanical influence of trimming and shoeing for therapeutic purposes is poorly understood by some farriers and veterinarians. Generally, traditional trimming and shoeing goals are focused on creating a normal-appearing, well-balanced foot. This concept serves the horse well as long as it meets the ever-changing maintenance requirements of the foot. However, the terms normal, balanced, and therapeutic are subjective at best and are relative terms. Compared with what? Foot problems frequently occur despite of the very best efforts of competent, experienced, and highly respected farriers, but are seldom resolved with more of the same well-shod, balanced appearance concept that if it looks good it must be so. Without consideration of the forces within the foot that influence the vital vascular supply routes to horn growth centers, the healing mode is handicapped, and problematic issues persist shoeing after shoeing.

Regardless of the many variables, such as breed, limb conformation, and environment, that will change the overall shape of the foot, the ill effects from the demand of

---

Disclosures: None.
[a] Podiatry Department, Rood and Riddle Equine Hospital, 2150 Georgetown Road, Lexington, KY 40511, USA; [b] PO Box 507, Versailles, KY 40388, USA
* Corresponding author.
E-mail address: rbras@roodandriddle.com

their athletic careers could end up with compromised performance. More importantly, it must be remembered that the foot is constantly changing due to growth, the rigors of training, and farrier influence. External alterations of the hoof capsule can be evident to the astute eye. However, many crucial changes go unnoticed until lameness or other problems are evident. The key to understanding the mechanical thought process lies in the awareness that the forces within the foot have a direct influence on the shape, strength, and durability of the hoof capsule, and likewise, these forces are altered as the capsule changes.

The equine veterinarian is responsible for the overall soundness of the horse. However, they share this responsibility equally with the farrier, who is responsible for maintaining the overall health of the hoof capsule, using farrier knowledge and skills. Collaborative efforts of each highly respected profession are required for best results when foot issues become evident. Both professions become proficient through years of experience and skill development using their respective education, knowledge, and dedication.

Equine podiatry is a blend of the 2 highly respected professions each contributing to the task at hand, but neither formally educated and trained as collaborative team members with a common thread of podiatry principles. Therefore, learning the art of podiatry from the perspective of each profession requires each individual to develop working knowledge of the combination of farrier science and veterinary medicine as it relates to the foot. A thorough knowledge of traditional horseshoeing enables the veterinarian to better interact with the farrier, ultimately enhancing communication and promoting better-quality hoof care. The farrier who develops an eye for radiographic information and learns to recognize the value of using it to assist strategic mechanical decisions greatly enhances the collaborative efforts as well as its success.

Trimming and shoeing has a direct effect on a variety of parameters associated with the hoof and the limb above it. Normal foot function, breakover, the manner in which the foot lands, the duration of the stance phase of the stride, and ill effects of injuries related to landing and weight-bearing are all affected by trimming and shoeing. Thus, the mechanical model is altered to some degree with each swipe of the rasp. A thorough knowledge of farrier science and mechanics within the foot provides a better understanding of how to change and improve abnormal foot conformation, and how to improve distal limb function. This article focuses on the principles of therapeutic shoeing based on the mechanical thought process of altering the internal forces as a means to aid preventing and/or treating the ill effects of capsule distortion that frequently occurs with the performance horse. Recognizing subtle changes in hoof conformation and understanding what has changed internally enable one to preserve the integrity of the hoof capsule, along with the structures enclosed within, and thus prevent many of the associated lameness in the performance horse.[4]

Understanding the forces at play that underlie the mechanical failure allows a more precise strategic management to be formulated. A key element relative to this discussion is the interconnectedness of all components of the digit. The interconnectedness of the digital structures allows the foot to function as an integrated unit, supporting the body and dissipating the forces of ground impact and loading to prevent overload and damage of any one particular component. Owing to the interconnectedness of the digital structures, when one component is weakened by genetic factors, overload, injury, disease, environmental factors, or human interference, the entire hoof capsule is weakened. A cascade of damage, altered growth, and hoof capsule distortion is inevitable, because all components are affected when one fails. As a result, the function of the entire digit is compromised.[5]

DEMANDS ON THE FOOT FOR THE PERFORMANCE HORSE

Regardless of breed, once horses go into training, the ill effects of training and shoeing along with sudden changes in nutrition and the environment demands on the foot quickly change the overall hoof capsule as well as the radiographic soft tissue parameters. Is the foot still normal as it goes through these noticeable changes? More importantly, how long can the horse remain sound or how much can the hoof capsule change before lameness is evident? An increase in training intensity often pushes the foot over the edge by significantly increasing the tensile, compressive, and shearing forces on the digital structures. A hoof capsule with adequate mass and resilience may be able to withstand these stresses without significant deleterious effects. A weakened hoof capsule has neither the strength nor the plasticity of a healthy horn. As a result, repeated compression during high-intensity exercise causes hoof capsule distortions.[6]

Once young horses go into training, most are confined to stalls or small pens and are inactive for most of the day. The germinal areas of the hoof capsule are dynamic tissues that respond and adapt to the forces placed on the horn; thus, inactivity can have a negative effect on the hoof capsule. The routine of most athletic horses is characterized by many hours of inactivity. This lifestyle has a negative effect on the foot. When the natural demand for toughness and durability of the protective capsule is not met, circulation of the foot is reduced due to inactivity and excessive moisture, which contributes to horn distortion more than any normal activity. Subtle but steady deterioration may be occurring in the horn, soft tissue, bone, and circulation of the foot, all while the horse is doing nothing. The weakened foot is then more susceptible to overload during athletic activity.[6] The tough durable hoof capsule is relatively rigid with limited distortion and natural recall that occur with each step. Excessive moisture that may be due to environmental conditions or man made with the practice of mudding feet to remove heat consistently weaken the horn integrity and make it more vulnerable to distortion that is incapable of natural recall. The cumulative ill effects are precursors to the crushed heel syndrome.

Unlimited exercise during turnout or intense exercise during training and competition can become a major trigger for overload and, ultimately, for distortion of the weakened hoof capsule. The hoof capsule with adequate mass (sole and horn), durability, and resilience has a much-improved chance to withstand the stresses placed upon it without significant deformation. The drawback of training a horse with steadily declining capsule strength is the risk of foot-related lameness. Repeated compression and strain during strenuous exercise cause hoof capsule distortions. The stronger feet will have natural recall and recover, whereas the weaker feet fall prey to the cumulative negative effects and soon lose the function of their natural shock absorbing, protective components.

MORPHOLOGY OF THE HOOF

Although certain generalities can be made, it is important to realize that there is a range of normal for hoof characteristics that is dependent on the horse's breed, age, environment, and discipline of use regardless of sport, breed, or discipline. The importance of understanding the variability in structure of the healthy foot lies in identifying subtle deviations from normal that are of clinical significance. One must overcome the "ideal" perception of the normal equine foot depicted in the veterinary and farrier literature for the past century as being symmetric and matching the opposite foot as well as that of other horses of similar breed. Matching toe and heel angles simply do not exist on healthy feet. Toe angles, once idealized as 45° for front feet and

50° for hindfeet, are a misconception because this combination only occurs with a very small population of horses that would have remarkably lower coffin bone angles than the average horse. The 45° hoof angle with a 50° to 52° bone angle would have a negative palmar angle (PA), crushed heel, and broken back pastern axis, a far cry from the ideal healthy foot[7] (**Fig. 1**). A rigid set of toe lengths, toe angles, and shoeing limitations can be problematic in disciplines that insist on recording toe angle measurements without regard to the coffin bone angle and shape that is the precursor of toe angles. It is also important to make the distinction between normal and healthy. Normal according to Webster is conforming to a standard, what is typical or expected, and it is this mindset that erroneously allows the belief that normal and healthy are one in the same. Most of the feet seen irrespective of breed with very similar shape are considered normal for that breed and discipline. However, this certainly does not mean the feet are healthy even though the horse appears sound and at the peak of their career. What may commonly be seen can be far from what is healthy for the individual foot on the individual horse. This leads to understanding podiatry principles.

SPECIFIC RADIOGRAPHIC PRINCIPLES

Being able to see, rationalize, and interpret what cannot be seen by observing the external capsule is one of the greatest benefits when studying the complex mechanical model because it allows veterinarians as well as farriers to develop better informed decisions relative to their respective roles as podiatry team members. This brings up an important point. The farrier world is vastly different from that of veterinarians because years of experience with multiple breeds puts literally thousands of feet in their hands with a great responsibility to keep them as healthy and sound as possible. The hands, eyes, and body language become programmed for small details and variations of normal concerning the unique characteristics of the external capsule, and

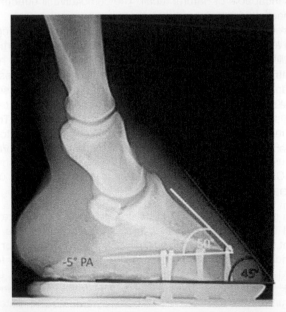

Fig. 1. Evidence of a 45° hoof angle with a 50° bone angle, which has a negative PA of 5°, crushed heel, and broken back pastern axis.

most spend their life working without the valuable information that is so easily produced with radiographs. Nevertheless, this does not negate their tremendous responsibility of enhancing the healing environment with therapeutic trimming and shoeing when foot issues occur.

Equine podiatry can be defined as a professional field of service that requires the efforts and dedicated responsibility of foot-focused veterinarians and pathologic focused farriers. The art of podiatry has an inherent learning curve that starts with knowledge of the inside of the foot. Important clinical decisions are made on the basis of measurements of only a few degrees of angulation in magnitude.[8] Digital radiography allows the most accurate and repeated measurements of certain parameters that are used as an important aid to trimming and the application of therapeutic shoes.[8] Specific radiographic information differs slightly from that produced with the traditional standard recommended views because the specific information sought is focused on particular areas of interest (**Fig. 2**). The new standard low-beam projection is the recommended standard when seeking answers for podiatry issues. This standard produces repeatable, comparative images from foot to foot and horse to horse, offering a reliable means of learning the large range of unique characteristics and the value of parameter alterations of greatest interest. This new standard also provides the farrier information that pertains to his or her decisions concerning mechanical therapeutic trimming and shoeing. The effects of altering hoof angles on distal limb joint angles have been described.[2,3,8] Adhering to the smallest details when taking radiographs and staying focused on positive mechanical benefits can assist farrier decisions and enhance the chances of success. Using specific beam/subject/cassette orientation focused on the particular area of interest, the clinician can produce consistent, comparable images that offer the best representation of the soft tissue parameters, the coffin bone, and the hoof capsule, thus enabling strategic decisions. This information is of utmost importance as a set of reference points for therapeutic trimming and shoeing decisions because they define the interconnectedness of the internal structures with external hoof-capsule characteristics.

The low-beam lateral-medial projection produces consistent, comparable images of the soft tissue parameters, which hold valuable information for the veterinarian-farrier team, for example, sole depth and cup (SD), PA, horn/lamellar zone, and digital breakover (DB) (**Fig. 3**). The low-beam dorsal-palmar (plantar) image reveals

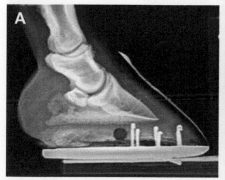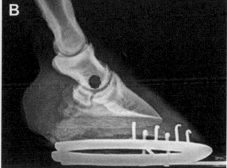

Fig. 2. (*A*) Low beam, horizontal to the ground, centered to the foot, 10 to 20 mm above the positioning blocks, perpendicular to the sagittal plane and cassette, producing one branch of the shoe. (*B*) High beam, positioned just below the coronary band, producing 2 branches of the shoe and both wings with an illusion of medial/lateral imbalance.

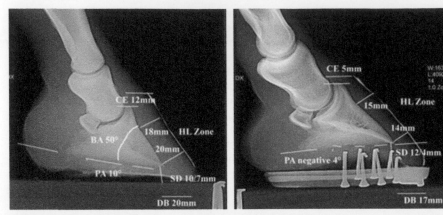

Fig. 3. Note the basic parameter information that can be consistently obtained from the low-beam projection. BA, Bone Angle; CE, Coronary band; HL, horn/lamellar zone.

medial-lateral coffin bone rim balance and should identify whether a higher projection is indicated to evaluate coffin and pastern joint articular symmetry (**Fig. 4**). These particular areas of interest are not distorted by oblique beam travel nor obscured by the shoe. They are of great interest because each can be altered by the rasp, farrier's knife, nippers, shoe style, and placement. The information that can be obtained from this low-beam protocol has diagnostic as well as prognostic value and is a reliable means of monitoring the efficiency of therapeutic trimming and shoeing, and

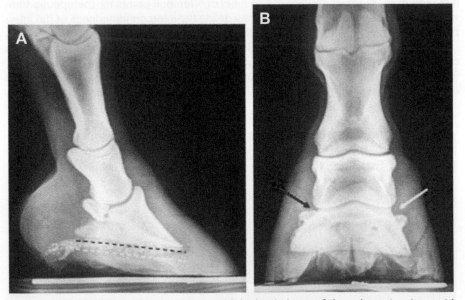

Fig. 4. (*A*) The low-beam lateral images reveal the load planes of the palmar rim along with associated soft tissue parameters and coffin-bone characteristics and allude to joint-plane symmetry. (*B*) The low-beam dorsal-palmar (plantar) image reveals medial-lateral coffin bone rim balance and should identify whether a higher projection is indicated to evaluate coffin and pastern joint articular symmetry.

preventive foot-maintenance programs. Veterinarians are responsible for obtaining the images that are useful guidelines for the trimming, shoe design, and application. Interpreting the parameters from even a medical standpoint requires good working knowledge of the foot. When those basic requirements are yet to be learned, the veterinarian must rely heavily on collaboration with the farrier. The farrier who has never had the opportunity to learn how to use radiographic information to help him or her fine-tune their efforts must then rely equally on the experience and dedication of the veterinarian. There are several parameters that are important for the farrier to know, because each is altered with every trim and shoeing procedure. The PA, SD, and DB are invariably altered with every trim and shoe application, because the farrier removes ground surface wall and sole. When pathologic condition and imbalance require specific mechanical realignment, it is vital that farriers know what they have to work with and what, if any, limitations need to be addressed before they start. When specific mechanical goals are to be achieved, it is important that the farrier be well aware of these parameters, especially when the horse is faced with career and life-threatening issues (**Fig. 5**).

Farriers have developed more confidence with complex cases by increasing their knowledge and skills through radiographic information that enables them to visualize what they have to work with and how well they can follow their goals. Veterinarians who have adopted this protocol also have gained knowledge, confidence, and skills as they become more involved with searching for useful information that before was not available to the team effort. Formerly generic recommendations, such as to raise or lower the heel, back the toe up, or tip the inside, can now be replaced with more specific reference points and parameters, and more favorable results can be expected as the farrier and veterinarian become more aligned with basic podiatry principles. The odds for success are greatly improved when farriers use radiographic information as it relates to their respective task at hand, and the veterinarian has working knowledge of the therapeutic trimming and shoeing process.

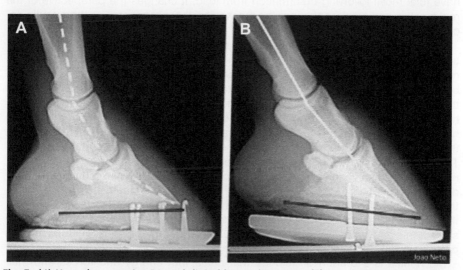

Fig. 5. (*A*) Note the negative PA and digital bone alignment. (*B*) Increasing the mechanical benefits resulted in a zero capsule PA and 6° ground PA with improved digital bone alignment. (*Courtesy of* Joao Neto, CF, APF, College Station, TX; with permission.)

MECHANICAL PRINCIPLES

The interconnectedness of the digital structures allows the foot to function as an integrated unit, supporting the body and dissipating the forces of the ground impact, and loading to prevent overload and damage of any one component. However, all components of the hoof capsule are connected to the muscles and tendons of the limb that are solely responsible for support and locomotion. Therefore, it can be said that without these controlling forces, the foot alone would be nonfunctional. Consistent and reliable clinical evidence supports the thought that the function of the deep digital flexor tendon (DDFT) plays a major role in equalizing the relationship between digital load and the vascular supply that is vital for the overall health of the foot. It is only prudent that the function of the DDFT is considered when attempting to maintain a healthy robust foot, preventing the proverbial crushed heel, quarter cracks, thin soles, bruises, shelly walls, and the associated ill effects. Distortion of one component is inevitably associated with distortion of adjoining components, albeit to a lesser degree in many cases.[7]

Breaking the complex foot model down into 2 basic zones with very different but complementing functions is a helpful means of developing the mechanical thought process for farriers and veterinarians. Visualizing the deep flexor muscle/tendon as a support component attached to the coffin bone that is statically attached to the laminae and the laminae in turn to the horn capsule completing the basic suspension of the digits. This unique arrangement makes the laminae and DDFT opposing antagonists. For every force, there is a resisting force, and these 2 very plastic but extremely strong components play a major role regulating the blood flow to this vital structure that is under constant alteration with the healthy foot as well as those suffering from a variety of conditions.[9] The support structures complement the suspension by acting as an energy sink as the digits descend under load and bottom out, so to speak, with ground contact. The support components consist of the digital cushion, frog, bars, sole, sole corium, and ground surface wall. If it is considered that a foot is balanced when the suspension and support components are in harmony and equilibrium, and have total recall following deformation from load, it changes the perspective of the real problem and greatly enhances the mechanical thought process as therapeutic decisions are contemplated (**Fig. 6**).

The biomechanics of the equine hoof are not well understood. Much of the information remains subjective, controversial, or unclear despite the abundance of new information related to various effects of therapeutic shoeing techniques and lower limb biomechanics. A major contributing factor to this is that most studies have evaluated the biomechanical effects of shoeing techniques on sound horses, and many others have been in vitro studies. In the case of performance research, most of the studies have evaluated horses not wearing tack or carrying a rider. It is only prudent to support the study with follow-up effect and outcome of proposed concepts and techniques. The absence of tissue response seriously limits the usefulness of in vitro and computer model data. Biomechanical studies of the foot could also be improved by requiring a detailed description of the external as well as internal characteristics of the feet in the study. Not one horse in any study will have matching symmetric feet; therefore, the conclusion data would most likely be remarkably different between feet on the same horse as well as between individuals. Therefore, the conclusion could also be different.

Mechanics is a branch of science that deals with energy and forces and their effect on bodies or the functional parts of an activity. Considering the complexity of the equine foot, it is only prudent that the forces at play and their influence on

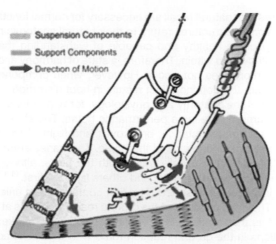

Fig. 6. Mechanical thought process: a foot is balanced when the suspension and support components are in harmony and equilibrium and have total recall following deformation from load.

all components are understood. There are significant gaps in the knowledge regarding how therapeutic trimming and shoeing interventions affect the function of the structures of the foot. Fortunately, there has been considerable progress in the current understanding of the biomechanical basis underlying the function of the digit. Over the years, countless types of shoes and techniques have been developed not only as a therapeutic aid to treat lameness but also to maintain or enhance functionality.[2]

FUNCTION, CONFORMATION, AND BALANCE

Understanding and observation of distal limb function, conformation, and balance is the basis of identifying where the greatest abnormal stresses within the distal limb are likely to occur.[6] This is a learned art that requires astute ongoing dedication and hands-on experience with the capsule as well as the relationship of internal components. Lameness is frequently the result of repeatedly applied stresses that exceed the capacity of the tissues; therefore, recognizing poor conformation or balance that might impair optimal function and contribute to lameness might suggest avenues for treatment.

It is important to understand distal limb function, because there is optimum balance for any given conformation, and a change in one plane influences the other. The terms conformation and balance are used frequently, and both refer, at least in part, to the shape and size of the distal limb, which in turn, is dependent on the shape and size of the individual elements of the distal limb and the spatial relations between them. Balance could be considered a subset of conformation, but balance refers not just to the appearance of the hoof but also by how dynamically the foot and its internal components interact with the ground. Conformation describes the static relations of the limb, including the foot, and balance describes both the static and the dynamic relations within the hoof, between the hoof and the ground, and the ground and the rest of the limb. This distinction has implications for treatment of lameness or poor performance in horses because balance can be manipulated in the adult horse, whereas conformation is relatively permanent.[6]

Durable structures with natural recall are necessary for normal function of the foot as well as for locomotion. All structures return to their natural anatomic relationship provided the hoof capsule is healthy and capable of withstanding the various forces placed on it from without and within. Therefore, a state of harmony and equilibrium exists, and hoof distortion does not occur. However, when components of the hoof capsule are weakened, the domino effect results in hoof distortion.

An understanding of the anatomy and physiology, form, and function of the foot is imperative when examining the lame performance horse. The stride is divided into 5 phases: initial contact, impact, stance, breakover, and flight.[10] The foot moves in a sagittal plane parallel to the long axis of the horse. This varies among horses due to conformation. Initial contact is usually made with the heels, although some horses land flatfooted, some on the lateral side, and others land toe first.[11,12] The propensity to land flatfooted increases with speed. Toe-first contact is rare unless there is foot-related lameness. The point of action of the ground reaction force is at the heels during initial contact, and its magnitude is low. The impact phase is marked by rapid high-frequency oscillations in the ground reaction force with a point of action toward the heels.[8] The oscillations are significantly reduced at the level of the first phalanx, indication that the soft tissues of the hoof, interposed articulations, and digital venous plexus are absorbing the energy impact. The vertical velocity and acceleration are greater in the forelimb than in the hind limbs, which may partially explain why the forefeet are more frequently injured.[13] The stance phase extends from the end of impact until the beginning of breakover. The point of action of the ground reaction force is centered in the foot, slightly medial to the dorsal third of the frog.[13] During the first half of the stride, the craniocaudal component of the ground reaction force of the foot is directed caudally, decelerating the limb; during the second half of the stride, it is directed cranially, propelling the horse forward. Toward the end of the stance phase, the point of action of the ground reaction force moves toward the toe.[11] With increasing speed, the ground reaction force increases, and the strain in the hoof wall and tension in the tendons increase. The breakover phase begins when the heels lift off the ground and ends when the toe leaves the ground. Once the heels are off the ground, the point of action of the ground reaction force is at the toe. The flight phase begins when the toe leaves the ground as the limb completes retraction and ends when the heel makes contact with the ground after protraction of the limb. The way in which a horse breaks over is influenced by conformation of the limb and foot, shoe styles and trim, and the influence of pain throughout the phases of the stride. These variables also contribute to the flight path of the foot, and the flight path of the foot contributes the way the foot lands. This relationship is used by farriers to correct interference problems and improve the appearance of the gait. Requesting radiographic information and input from the veterinarian teamed up with a farrier complements suggestions, and recommendations can often enhance therapeutic shoeing success.

INFLUENCE OF THE DEEP DIGITAL FLEXOR TENDON

Appropriate tension in the DDFT is necessary for normal digital structure and function as well as for locomotion. Provided the hoof capsule is healthy and able to withstand the various forces placed on it from without and within, normal and appropriate tension in the DDFT does not unduly distort the hoof capsule. When any component of the hoof capsule is weakened by genetics, overload, injury, disease, environmental factors, or human interference, however, the pull of the DDFT can cause or exacerbate distortion of the hoof capsule.[7]

Radiographic contrast studies, known as venograms, on healthy and pathologic issues clearly reveal the relationship between load, laminae, sole corium, and vascular patency, which helps to explain the disparity in wall growth.[11] They graphically illustrate the influence of the DDFT on the laminar attachment and thus on the hoof wall (**Fig. 7**). If the limb is fully loaded during injection of the contrast agent into the digital vein, vascular filling of the laminar corium is limited. However, relieving tension in the DDFT by slightly flexing the horse's carpus during dye injection allows normal filling of the laminar corium. This finding indicates that when the DDFT is under tension, so too is the laminar attachment, particularly in the dorsal aspect of the hoof wall. This tension is transferred via the dermal-epidermal laminar connection to the horn of the wall.

INFLUENCES OF SHOEING

Shoeing horses has several influences on normal foot function. The weight of a shoe increases the moment about the distal joints of the limb.[6] In the performance horse, this increases animation, which is considered desirable in some disciplines. It increases stride duration, but does not increase stride length.[14] However, increasing the weight of the distal limb is likely to result in increased fatigue. The flat surface of a shoe can cause a horse to slide further after impact on a hard surface than if the horse was barefoot.[15] Also, the ability of the hoof to accommodate to an uneven surface because of its viscoelastic nature maybe reduced as a result of the rigid nature of the shoe. The attachment of a shoe to a foot reduces expansion of the hoof capsule, but it does not prevent the heels from expanding.[16] It also increases the maximum deceleration of the foot and increases the frequency of vibrations as the foot impacts the ground and the maximum ground reaction force.[17] This effect on reduced damping of impact forces by the hoof is negligible at the level of the metacarpophalangeal joint.[18] Shoes reduce the decrease in pressure within the digital cushion associated with weight-bearing during the stride and increase pressure on the navicular bone from the DDFT.[19] Interestingly, shoes do not change the point of application of the ground reaction force nor do they change the stresses within the hoof wall, although

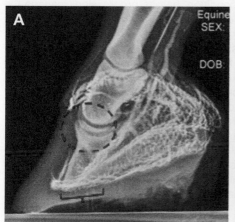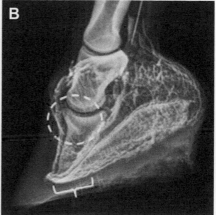

Fig. 7. Venograms. Influence of the DDFT on the laminar attachment. (*A*) When the limb is fully loaded during injection of the contrast agent into the digital vein, vascular filling of the laminar corium is limited. (*B*) Relieving tension in the DDFT during dye injection allows normal filling of the laminar corium.

they do cause some reorientation of these stresses.[20] In addition to altering the kinematics of the distal limb and biomechanics of hoof function, shoes influence the rate of wear and growth of the foot. A shoe prevents natural wear from the weight-bearing of the foot. Therefore, instead of maintaining a consistent length, the length of the foot fluctuates with the shoeing cycle, causing changes in the moment about the distal interphalangeal joint.[6]

HOOF CAPSULE DISTORTIONS

Many foot-related lameness issues involve hoof capsule distortions. Hoof capsule distortions occur when the tensile, compressive, or shearing forces on the hoof exceed the capacity of the hoof capsule components to withstand them. There are 3 basic situations in which the loading capacity of a structure can be exceeded: normal load on an abnormal structure, abnormal load on a normal structure, and abnormal load on an abnormal structure. The latter is a more reliable recipe for distortion and perhaps outright destruction of the compromised component.[7]

Understanding the basic mechanisms of hoof capsule distortions and foot-related lameness enables the clinician to unravel the sometimes complex mix of abnormalities, identify early warning signs, and manage existing problems more effectively. Evaluating each of the components of the hoof capsule, both individually and as an integrated unit, allows the clinician to address the primary and secondary problems and come up with effective options for countering or attenuating the forces responsible for the distortion. The shape of the distorted hoof capsule reflects the distribution of loads across the foot. The severity of the defects thus depends on the severity and duration of the imbalance. One must bear in mind that the normal equine limb is not evenly loaded with the medial side normally bearing proportionately more load than the lateral side. This fact is reflected in the subtle but important differences in shape and density of the horn, soft tissues, bone, and vasculature between medial and lateral sides of the digit. These abnormalities compromise circulation to the germinal layers of the hoof capsule, thus retarding horn growth in affected areas, which further distorts the hoof capsule. A perfectly symmetric foot does not exist, and one should not be attempting to create such a foot with manipulations.

Although we may able to improve the condition, halt its progression, manage the secondary effects, and improve the appearance of the foot, it must be accepted that the misunderstood distortion cannot be prevented or completely resolved. Attempting to do so can have deleterious effects on other components of the digit. As we attempt to deal with one area of the foot, we must remain aware of the ill effects our manipulations may have on related structures. One must bear in mind that there is an interrelated network of structures involved: DDFT, P3, laminar attachment, solar corium, and hoof capsule. When altering one component, it is important to consider the effect that action is likely to have on the other structures.

Failure to understand the normal structure and function of the equine foot and to manage the foot and the horse accordingly has deleterious effects. With existing problems, developing these skills enhances the clinician's ability to interpret the degree of damage accurately and to devise mechanical solutions that create an environment in which healing and restoration of function are maximized.

GOALS AND PRINCIPLES OF THERAPEUTIC TRIMMING AND SHOEING

The function of the hoof can be affected by environment, discipline, exercise, and farriers to mention just a few. The hoof has the ability to respond relative to its structural characteristics and its natural tolerance of the mechanical challenges, or by adaptation with changes in growth rate and shape.[1] The stance phase is considered the most critical part of the stride for developing injuries of the musculoskeletal system.[21] The stance phase is when the foot is in contact with the ground and the limb is therefore subjected to an external impact force by the ground. This external impact is termed the ground reaction force, the magnitude of which depends on the horse's weight, speed of movement, and the surface on which the horse moves.[22] Lameness during the loading phase will alter the landing as well as breakover and influence the stride phase of the support limb as the horse becomes reluctant to load and prematurely unloads the painful foot. The horse must surely feel the discomfort from folded heel tubules, drastic loss of digital cushion, medial unnatural listing, joint imbalance, thin soles, and a negative PA long before showing detectable soreness. This may explain why these common signs of hoof distortion are often not taken seriously until it is very obvious something is wrong with the foot.

Mechanical therapeutic trimming and shoeing techniques attempt to unload a specific painful or compromised area by shifting the load to more healthy components. When considering therapeutic shoeing to enhance soundness or to prevent further capsule distortion to, it is hoped, ward off future problems, it is useful to keep in mind the type of horse, hoof, conformation, internal parameters, discipline, exercise regimen, environment, surface the horse works on, and extent of the distortion and associated unsoundness. The latter is important, because the therapeutic shoe-ground interaction is often at the heart of the success or failure of the intended treatment.

In general, the goals of mechanical therapeutic shoeing are based on the relationship of the suspension and support components. Remarkably, reducing the tension of the DDFT relative to the intensity of the tissue lesion or hoof distortion using a variety of breakover enhanced trims and/or shoes is the basis for mechanical shoeing. This can be broken down into 4 basic goals: (1) reducing concussion to the foot in general with focus on specific areas, (2) shifting load away from painful or compromised components to healthier areas, (3) altering the distribution of force, and (4) changing the ease of movement about the distal interphalangeal joint. Preventive maintenance is the key; however, there are many variables that we cannot control that lead to foot injury despite having durable robust feet.

In general, the goals of mechanical therapeutic trimming and shoeing will be quite different than goals set forth with guidelines for flat trims and application of flat shoes. There are advantages and disadvantages of both shoeing concepts that need to be taken into consideration relative to the nature of the condition affecting the foot, the severity of the problem, immediate and long-term goals of the client, and the level of knowledge and experience of the farrier using focused, radiographic-guided mechanics. Fine tuning the mechanics requires working knowledge of the function of the suspension, support components, radiographic parameter interpretation, and working knowledge of how mechanics can enhance the healing environment. This is one of the disadvantages because there is a learning curve required for all farriers as they step into a totally different dimension of therapeutic shoeing. It is also more time consuming than flat shoeing because it requires close attention to the effect of the trim, shoe features, and how they relate to internal structures relative to the level of mechanics to be achieved.

Basic goals for the crushed heel, negative PA are to reestablish digital alignment, a zero to slightly positive PA, coffin joint symmetry, and preserve sole mass distal to the apex of the coffin bone. The trim lines are determined from the radiographic parameters, for example, sole depth PA, DB, and coffin joint medial, lateral spacing. These basic goals are met by trimming the ground surface to a slightly positive PA from toe to just caudal to the widest point of the foot. The crushed, folded heel tubules are trimmed in a manner that removes the distorted wall down to solid relatively straight horn tubules (**Fig. 8**). Various styles of rocker shoes can then be forged to meet the trimmed profile. The peak of the breakover should be directly distal to the center of articulation. This mechanical benefit remarkably increases the PA, loads the heel to the widest part of the frog, has a significant degree of self-adjustment, and allows most horses to remain in training relative to the degree of soft tissue damage.

Hindfeet notoriously have crushed heels, bull-nosed dorsal wall, and negative plantar angles on a large population of performance horses. Close observation reveals hindfeet are mismatched just as frequently as front feet, and most probably there is a connection. The hindfoot that is directly behind the steeper foot in front routinely has a lower profile heel than its opposite. This asymmetry can be detected by observing the heel height from behind, the relationship of the coronary band angle with the ground, and the plantar angle viewed on the low-beam lateral radiograph. The big advantage with rocker mechanics is the ability to remarkably reestablish digital alignment and a positive PA, each enhancing in a favorable tissue response (**Fig. 9**).

PREVENTION

Mechanical benefits that can produce medical benefits appear to be a major key to therapeutic and pathologic shoeing. A well-made strategic plan based on the basic mechanical requirements of the foot can greatly improve the outcome and success of many podiatry cases. Understanding the basic principles of podiatry allows the veterinarian and farrier to manage the hoof in such a manner to aid the prevention of foot-related lameness, maintain a sounder horse, and implement therapeutic shoeing when necessary.

As with many other types of foot-related lameness, prevention is much more effective than treatment. Prevention begins with careful observation. It is important that detrimental changes in the foot be recognized early and dealt with appropriately while there is still a chance to preserve the integrity of the foot.

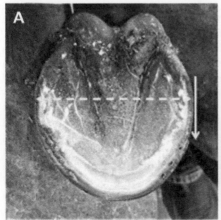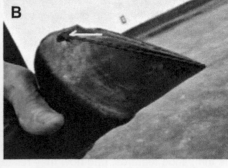

Fig. 8. (*A*) Basic goals for the crushed heel, negative PA are met by trimming the ground surface to a slightly positive PA from toe to just caudal to the widest point of the foot. (*B*) The folded heel tubules are trimmed in a manner that removes the distorted wall down to solid relatively straight horn tubules and back to the base of the frog. Note the red line represents traditional flat trim concepts that would leave excessive toe length and a negative PA.

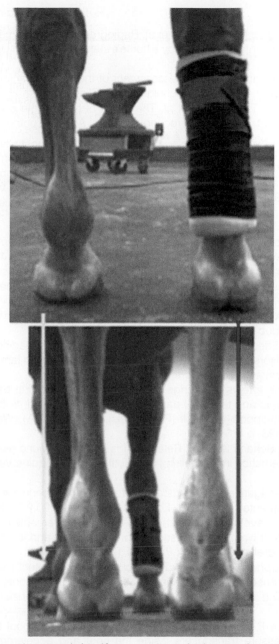

Fig. 9. Close observation reveals hindfeet are mismatched just as frequently as front feet. The hindfoot that is directly behind the steeper foot in front routinely has a lower profile heel than its opposite.

REFERENCES

1. Pauwels F, Rogers C, Wharton H, et al. Radiographic measurements of hoof balance are significantly influenced by a horse's stance. Vet Radiol Ultrasound 2017; 58(1):10–7.
2. Eliashar E. An evidence-based assessment of the biomechanical effects of the common shoeing and farriery techniques. Vet Clin North Am 2007;23:425–42.
3. Bushe T, Turner T, Poulos P, et al. The effect of hoof angle on coffin, pastern and fetlock joint angles, in proceedings. Am Assoc Equine Pract 1988;33: 729–38.
4. Meriam JG. The role and importance of farriery in equine veterinary practice. Vet Clin North Am 2003;19:273–83.
5. Redden R. Radiographic imaging of the equine foot. Vet Clin North Am Equine Pract 2003;19:379–92.
6. Parks A. Form and function of the equine digit. Vet Clin North Am 2003;19: 285–307.
7. Redden R. Hoof capsule distortion: understanding the mechanisms as a basis for rational management. Vet Clin North Am Equine Pract 2003;19:443–62.
8. Back W, Schamhardt HC, Hartman W, et al. Kinematic differences between the distal portions of the forelimbs and hind limbs of horses at the trot. Am J Vet Res 1995;56:1552–8.
9. Redden RF. A technique for performing digital venography in the standing horse. Equine Vet Educ 2001;3(3):172–8.
10. Clayton HM. Effects of hoof angle on locomotion and limb loading. In: White NA, Moore JN, editors. Current techniques in equine surgery and lameness. 2nd edition. Philadelphia: WB Saunders; 1998. p. 504–9.
11. Balch OK. The effects of change in hoof angle, mediolateral balance, and toe length on kinetic and temporal parameters of horse walking, trotting and cantering on a high-speed treadmill [PhD thesis]. Pullman (WA): Washington State University; 1993. p. 21–30.
12. Merkens HW, Schamhardt HC. Relationships between ground reaction force patterns and kinematics in the walking and trotting horse. Equine Vet J Suppl 1994; 17:67–70.
13. Barrey E. Investigation of the vertical hoof force distribution in the equine forelimb with an instrumented horseboot. Equine Vet J Suppl 1990;9:35–8.
14. Willeman MA, Savelberg HH, Barneveld A. The improvements of the gait quality of sound trotting warmblood horses by normal shoeing and its effect on the load on the lower forelimb. Livestock Prod Sci 1997;52:145–53.
15. Hertch B, Hoppner S, Dallmer H. The hoof and how to protect it without nails. 1st edition. Salzhausen-Puetensen (Germany): Dallmer Publications; 1996. p. 14–43.
16. Colles CM. The relationship of frog pressure to heel expansion. Equine Vet J 1989;21:13–6.
17. Dyhre-Poulsen P, Smedegaard HH, Roed J, et al. Equine hoof function investigated by pressure transducers inside the hoof and accelerometers mounted on the first phalanx. Equine Vet J 1994;26:362–6.
18. Benoit P, Barrey E, Regnault JC, et al. Comparison of the damping effect of different shoeing by the measurement of hoof acceleration. Acta Anat 1993; 146:109–13.
19. Willemen MA, Savelberg HH, Barneveld A. The effect of orthopedic shoeing on the force exerted by the deep digital flexor tendon on the navicular bone in horses. Equine Vet J 1999;31:25–30.

20. Thomason JJ. Variation in surface strain on the equine hoof wall at the midstep with shoeing gait, substrate, direction of travel, and hoof shape. Equine Vet J Suppl 1998;26:86–95.
21. Pratt GW. Model for injury to the foreleg of the thoroughbred racehorse. Equine Vet J Suppl 1997;23:30–2.
22. Crevier-Denoix N, Robin D, Pourcelot P, et al. Ground reaction force and kinematic analysis of limb loading on two different beach sands tracks in harness trotters. Equine Vet J Suppl 2010;42:530–7.

Cardiac/Cardiovascular Conditions Affecting Sport Horses

Katherine B. Chope, VMD

KEYWORDS

- Sport horse • Murmur • Valvular regurgitation • Arrhythmia • Echocardiogram
- ECG • Exercising ECG

KEY POINTS

- Auscultation should be performed once to twice yearly in performance horses.
- A grade 3/6 or above left-sided systolic murmur, grade 4/6 or above right-sided systolic murmur, grade 3/6 or above diastolic murmur or nonphysiologic arrythmia should prompt echocardiographic or ECG evaluation.
- Moderate to severe aortic regurgitation has been associated with ventricular arrhythmis at exercise.
- Exercising radiotelemetry is indicated in moderate to severe mitral regurgitation, moderate to severe aortic regurgitation, atrial fibrillation, history of collapse during exercise, or unexplained poor performance.
- Sport horses undergoing exercise radiotelemetry should be evaluated performing in their intended discipline whenever possible.

INTRODUCTION

Low-grade heart murmurs and arrhythmias due to vagal tone are not uncommonly detected in horses. In most cases, low-grade murmurs are physiologic murmurs with no effect on performance or life expectancy. Atrioventricular (AV) or aortic valvular regurgitation, however, can develop with age and may be progressive. In the milder forms, little to no effect maybe observed; however, in more severe cases, valvular regurgitation may be implicated in decreased performance or in the development of secondary arrhythmias, which may in turn affect performance or ridden safety. Arrhythmias may present as a clinically insignificant finding, such as in second-degree AV block, a performance limitation, or a safety concern, such as can occur in unstable ventricular arrhythmias (VAs). Sport horses typically peak in performance at a later age than their racing counterparts and are expected

Disclosure Statement: No conflicts or commercial affiliations to disclose.
Department of Clinical Sciences, Tufts University Cummings School of Veterinary Medicine, 200 Westboro Road, North Grafton, MA 01536, USA
E-mail address: katherine.chope@tufts.edu

to be used athletically well into their late teens or beyond, when age-related cardiac changes are more likely to manifest. Given the variety of types of athletic work the sport horse moniker encompasses and the variability in rider ages and expertise, it is important that the equine sport horse veterinarian understand which conditions are most likely to be of performance, safety, or prepurchase concern. This article discusses the physical findings, diagnostic options, and presentation of commonly encountered cardiac conditions in the sport horse. Infectious, inflammatory, toxic, congenital, and less frequent causes of cardiovascular disease less specific to the competing athlete are outside the scope of this article. They may occur, however, and should be considered as differentials if clinical signs warrant.

PATIENT EVALUATION

A careful, thorough physical examination of the cardiovascular and respiratory systems should be performed in any horse in which a cardiovascular abnormality is suspected. Auscultation should be performed in a quiet environment with minimal external stimuli to enhance detection of murmurs and accurately obtain resting values. Mucous membranes, capillary refill time, jugular refill, jugular pulse and arterial pulse quality should be evaluated. Thoracic auscultation is recommended as an aid in determining the respiratory contribution in cases of exercise intolerance.

Auscultation

Auscultation should be performed over the pulmonic, aortic, and mitral valve regions on the left side of the chest (**Fig. 1**) and the tricuspid region on the right side of the chest (**Fig. 2**). It is necessary to place the stethoscope cranially on each side underneath the triceps muscle or move the leg forward to perform proper auscultation; otherwise, cranial or soft murmurs can be missed (**Fig. 3**). Further evaluation immediately postexercise or during physical stimulation to increase heart rate may be indicated help differentiate between a physiologic flow murmur

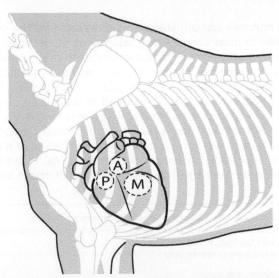

Fig. 1. Schematic of the pulmonic (*P*), aortic (*A*) and mitral (*M*) valve regions for auscultation. (*Courtesy of* Katherine Chope, VMD. North Grafton, MA; with permission.)

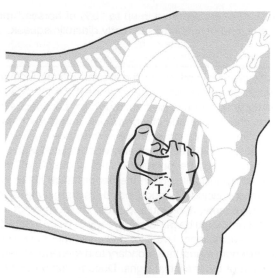

Fig. 2. Schematic of the tricuspid (*T*) valve region for auscultation. (*Courtesy of* Katherine Chope, VMD. North Grafton, MA; with permission.)

and murmur due to valvular regurgitation or to document abolishment of a suspected second-degree AV block.

The heart rate, rhythm, and presence or absence of any murmurs should be identified and recorded. Murmurs should be characterized as to timing, pitch, character, point of maximal intensity, and radiation.

Typical Findings

In normal horses, 2, 3, or 4 heart sounds maybe audible (S1, S2, S3, and S4). Physiologic or functional flow murmurs are common, audible in up to 50% of horses.[1] They are typically early systolic to midsystolic, crescendo-decrescendo in pitch, and with a point of maximal intensity over the pulmonic valve region (see **Fig. 1**). They may vary with heart rate, often becoming louder with increasing heart rate. Benign murmurs of

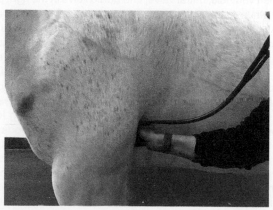

Fig. 3. Photograph of stethoscope placement for auscultation cranially on the left side of the chest.

ventricular filling (diastolic) are reported in up to 15% of horses,[1] most commonly in young Thoroughbreds, and described as an early diastolic squeak.

Indications

Indications for cardiovascular work-up in the equine athlete include auscultation of grade 3/6 or above left-sided systolic murmur, grade 4/6 right-sided systolic murmur, grade 3/6 or above diastolic murmur, bilateral murmurs, continuous murmur, development of new murmur, change in grade of a previously detected murmur, detection of a resting or postexercise arrhythmia, exercise intolerance, prolonged recovery, or collapse. Murmur intensity, however, is not always correlated with severity of the disease process; work-up should be pursued if clinical suspicion indicates. Although less commonly seen as an initial finding in the performance horse, signs of left-sided or right-sided heart failure, including cough, nasal discharge, elevated resting heart or respiratory rate, ventral edema, and jugular pulses, should prompt immediate evaluation. Cardiac auscultation should be performed yearly or twice yearly during routine veterinary evaluations or vaccinations. This is of particular importance in the middle-aged to older sport horse in whom murmurs secondary to degenerative valvular disease may develop in the absence of other clinical signs. Documentation and description of any murmurs found can be helpful for diagnostic, prognostic, and prepurchase purposes.

DIAGNOSTICS
Echocardiography

Echocardiography is the test of choice for evaluating cardiac disease in the horse. It provides semiquantitative and quantitative information on cardiac structure, size, function, and severity of disease if present.

Proper echocardiographic examination requires a phased array scanner (2.5–5.0 MHz) and ultrasound unit with ECG, M-mode, color Doppler, continuous wave Doppler, and pulsed wave Doppler capabilities. The echocardiogram should be performed by a sonographer with training and experience in equine echocardiography. Poor image quality, incorrect placement of calipers for measurement, and misalignment of Doppler beam can result in erroneous conclusions. Repeatability of measurements over serial examinations is critical in assessing progression and prognosis. The examination should include B-mode images in right outflow, left outflow, and 4-chamber views in the right parasternal long axis window; left ventricle, mitral valve, and aortic valve in the right parasternal short-axis view; and left atrium/mitral valvular evaluation in the left parasternal long-axis view. M-mode images should be taken at the level of the left ventricle, mitral valve, and aortic valve for measurement purpose and analysis of valvular and wall motion.

Two dimensional and M-Mode measurements should be compared with breed or published normal measurements if available and any previous evaluations. This is of particular relevance in sport horses given their expected career longevity. Published normal 2-D and M-mode measurements exist for Thoroughbred racehorses[2,3] and Standardbred racehorses,[4] with a few additional studies controlling for weight or type in horses and ponies.[5,6] Limited information exists for warmbloods and other sport horse breeds and there is variation within these breeds themselves as to size and bloodlines. The sonographer should be careful not to rule out left ventricular enlargement based on measurements alone if there is clinical or echocardiographic evidence suggestive of an increased left ventricular internal diameter. Myocardial function should be evaluated and in compensated cases of left ventricular enlargement should increase; in left ventricular dysfunction or progression toward uncompensated cardiac disease, the fractional shortening may decrease.

All valves should be interrogated with color Doppler. Severity of regurgitation is based on the size of the jet, width at valve orifice, timing, duration, and direction. Grading severity of the regurgitant jet size based on percent area within the atrium or width at valve orifice has also been described.[7] Reproducibility can be difficult, however, and it has been suggested that greater than a 25% change in color flow Doppler characteristic on successive examinations is required to be significant.[8] Continuous wave Doppler should be used to further quantify the severity of any aortic regurgitation (AR) as it relates to left ventricular filling pressures and evaluation of shunts due to ventricular septal defects.

In healthy horses, correlation of heart size with racing/performance success are conflicting outside of high-level endurance horses.[9,10]

ECG

A standard base apex resting ECG should be performed on all horses with arrhythmia not easily attributable to second-degree AV block, an episode of syncope or collapse, or sudden onset of poor performance not attributable to respiratory or musculoskeletal conditions. In ambulatory settings, a smartphone-based portable heart monitor is available (www.alivecor.com) and has been validated for diagnostic use at rest on the horse for use ambulatory conditions.[11] Digital telemetric ECG systems (www.televet.de) are readily portable and can be used to obtain real time digital monitoring and recording at rest or during exercise. A 24-hour Holter monitor is recommended to determine frequency of atrial premature complexes (APCs) or ventricular premature complexes (VPCs), in cases of suspected but unconfirmed arrhythmia or as part of the evaluation of collapse or other behavior in which may have a cardiac etiology. It is the most thorough method to qualify and quantify resting arrhythmias. Holter units are available for order through select academic institutions and referral practices; they are placed on the horse in its home environment for 24 hours and returned to the provider for clinical interpretation of results and recommendations. Holter monitor functionality is also available in some portable digital telemetric units; recordings may be sent out for evaluation.

On a standard base-apex configuration, a clear P wave, QRS and T wave should be able to be identified in every beat. R-R intervals should be regular with a P wave for every QRS and a QRS for every P wave. Manual or digital calipers should be used for measurements of cardiac intervals and durations of complexes. Mild variations in PR and RR intervals can occur with vagal tone. The most common normal variation seen is second-degree AV block. Documentation of second-degree AV block via ECG is not typically necessary but can be helpful for the medical record.

Exercising ECG

An exercising ECG is indicated in horses with moderate to severe AR, moderate to severe mitral regurgitation (MR),[12] atrial fibrillation (AF), APCs or VPCs, collapse or unexplained poor performance during exercise, or bradyarrhythmias at rest. The exercising ECG allows a veterinarian to evaluate heart rate and rhythm during each stage of exercise. With the availability of portable and affordable digital telemetric systems, exercising ECGs can be performed in the field allowing clinicians to observe a horse performing at its intended use in the varied field conditions the sport horse may encounter. In some units, GPS speed data are also available. Heart rate monitors, which record rate but not rhythm, are commercially available for the evaluation of fitness in the equine athlete (https://ker.com). These can be a useful monitoring tool in horses with AF or moderate cardiac disease in whom alterations in baseline exercising heart rates may portend deterioration.

With telemetric ECG systems adhesive, electrode attachments are placed in a modified base-apex configuration, on the left and right hemithorax and sternum (**Fig. 4**). Leads can be secured via elastic adhesive tape under a surcingle or saddle

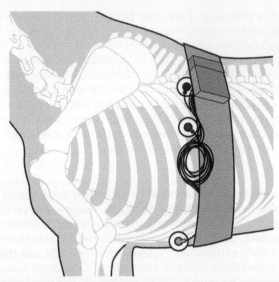

Fig. 4. Example of placement of radiotelemetry unit in a modified bas apex configuration, left side. (*Courtesy of* Katherine Chope, VMD. North Grafton, MA; with permission.)

and girth and attached to a transmitter box onto the surcingle or saddle. The signal can be stored or relayed via Bluetooth technology to a computer with appropriate software package. Real-time information is displayed. The entire exercising ECG with cool-down period should be saved for analysis and record keeping. Program software allows for computerized analysis of R-R intervals; however, this should not replace critical evaluation by the veterinarian.

Standardized field tests have been proposed for sport horses[13] and most encompass approximately 20 minutes of warm-up, trot, canter, hand gallop, and cooldown exercise. Data obtained in studies on jumpers[14] and dressage horses[15] suggest that it is probably most informative to observe the horse perform in as close to normal type of work as possible, including upward and downward gait changes to mimic the changes in autonomic tone, which may occur in the course of training and competition.

Rate

Table 1 indicates normal heart rate ranges for each level of exercise. Heart rate range by discipline is illustrated in **Table 2**. Heart rates tend to be initially higher for a given level of

Table 1	
Normal heart rates for each level of exercise	
Gait	**Heart Rate (Beats per Minute)**
Walk	60–80
Trot	80–120
Canter	120–150
Hand gallop	150–180
Gallop	180
Maximal heart rate	220–240

Data from Patteson M. Clinical examination. In: Cardiology of the horse. Cambridge (MA): Blackwell Science; 1996. p. 69; and Durando M. Exercise and stress testing. In: Marr CM, Bowen M, editors. Cardiology of the horse. 2nd edition. New York: Saunders Elsevier; 2010. p. 141.

Table 2 Heart rates by discipline		
	Mean (Beats per Minute)	Range/Peak Range (Beats per Minute)
Show jumping	—	90–180
Dressage	140	125–193
Eventing: cross country	—	Up to 170–200
Polo	—	Up to 215–225
Thoroughbred racing	—	220–240

Data from Refs.[9,14–16]

exercise in the first 2 minutes to 3 minutes of exercise and decrease to a steady state thereafter. Mean maximal heart can gradually increase over periods of prolonged submaximal exercise[9] This is most likely due to effects of dehydration and environment. Heart rate recovery is typically rapid in the first minute after exercise stops. Heart rate should decrease below 100 beats per minutes (bpm) in the first 5 minutes after maximal exercise and to normal by 30 minutes to 45 minutes thereafter.[9,17] After light exercise, it has been suggested that heart rate should return to 15% of normal within 15 minutes.

If cardiac disease is severe enough to affect output, then the heart rate for each level of work increases. In determining what is maximal level of work for these horses, the level of exercise which produces a consistent heart rate of 180 bpm, has been suggested as the maximumExcitement, inadequate fitness, lameness, pain, respiratory disease, dehydration, heat, or humidity, however, may result in a higher heart rate for each level of exercise than expected. Heart rate recovery can also be monitored as a presumed indicator of fitness or cardiac disease.

Rhythm
Evaluation of the cardiac rhythm is important for identification of arrhythmias, which may contribute to poor performance, collapse, or sudden cardiac death (SCD). A single exercising ECG, however, is only 1 point in time and a single normal exercising ECG does not definitely rule out arrhythmias as a contributing factor or rule out the development of future arrhythmias.[18] Criteria for diagnosis of premature depolarizations are a 20% reduction in R-R interval at rest and 10% reduction during maximal exercise.[15] At below maximal heart rates, however, there is more variability in R-R interval, meaning criteria for sport horses may need to be considered differently, and some investigators suggest 8% reduction during exercise.[19]

Occasional single supraventricular premature complexes (SVPCs) and VPCs in the absence of underlying structural disease are generally accepted as clinically irrelevant in equine exercising ECGs.[20] Implications of exercising arrhythmias are discussed later.

Cardiac Stress Echocardiography
Cardiac stress tests with pre-exercising and postexercising echocardiography and concurrent exercising radiotelemetric ECG has been used in horses to diagnose cardiac dysfunction.[21] To gain a true estimate of exercising function, wall motion should be evaluated within 1-minute postmaximal exercise in horses that are exercising at or near maximal cardiac output. If the heart rate decreases below 100 bpm, fractional shortening decreases and interpretation of results is difficult. Pre-echocardiography and postechocardiography are best applied to racing populations or horses that may have subtle high-level cardiac output abnormalities and can undergo a rigorous exercise test near maximal cardiac output.

Laboratory Tests

- Elevations in serum and plasma concentrations of cardiac troponin can be diagnostic and prognostic for myocardial damage in horses. Indications include suspected recent-onset myocardial disease and VAs. Elevations in cardiac troponin can also occur in other disease states, however, such as renal disease, acute severe hypoxia, and systemic inflammation. Mild elevations may also be seen after racing, endurance racing, and treadmill exercise.[22,23]
- Serum levels of potassium and magnesium and fractional excretion of potassium are recommended in horses with paroxysmal or recent-onset AF.
- A complete blood cell count/blood chemistry screen is recommended in horses with persistent unexplained arrhythmias or prior to administration of pharmacologic therapies.
- Elevations in atrial natriuretic peptide has more recently been reported as an indicator of left atrial dilation in horses.[24]

VALVULAR REGURGITATION

Physiologic valvular regurgitation occurs not uncommonly. It is seen in higher incidence in race horses than in the general population but has been described in other equine athletes. Physiologic regurgitation is defined as regurgitation that occurs in structurally normal valves, with no secondary cardiac changes and is regarded as a training effect. Pathologic regurgitation is associated with hemodynamic and structural changes and abnormalities of the valve.

Mitral Regurgitation

Murmurs associated with MR can be holosystolic, pansystolic or midsystolic to late systolic and are generally crescendo or band-shaped in character. MR can be due to degenerative or inflammatory changes, mitral valve prolapse, dysplasia, ruptured chordae tendineae, and flail leaflet. MR can also be present in valves that appear to be structurally normal. Horses with mild MR, no changes in cardiac size, and no overt valvular changes can have normal performance and life expectancy.[8,12] In these cases the MR may represent a training-associated phenomenon and may not be progressive. Otherwise, prognosis depends on the underlying cause and severity at time of detection. Ruptured chordae tendineae and flail leaflets represent more severe disease and a worse prognosis. Occasionally, the chordal rupture involves a smaller accessory leaflet progression and maybe somewhat better tolerated.

Echocardiographically the mitral valve should be examined carefully for changes in structure and motion. Detection of mild age-related degenerative changes, however, is often relatively subjective.[12] The size and shape of the left atrium and left ventricle help determine the severity of the MR, although in acute cases significant changes in chamber sizes may not have had time to develop. Myocardial function should be evaluated and in compensated cases of left ventricular enlargement should increase; in left ventricular dysfunction or progression toward uncompensated cardiac disease, the fractional shortening may decrease. Left atrial size is of particular importance because enlargement is a predisposing factor to the development of AF. A jet of regurgitant flow on color Doppler confirms the presence of MR. Due to angle of interrogation in the horse, however, it is often an underestimation of the true amount of regurgitation.

Prognosis

The prognosis for horses with mild MR or mitral valve prolapse is normal function and life expectancy. Horses with moderate MR and mild size changes may have a fairer prognosis. The prognosis is more guarded in horses with moderate to severe MR and moderate to severe size changes in the size of the left ventricle.[12] In severe cases of left ventricular failure, signs of left-sided failure and enlargement of the pulmonary artery occur. Concomitant aortic or tricuspid valvular dysfunction can worsen prognosis. Increase in left atrial size presents an increased risk for the development of AF.

Recommendations

Horses with MR should be re-evaluated echocardiographically once a year, or in cases of established mild MR once every 2 years.[12] Horses with moderate to severe MR should be auscultated for heart rate and rhythm periodically. Exercise testing is recommended in horses with moderate to severe MR, horses in which AF has developed or horses with unexpected progression of MR.

Aortic Regurgitation

AR is a common finding in older horses. Murmurs associated with AR are left-sided holodiastolic murmurs in which grade, pitch, character, and radiation can vary widely. If sufficiently loud, these murmurs may radiate to the right side. It is particularly important to be aware in murmurs of AR that the intensity of the murmur is not necessarily related to the severity of regurgitation and that a decrease or increase in intensity is not synonymous with improvement or worsening. Arterial pulse quality is an important indicator of clinical status in horses with AR and should be carefully evaluated in horses with a diastolic murmur. Bounding or hyperdynamic pulses suggest more hemodynamically severe AR with left ventricular volume overload.

AR is most commonly due to age-related degenerative changes or valvular prolapse. Less commonly, congenital and infectious changes can occur. Echocardiographically, degenerative changes of the aortic valve can be fairly readily identified as thickening, nodules, fenestration, or prolapse. Fluttering or vibrations can be seen with musical murmurs. The left ventricle should be carefully assessed for size, shape, and function. Left ventricular enlargement is correlated with increasing disease severity. Myocardial function should be evaluated and in compensated cases of left ventricular enlargement should increase; In left ventricular dysfunction or progression toward uncompensated cardiac disease, the fractional shortening may decrease. A regurgitant jet can be identified on color Doppler with width, extent, and ratio[22] of AR to the aortic valve measurements obtained. Jets can be directed toward the mitral valve resulting in degenerative changes on the mitral valve. Continuous wave Doppler with pressure half-time measurement should be used to help estimate left ventricular pressures.

Prognosis

AR is typically well tolerated and slowly progressive. Mild AR is associated with a normal life and performance expectancy.[12] Moderate to severe AR is associated with reduced performance life and longevity. If AR is detected in a horse less than 10 years of age, the likelihood of reduced performance and life span increases.[12] SCD associated with fatal VAs has been reported in horses with moderate to severe AR. Horses with AR are considered at a higher risk for development of VAs.

Recommendations

Horses with mild AR should be re-evaluated echocardiographically once a year. This interval can be extended if there is documented lack of progression over time. Horses with moderate to severe AR should be re-evaluated twice yearly with echocardiography and exercising ECG. All horses with moderate to severe AR or performance issues and AR are recommended to have an exercising ECG[12] to determine the presence of any VPCs or arrhythmias and appropriate exercising heart rates. Horses with AR and

VPCs during exercise are considered less safe to ride.[12] It is generally held that horses with moderate to severe AR should be ridden by consenting adults only. Regular auscultation should be performed to evaluate murmur, heart rate, and rhythm. Changes in murmur quality, elevated resting heart rate, or APCs/VPCs may indicate progression.

Tricuspid Regurgitation

Triscuspid regurgitation (TR) is a common finding in equine athletes. Most commonly it is associated with training effects and is considered benign and nonprogressive. Less commonly tricuspid regurgitation can occur due degenerative changes, or secondary to congestive heart failure, pulmonary hypertension, or bacterial endocarditis. The murmur associated with TR is a right-sided holosystolic or pansystolic murmur of varying grade, the main differential being ventricular septal defect. Echocardiographic evaluation is mainly indicated for grade 4/6 or louder right-sided systolic murmur, concurrent thrombophlebitis, or fever of unknown origin. On echocardiographic evaluation of benign or training-related TR, no abnormalities are detected on the tricuspid valve and chamber sizes are within normal limits. With more clinically significant TR, abnormalities of the valve or increases in chamber size can be identified. The jet is described as wider.[12] If TR jet velocity is greater than 3.5 m/s, pulmonary hypertension should be suspected and the horse further evaluated for pulmonary disease or left-sided heart disease. TR with right atrial enlargement may likewise predispose to AF, although less commonly than with MR.

Prognosis

Horses with TR most commonly have a normal performance and life expectancy; structural valve lesions, right-sided failure, and severe MR with pulmonary hypertension are negative prognostic indicators.

Recommendations

Horses with moderate to severe TR should have a yearly echocardiogram.

Treatment

In a joint American College of Veterinary Internal Medicine–European College of Equine Internal Medicine statement on cardiovascular disease in the horse in 2014,[12] a consensus could not be reached on the use of angiotensin-converting enzyme (ACE) inhibitors in horses with MR or AR in the absence of heart failure. More recently a prospective, randomized, double-blinded, placebo-controlled trial looking at benazepril, at a dose of 1 mg/kg twice a day for 28 days, demonstrated improvement in echocardiographic indices in horses with left-sided valvular regurgitation,[25] supporting arguments for their use prior to the onset of signs of congestive heart failure. Side effects include inappetence, lethargy, and low blood pressure.

Hydralazine has been used as an afterload reducer in horses with questionable renal function that may not tolerate an ACE inhibitor. Otherwise, at this time, no treatment is recommended prior to the onset of congestive heart failure. If signs of congestive heart failure are present, appropriate medical management should be instituted, including positive inotropic support, the use of an ACE inhibitor, and diuretics if indicated.

ARRHYTHMIAS

An extensive discussion of all potential arrhythmias and their causes are outside the scope of this article. Discussion is limited to AF and arrhythmias encountered during exercise. Arrhythmias, however, can be isolated or secondary to several factors unrelated to structural heart disease, including metabolic or endocrine disorders, systemic inflammation, hemorrhage, autonomic influences, toxicosis, and drugs[12]; any of these may occur in the sport horse and should be included in the differential of an unexplained arrhythmia. Arrhythmias in horses that are ridden or driven may result in decreased performance or may contribute to episodes of collapse or SCD, presenting a risk to horse and rider.

Atrial Fibrillation

AF is the most common performance affecting arrhythmia in horses. The effect of AF on exercise tolerance in the sport horse depends on the cardiovascular demands of its intended use and individual tolerances. Disorganized atrial contraction results in inadequate ventricular filling, reduced stroke volume, and increased heart rate during exercise. Horses in AF tend to have heart rates of 40 bpm to 60 bpm[26] higher than expected normal for each level of exercise. This results in a dramatic drop-off in performance in horses that operate at or near maximal cardiac output, such as racehorses. Upper-level event horses and other horses undergoing exertions that require near-sustained maximal heart rates may also experience performance issues. Performance may be unaffected in other sport disciplines, however, with lower cardiovascular demand and it may be clinically inapparent until detected on routine auscultation.

AF can be paroxysmal, in which spontaneous conversion to a normal sinus rhythm occurs in 24 hours to 48 hours, or persistent. Lone AF is defined as AF in the absence of detectable heart disease. Left atrial enlargement predisposes to the development of persistent AF, reduces likelihood of conversion, and increases the risk for recurrence. Over time, electrical and structural remodeling within the atria occurs, decreasing the chances for successful cardioversion and promoting risk of persistent or recurrent AF.

On auscultation, AF is an irregularly irregular rhythm with no discernible S4 sound. Horses should be carefully evaluated for any concurrent murmurs suggestive of structural heart disease. ECG evaluation is confirmed by baseline fibrillation waves, no discernible P wave associated with a QRS complex, and irregularly irregular RR intervals. Serum potassium and magnesium and a fractional excretion of potassium should be obtained in acute cases and in high-level athletes.[12] An echocardiogram should be performed with emphasis on evaluation of left atrial size, the presence of MR, and left ventricular function.

An exercising ECG is recommended to assess exercise tolerance and safety in horses for in which conversion is not indicated or not under immediate consideration. If the heart rate is more elevated than expected for AF at each level of exercise, this suggests that the AF is limit performance or necessitate use at a lower level. Conversion is recommended if the average maximal heart rate during exercise is 220 bpm at equal to or slightly greater than the horse's normal exercise level[12] **(Fig. 5)**. Commercial heart rate monitors may be useful for monitoring heart rate during training on a regular basis.

Careful screening of the exercising ECG should also be performed for evidence of ventricular tachycardia (VT) or VPCs, which could in turn predispose to an unstable VA. In a lunging exercise study of largely warmblood horses with lone AF and clinical signs of exercise intolerance, VPCs were identified in 69% of the horses during exercise with 73% having 2 or more morphologies and 33% having R-on-T morphology. Disproportionate tachycardia and QRS broadening were also present and occurred during hand gallop and when startled.[27] Although this group represents horses with clinical performance issues as opposed to those in AF without overt clinical signs, it is important to be aware of the potential for occurrence in horses with lone AF even if used for lower level exercise. It is recommended that

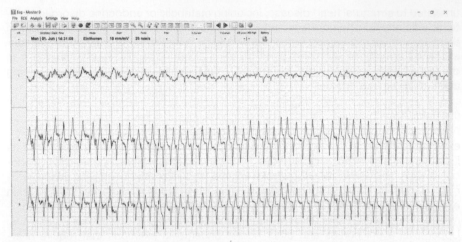

Fig. 5. Exercising ECG from a high-level warmblood show jumper in lone AF with signs of exercise intolerance. Heart rates were 200 bpm to 210 bpm at a strong trot/slow canter. Horse successfully returned to previous level of show jumping postconversion to a normal sinus rhythm; 25 mm/s paper speed displayed.

conversion be attempted if VAs are observed; if conversion is not indicated or not an option, then the owner should be cautioned as to concerns for development of unstable VAs.

Options for horses in AF include no treatment (with periodic monitoring recommended), pharmacologic conversion with oral quinidine sulfate gluconate, and transvenous electrocardioversion (TVEC). Conversion is recommended for all horses performing rigorous work, horses that demonstrate VAs during exercise testing, and horses whose sustained maximal heart rate is 220 bpm or greater during the horse's normal level of exercise.[12] Quinidine sulfate is reported to have a 70% to 89% success rate and TVEC a 94% to 99% success rate, although direct comparison is difficult due to differing study populations.[26]

Treatment with quinidine sulfate should only be performed in a hospital setting with continuous ECG monitoring and observation. It is indicated in lone AF, AF with mild LA, and horses having contraindications to general anesthesia.[12] Risks of quinidine treatment include rapid ventricular response rate, ventricular ectopy, and risk of polymorphic VT. Adverse drug effects, which may necessitate discontinuation of treatment, or administration of other drugs to control ventricular response rate can occur.

TVEC is available in select referral centers. It is indicated in lone AF, AF with mild atrial enlargement, and horses intolerant of or not responsive to quinidine.[12] Risks of TVEC include risks associated with general anesthesia and development of fatal arrhythmia, although both are rare. Recurrence rates are believed similar between the 2 forms of treatment.[12,26] A complete postconversion echocardiogram should be performed to assess function and size. Left ventricular function should return to normal within 3 days[12]; left atrial return to function may take a week or longer in long-standing cases.[12] A rest period postconversion is recommended. One-week rest post-cardioversion is suggested for acute cases, but 4 weeks' rest postconversion is recommended if the AF is long standing or contractile dysfunction persists.[12] A 24-hour Holter monitor should be performed postconversion to assess the frequency of any atrial ectopy.

Recurrence rates of 15% to 40% have been reported. Recurrence is 15% in lone AF or recent onset of less than 1 month.[12] In a study evaluating horses with successful conversion of a first AF episode, recurrence rate was 39%; risk factors for recurrence were mild regurgitation and a previous unsuccessful attempt.[26] Recurrence rate of AF increases in horses with underlying heart disease, chronic mitral valvular disease, atrial enlargement, high numbers of APCs postconversion, previous unsuccessful attempt, and evidence of left atrial dysfunction postconversion. Persistent left atrial dysfunction is believed to indicate irreversible atrial remodeling.

Exercising Arrhythmias

SVPCs and VPCs have been documented during exercise and immediately postexercise in normally performing racehorses (training, racing, and treadmill) and normally performing show jumping and dressage horses.[14,15,28] During exercise and postexercise, infrequent isolated APCs and VPCs postexercise are generally accepted as clinically insignificant.[17,20,28] Evidence-based criteria, however, are lacking for what frequency maybe considered clinically significant.

Arrhythmias during exercise in horses without structural disease are suspected to be due to training-related cardiac remodeling and amplified severity of the metabolic imbalances,[29–35] which occur during strenuous exercise and hypoxia in horses with altered respiratory function.[21] Changing autonomic tone[19] is likely a contributor to the increased number of arrhythmias seen on cooldown.

Incidence in sport horses
In looking at the prevalence of cardiac arrhythmias in clinically healthy show jumpers, Buhl and colleagues[14] found SVPCs in 89% of horses during exercise and 54% during recovery. Most SVPCs occurred at lower heart rates of 40 bpm to 98 bpm, which correlated to time between jumps and decelerations during warm-up. VPCs were demonstrated in 18% of horses during exercise and 7% during recovery with less than 2 per horse. In a study of normal performing dressage horses, SVPCs occurred in 28.6% of horses during exercise and 61.9% during recovery. VPCs were only identified in 1 horse; 39% of show jumpers had mild valvular regurgitation and 52% of dressage horses; no association between arrhythmias and mild regurgitation was seen in either study. The incidence of arrhythmias at the lower heart rate that occurred between jumps and during warm-up in jumpers and during postexercise period in dressage horses further indicates that arrhythmias are likely influenced by fluctuations autonomic tone.[14]

Poor performance and sport horse considerations
Nonmalignant cardiac arrhythmias are suspected to affect performance by contributing to reduced cardiac output. The effect of premature contractions and less malignant arrhythmias on performance in sport horses that operate at lower levels of cardiac output is difficult to ascertain. It is reasonable to assume that horses with higher demand or concomitant respiratory disease may be more affected. More research needs to be done to evaluate the significance of SVPCs and VPCs in normal sport horses and those with structural cardiac changes or symptoms suggestive of cardiac dysfunction. Findings in discipline-specific studies suggest the importance conducting an exercise test that mimics the work typically encountered during training and competition.

Supraventricular premature complexes
- Premature beats in an otherwise regular rhythm
- Diagnosis via ECG: decrease in R-R interval by 20% at rest or 10% during exercise, no change in configuration of QRS

- Considered supraventricular tachycardia if 3 or more consecutive SVPCs
- Uncommon cause for poor performance
- Consider safe to ride or use athletically
- May predispose to atrial flutter or AF; if identified postconversion, risk factor for recurrence of AF
- If more than 1 per hour at rest, evaluate for underlying metabolic causes.

Ventricular premature complexes

- Premature beats in an otherwise regular rhythm
- Diagnosis via ECG: QRS with no P wave; taller, wider, unusual QRS morphology followed by a compensatory pause (**Fig. 6**)
- Decrease in R-R interval by 20% at rest or 10% at exercise
- Pulse deficit and/or jugular pulses may be present
- Can occur as isolated beats, couplets, or triplets; 3[12] to 4[19] or more is VT
- May present a safety risk to horse or rider (discussed later)

Collapse or sudden cardiac death

Determination of the risk of collapse or SCD due to arrhythmias in horses used for athletic endeavors is of considerable importance for the well-being of rider, horse, and sport. Due to difficulties in establishing definitive diagnosis and varied reporting techniques, the incidence of collapse death due to a sudden cardiac cause in horses is difficult to accurately determine, although relatively low overall. Most reporting involves evaluating causes of sudden death in racehorse, of which SCD is 1 category. SCD has been reported, however, in eventers and elite show jumpers.[19] Navas de Solis, in a review of exercising arrhythmias and SCD in horses,[20] summarizes cardiac disease as the cause of death in 14% of equine sudden death cases and 24% of collapse cases. The immediate postexercise period seems most vulnerable time for the genesis of cardiac arrhythmias and SCD presumably due to a combination of changing autonomic influences and metabolic factors.[16,19,36] It has been proposed

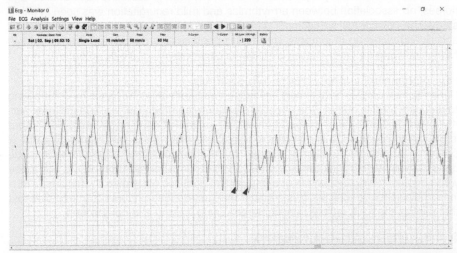

Fig. 6. Example of VPC couplet during exercise. Displayed paper speed 50 mm/s. Displayed paper speed can be adjusted for purpose of analysis. The two arrowheads indicated as abnormal beats. (*Courtesy of* Dr Mary Durando, Newark, DE; with permission.)

that exercise-induced arrhythmias may be lessened by a sustained and gradual warm-down at the end of exercise to moderate changes in autonomic tone.[36]

Ventricular ectopy

Ventricular ectopy is presumed the main concern for safety of horse or rider due to the risk of development of unstable VAs. Multiform VT, short coupling intervals, R-on-T timing, sustained VT, ventricular rate of 120 bpm or greater, and couplet or triplet activity are referred to as complex VAs and are considered potentially malignant. Complex VT or multiform VT is presumed to relate to the risk of hypotension and SCD due to the development of ventricular fibrillation.[12] Risk stratification, however, for VA is imperfect.[12] A history of PVCs in association with collapse, structural heart disease, or AF is suggestive of an increased risk of the development of unstable VA (see **Fig. 6**).

Recommendations: horses with VT or complex VA or VA in conjunction with poor performance, collapse, or relevant cardiac murmur should undergo echocardiographic evaluation, measurement of serum or plasma cardiac troponin levels, and 24-hour Holter monitor. Horses with known VT or complex VA at rest should not be exercise tested. Horses with monomorphic VT that responds to treatment should demonstrate 4 weeks with no evidence of ectopy and then may return to work based on a normal echocardiogram, 24-hour Holter monitor, and exercising ECG.[12] Horses with symptomatic or complex VA that are rested and treated remain of uncertain safety risk for athletic use.[12]

REFERENCES

1. Blissitt K. Auscultation. In: Marr CM, Bowen M, editors. Cardiology of the horse. 2nd edition. New York: Saunders Elsevier; 2010. p. 92.
2. Patteson M. Diagnostic aids in equine cardiology. In: Cardiology of the horse. Cambridge (MA): Blackwell Science, Ltd; 1996. p. 98.
3. Reef V. Echocardiography. In: Reef VB, editor. Equine diagnostic ultrasound. 1st edition. Philadelphia: WB Saunders and Company; 1998. p. 222.
4. Zucca E, Ferrucci F, Croci C, et al. Echocardiographic measurements of cardiac dimensions in normal Standardbred racehorses. J Vet Cardiol 2008; 10(1):45–51.
5. Slater JD, Herrtage ME. Echocardiographic measurements of cardiac dimensions in normal ponies and horses. Equine Vet J Suppl 1995;19:28–32.
6. Available at: http://cal.vet.upenn.edu/projects/lgcardiac/index.html.
7. Buhl R, Ersbøll AK, Eriksen L, et al. Use of color Doppler echocardiography to assess the development of valvular regurgitation in Standardbred trotters. J Am Vet Med Assoc 2005;227:1630–5.
8. Marr CM, Patteson M. Echocardiography. In: Marr CM, Bowen M, editors. Cardiology of the horse. 2nd edition. New York: Saunders Elsevier; 2010. p. 119.
9. Marr CM, Patteson M. Cardiac responses to exercise and training. In: Marr CM, Bowen M, editors. Cardiology of the horse. 2nd edition. New York: Saunders Elsevier; 2010. p. 36, 43, 36–7.
10. Trachsel D, Giraudet A, Maso D, et al. Relationships between body dimensions, body weight, age, gender, breed and echocardiographic dimensions in young endurance horses. BMC Vet Res 2016;12:226.
11. Gilsenan WF. How to diagnose cardiac arrhythmias in the field. In Proceedings. Am Assoc Equine Pract 2017;413–8.
12. Reef VB, Bonagura J, Buhl R, et al. Recommendations for management of equine athletes with cardiovascular abnormalities: joint ACVIM/ECEIM consensus statement. J Vet Intern Med 2014;28:749–61.

13. Van Erck Westergren E. Value of field trials to investigate poor performance in sport horses. Scientific Abstracts, International Conference on Equine Exercise Physiology. 2014;46(s46).

14. Buhl R, Meldgaard C, Barbesgaard L. Cardiac arrhythmias in clinically healthy show jumping horses. Equine Vet J 2010;42(S38):196–201.

15. Barbesgaard L, Buhl R, Meldgaard C. Prevalence of exercise associated arrhythmias in normal performing dressage horses. Equine Vet J 2010;42(s38):202–7.

16. Allen KJ, Van Erck-Westergren E, Franklin SH. Exercise testing in the equine athlete. EVE 2016;28(2):89–98.

17. Durando M. Exercise and stress testing. In: Marr CM, Bowen M, editors. Cardiology of the horse. 2nd edition. New York: Saunders Elsevier; 2010. p. 141.

18. Navas de Solis C, Green C, Slides R, et al. Arrhythmias in thoroughbred racehorses during and after treadmill and racehorse exercise. J Equine Vet Sci 2016;18:19–24.

19. Allen K, Young L, Franklin H. Evaluation of heart rate and rhythm during exercise. Equine Vet Educ 2016;28(2):99–112.

20. Navas de Solis C. Exercising arrhythmias and sudden cardiac death in horses: review of the literature and comparative aspects. Equine Vet J 2016;48:406–13.

21. Martin B, Reef V, Parente E, et al. Causes of poor performance in horses during training, racing or showing: 348 cases 1992-1996. J Am Vet Med Assoc 2000; 216(4):554–8.

22. Buhl R, Ekkelund Peterson E, Lindholm M. Cardiac arrhythmias in standardbreds during and after racing. Possible association between heart size, valvular regurgitations, and arrhythmias. J Equine Vet Sci 2013;33:590–6.

23. Seco Diaz O, Durando M, Birks K, et al. Cardiac troponin I concentrations in horses with colic. J Am Vet Med Assoc 2014;245(1):118–25.

24. van der Vekens A, Decloedt D, de Clercq S, et al. Atrial Natriuretic peptide vs. N-terminal-pro-atrial Natriuretic peptide for the detection of left atrial dilatation in horses. Equine Vet J 2016;48(1):15–20.

25. Alfonso T, Giguere S, Brown S, et al. Preliminary investigation of orally administered benazepril in horses with left-sided valvular regurgitation. Equine Vet J 2017;45:1–6.

26. Decloedt A, Schwarzwald C, De Clercq D, et al. Risk factors for recurrence of atrial fibrillation in horses after conversion to sinus rhythm. J Vet Intern Med 2015;29:946–53.

27. Verheyen T, Decloedt A, van Der Vekens N, et al. Ventricular response during lungeing exercise in horses with lone atrial fibrillation. Equine Vet J 2013;45:309–13.

28. Ryan N, Marr C, McGladdery A. Survey of cardiac arrhythmias during submaximal and maximal exercise in thoroughbred racehorses. Equine Vet J 2005;37(3):265–8.

29. Lyle C, Blissit K, Kennedy C. Risk factors for race associated deaths in thoroughbred racehorse in the UK (2000-2007). Equine Vet J 2012;44:469–75.

30. Lyle C, Uzal F, McGorum B. Sudden death in racing thoroughbred horses: an international multicenter study of post mortem findings. Equine Vet J 2011;43(3): 324–31.

31. Munsters CC, van Iwaarden A, van Weeren R, et al. Exercise testing in warmblood sport horses under field conditions. Vet J 2014;202(1):11–9.

32. Van Erck Westergren E, Richard E, Audrey A, et al. Field investigation of poor performance in TB racehorse. Scientific Abstracts, International Conference on Equine Exercise Physiology. 2014;46(s46).

33. Vincent TL, Newton JR, Deaton CM. Retrospective study of predictive variables for maximal heart rate (HR Max) in horses undergoing strenuous exercise. Equine Vet J 2006;(s36):146–52.
34. Decloedt A, Verheyen T, Van Der Vekens N. Long-term follow up of atrial function after cardioversion of atrial fibrillation in horses. Vet J 2013;197:583–8.
35. Lorello O, Ramseye A, Burger D. Repeated measurements of markers of autonomic tone over a training season in eventing horses. J Equine Vet Sci 2017; 53:38–44.
36. Physick-shear P, McGurrin M. Ventricular arrhythmias during race recovery in Standardbred racehorses and associations with autonomic activity. J Vet Intern Med 2010;24:1158–66.

Upper Airway Conditions Affecting the Equine Athlete

Eric J. Parente, DVM

KEYWORDS

- Upper airway • Performance • Larynx

KEY POINTS

- There are multiple different causes of upper airway dysfunction that can negatively impact performance.
- With history and physical examination findings, a critical resting endoscopic evaluation can reveal most abnormalities, but on occasion further diagnostic evaluations are important.
- Exercising endoscopy and ultrasound of the larynx can help determine abnormalities that are not easily determined otherwise.

INTRODUCTION

A primary purpose of the upper airway is to provide a large stable conduit for respiration. However, the simplicity stops there. Although either static or dynamic obstructions can compromise the flow of respiratory gases, determining the clinical significance of an abnormality relative to performance is challenging because there are so many factors that impact performance and so many different types of performance. Thus, any abnormality found on a resting endoscopic examination should always be considered in the context of the type of performance before reaching conclusions about performance limitations (eg, a moderate recurrent laryngeal neuropathy [RLN] may be totally irrelevant in a show jumper but significant for a flat racehorse). Furthermore, many of the abnormalities affecting performance horses are just appreciated under dynamic conditions and cannot be appreciated unless the horse is evaluated while performing. Therefore, any speculation after a resting endoscopic examination about a performance limiting respiratory problem should only be made if there is other corroborating evidence with history, clinical examination, and/or other diagnostics.

To add further complexity to the problem, because the respiratory tract intersects the digestive tract at the pharynx, almost any action taken on the respiratory tract can have an adverse effect on the functional separation of the two tracts. Thus, although the respiratory tract is the focus of the performance limitation, any intervention to improve the respiratory tract that inadvertently compromises the functional

Disclosure Statement: There is no conflict of interest.
Department of Clinical Sciences, New Bolton Center, University of Pennsylvania, 382 West Street Road, Kennett Square, PA 19348, USA
E-mail address: ejp@vet.upenn.edu

flexibility to manage feed material passed the respiratory tract results in contamination of the respiratory tract and likely a negative impact on performance.

This article elucidates the appropriate diagnostic techniques to arrive at a valid conclusion about performance-limiting respiratory problems and discusses potential treatments. Although the greatest area of resistance to airflow is nasal, it is uncommonly a site of obstruction in the performance horse and is not addressed in more detail.

THE EVALUATION

Any horse that makes an abnormal respiratory noise during exercise is likely experiencing some type of airflow obstruction and should be evaluated. The intensity of the abnormal noise is usually coincident with the intensity of exercise, so any variations in noise appreciated by the owner may just be a reflection of the noise associated with a different level of exercise and not a reflection of a change in the problem within the upper airway. Regardless, every initial evaluation should begin with history and physical examination. Palpation of the larynx for asymmetry or surgical scars may provide the clinician with valuable information. After this a resting endoscopic evaluation should be performed. It is always best to develop a standard routine for an examination to ensure that it is comprehensive and performed efficiently. A twitch for restraint is always recommended to give greater control over the horse's head position, and no sedatives should be given that would falsely alter the functional assessment of the upper airway. Although many practitioners perform the examination by passing and directing the scope themselves with just one person holding the horse, it is beneficial to have a different person pass the endoscope so there is greater control maintaining the position of the endoscope in the nasal passage.

The endoscope should be passed quickly through the rostral nasal passage and the endoscope should be directed ventral and medial to make certain it slides down the ventral meatus. Horses object the greatest when the endoscope is first passed. It is also important to not initially pass the endoscope more than 30 to 35 cm in the average adult. Passing it further may result in stimulating the pharyngeal wall and causing the horse to swallow or displace only because of the scope stimulation. This is often misinterpreted as a problem, when in many cases it is just because of the stimulation from the endoscope.

An initial overall assessment should be made of the pharyngeal vault. The epiglottis should be positioned dorsal to the palate and have a distinctly "serrated" edge with a clear vascular pattern. This pattern may not be seen in cases of epiglottitis or epiglottic entrapment. In either case the epiglottis remains dorsal to the palate and these conditions should not be confused with dorsal displacement of the soft palate. The arytenoids should be evaluated for their overall appearance and symmetry. Disruption of the arytenoid mucosa, or areas of granulation tissue on the axial surface with any enlargement of the arytenoid, may indicate an early chondrosis. A smaller misshapen corniculate, especially associated with decreased abduction, may indicate dysplasia. The movement/abduction of the arytenoids should initially be assessed with the horse at rest and immediately after stimulation of a swallow to determine maximum abduction on either side. Some clinicians prefer assessment of abduction during nasal occlusion but attaining full abduction this way is extremely variable depending on the tractability of the horse and the experience of the clinician. During swallowing there should be full symmetric midline adduction (that often cannot be seen because of pharyngeal contraction) followed by a fleeting full symmetric abduction of both arytenoids. Any asymmetry, particularly a lack of full abduction of the left relative to the right, is likely an indication of some degree of RLN. There are multiple grading systems to categorize laryngeal function during resting endoscopy[1–3] so correlations can be made between resting and exercising endoscopy[4–7] primarily for racehorses, but generally speaking any racehorse with even mild RLN likely suffers some dynamic collapse during strenuous exercise. Any other performance horse has to be evaluated during exercise on an individual basis to determine the impact on that specific horse.

Close inspection of the vocal cords and the ventricles of the larynx should always be performed. Because laser ablation/resection of the cord or ventricle has become commonplace for the treatment of RLN, an abnormal appearance of these structures may be a clue to a previous problem and treatment. Depending on how the previous procedure was performed, all that may be noticed is a loss of normal mucosa and a scarred appearance without complete absence of the cord (**Fig. 1**).

Before concluding the examination, it is worthwhile to pass the endoscope into the trachea and withdraw it. When the endoscope is withdrawn from the trachea it is common for the soft palate to be displaced dorsally. Normally, the horse should swallow quickly and replace the palate on the first attempt. Occasionally the swallow takes place just as the endoscope comes out of the larynx so that the free edge of the palate is never observed. If the horse does not replace the palate to normal position without prompting, the horse should be made to swallow by stimulating the pharynx with water from the endoscope or bumping the pharyngeal wall with the endoscope. Abnormalities of pharyngeal function, or abnormalities below the epiglottis, such as a cyst, may manifest themselves during these maneuvers. A horse with normal pharyngeal function should always have the epiglottis above the palate after swallowing.

RECURRENT LARYNGEAL NEUROPATHY

RLN is one of the most common abnormalities seen in performance horses. These horses typically make an inspiratory noise that becomes higher pitch and louder with increasing exercise and fatigue. It is typically progressive, so rest does not yield any

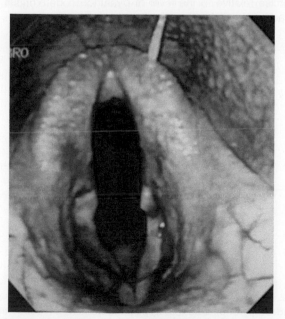

Fig. 1. Evidence of incomplete laser ablation of both vocal cords.

improvement. Arriving at a correct diagnosis of RLN is critical because the milder cases can easily be missed, or other disorders are easily misinterpreted as RLN potentially resulting in inappropriate treatment that is not effective (eg, a laryngoplasty being performed on a horse with a chondropathy or dysplasia, not a neuropathy) (**Fig. 2**). History, physical examination findings (asymmetrically palpable muscular process), resting endoscopy, and potentially dynamic endoscopy or ultrasound of the larynx are all critical components of ensuring an appropriate diagnosis. Asymmetric (incomplete) abduction of one arytenoid on resting endoscopy in conjunction with a horse that makes an abnormal inspiratory noise during exercise and an asymmetrically prominent muscular process on palpation of the larynx is typically all that is required to conclude the horse is experiencing dynamic collapse of that arytenoid during exercise. Although it is possible other soft tissue structures are also collapsing into the airway and some clinicians would advocate a dynamic endoscopic examination to determine what those structures might be, the airflow conditions before any treatment are different after treatment and thus the dynamics that affected those other tissues initially may no longer be present. Furthermore, if any one component of the initial examination is not consistent with the diagnosis then further diagnostics should be pursued.

If a diagnosis is not clear based on the history and resting examination an exercising examination or ultrasound of the larynx should be pursued. If performed appropriately an exercising examination should be conclusive. When head and neck position play an important role in how the horse performs or is noted to impact the presence of an abnormal noise, especially in certain breeds, an overground endoscopy rather than treadmill endoscopy is warranted.[8] If an exercising examination cannot be performed ultrasound of the larynx is reliable.[9] By some accounts ultrasound of the larynx was a better predictor of dynamic arytenoid collapse than resting endoscopy in racehorses.[10] This distinction on which horses this is applied to is important because although laryngeal ultrasound can determine the presence or absence of RLN in any horse, it cannot determine if dynamic laryngeal collapse will occur in any nonracehorses because the only level of exercise relative to the level of dysfunction determines if the arytenoid cannot maintain adequate abduction or not.

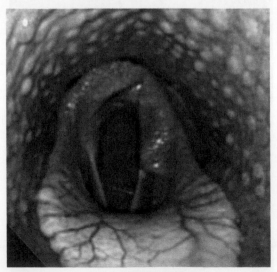

Fig. 2. Resting endoscopy of a horse that appears to be RLN, but subtle endoscopic abnormalities raised suspicion of chondropathy that was confirmed ultrasonographically.

The next principle is to target treatment to resolve the primary clinical problem. There is no single treatment that is the best for all horses because horses of different disciplines have different clinical problems. In the racehorse the primary problem is exercise intolerance, not abnormal noise. Although the noise is a clinical abnormality indicative of the problem, the abnormal noise is not the most relevant problem. Thus, the primary goal is to improve exercise tolerance by preventing obstruction of the collapsing arytenoid and associated soft tissue. Treatment by ventriculocordectomy solely is likely insufficient in most racehorses, although some evidence may suggest otherwise.[11] Pursuing a vocal cordectomy alone for a nonracehorse that is making an abnormal noise without exercise intolerance (not experiencing complete dynamic collapse of the arytenoid during exercise) is reasonable to consider and likely efficacious. The only caveat is that the progressive nature of the disease will likely result in greater dynamic collapse in the future and more significant respiratory compromise that warrants techniques that yield greater arytenoid abduction/stabilization later. The surgical options to create greater abduction/stabilization or just a larger opening to the glottis when a horse is experiencing dynamic collapse of the arytenoid are arytenoidectomy or laryngoplasty.

Horses can race/perform well after arytenoidectomy and the overall "return to racing" percentage may be similar to the return to racing percentage in horses after traditional laryngoplasty,[12,13] yet the career length seems shorter after arytenoidectomy compared with laryngoplasty.[14] Although it is not identified why the career length is shorter, it is most likely because the upper airway mechanics are improved but still insufficient to race successfully or there is secondary lower airway inflammation that is compromising performance. Experimental data support this concept.[15] Radcliffe and colleagues[15] showed in a recurrent laryngeal neurectomy model that the upper airway mechanics after arytenoidectomy were improved but greater improvement was achieved with a laryngoplasty, and contamination of the lower airway was confirmed via tracheobronchial aspirate analysis. Thus, the laryngoplasty is the preferred method of treatment of RLN with dynamic arytenoid collapse and the surgery is performed no differently for a racehorse than any other horse, although the surgeon may be less likely to attempt as much abduction with the nonracehorse as they do with the racehorse. Based on experimental evidence, 90% abduction is the ideal target.[16] Depending on the experience and specific technique the surgeon chooses, a certain amount of abduction loss may be expected postoperatively and this should be taken into account at the time of surgery so the long-term result is still 80% to 90% abduction.

Clinical success after laryngoplasty in racehorses has been modest, ranging from 45% to 70%.[17–19] There is no evidence that the preoperative degree of arytenoid dysfunction limits the success of the surgery. Postoperative loss of abduction likely has the greatest impact on the limited success. Loss of abduction after laryngoplasty has been documented clinically[17–21] and experimentally.[15,22] The most dramatic loss is within the first few weeks but can continue 6 weeks or more, and the amount of abduction loss is not uniform for every horse.[20] There is also controversial evidence that the resting degree of abduction after surgery has any bearing on the stability of the arytenoid during exercise or on postoperative performance.[23,24] A conclusion made by some clinicians that stability is more important than the amount of abduction is misleading because these two factors are not exclusive of each other, and ideally a stable opening with greater abduction is the most favorable physiologic condition that provides the greatest airflow.

Resting postoperative endoscopic evaluations are recommended 1 day and 4 weeks after surgery to assess the resting position of the arytenoid, healing of the cordectomy (if performed), and any unanticipated abnormalities. Greater abduction increases the risk of aspiration, but the amount of abduction is not directly correlated to the amount of aspiration. Greater than 80% abduction long term seems to also increase the risk of long-term chondropathy even without any gross evidence of aspiration.

Coughing secondary to aspiration is another potential complication postoperatively. Gross feed material should never be seen within the nasopharynx or larynx, yet some clinicians expect horses will cough for several days after surgery associated with maximal arytenoid abduction from the time of surgery, and anticipate the coughing will stop as the horse loses some abduction. Although this may be true, postoperative coughing can virtually be eliminated by minimizing surgical trauma during the laryngoplasty, by more deliberate positioning of arytenoid abduction with intraoperative endoscopy, and by using a technique that minimizes postoperative abduction loss. Thus "overabduction" is avoided at surgery. If abduction seems excessive on resting endoscopic examination and coughing persists beyond several weeks, revision is recommended.

There are many differences among surgeons in how they perform laryngoplasties. The modified laryngoplasty was developed to minimize abduction loss in the immediate postoperative period and to enhance the long-term stability of the abduction created at surgery.[25] In earlier studies only 70% to 80% of horses treated by traditionally laryngoplasty returned to racing,[14,17,18] and even those that raced had limited career lengths. In a recent retrospective using quarterly earnings to assess success the results showed that 100% of the horses undergoing a modified laryngoplasty returned to racing,[26] they had similar earnings over all quarters (except the first during the immediate postoperative period) and had a competitive career of similar length to cohort controls. This contrasts with other studies[14,23] that demonstrated a shortened career length of the traditional laryngoplasty horses versus control animals, and this refutes a common perception that horses having undergone a laryngoplasty have a shorter racing career with decreased earnings relative to their peers.

Horses that continue to make abnormal respiratory noise or experience continued poor performance after laryngoplasty should warrant further diagnostic examinations to determine the cause. A resting endoscopic examination should be performed first to assess the amount of arytenoid abduction and shape/appearance of the corniculate. Horses with well abducted arytenoids (>70%) should undergo exercising endoscopy overground or on a treadmill to determine if there is dynamic collapse of the arytenoid or other soft tissues.[24,27] If the left arytenoid is not collapsing, the other likely potential offenders are the right aryepiglottic fold or right vocal cord (assuming the left vocal cord is no longer present). If the glottic opening is obviously compromised at rest from an unabducted arytenoid or arytenoid chondropathy then revision surgery or retirement from racing must be considered.

ARYTENOID ABNORMALITIES (CHONDROPATHIES/DYSPLASIAS)

Chondropathies and dysplasias are functionally more similar to each other than RLN because the cricoarytenoideus dorsalis muscle is often normal with chondropathies/dysplasias but the inability to attain a large glottis is secondary to structural abnormalities of the laryngeal cartilages themselves and the anatomic relationship to each other. The difference between chondropathies and dysplasias is that dysplasias are congenital and rarely worsen over time, yet chondropathies typically develop secondary to an infectious process and can reach periods of stasis but often worsen over time.

The specific cartilage and articular abnormalities of laryngeal dysplasias vary between horses.[28] Although the more common abnormalities noted endoscopically are incomplete right-sided abduction, palatopharyngeal arch displacements, and corniculate incongruity, there are occasions that abnormalities are not appreciated on resting endoscopy (**Fig. 3**) or even mimic the resting endoscopic appearance of

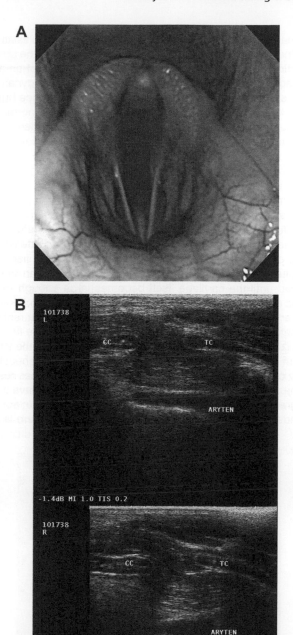

Fig. 3. (*A*) Endoscopic image of maximal abduction of a horse that made an abnormal noise during exercise associated with poor bilateral abduction. (*B*) The associated ultrasound images of the same horse with separation of the thyroid and cricoid cartilages. CC, cricoid cartilage; TC, thyroid cartilage.

RLN. The significant functional difference between RLN and dysplasias is that dysplasias often have the inability to attain full abduction but may have the ability to maintain whatever abduction they can attain. The lack of full abduction of an arytenoid often precipitates adjacent soft tissue structure to collapse under dynamic conditions. The diagnosis is suspected by the resting endoscopic appearance but confirmed by ultrasound or MRI.[28] The most consistent ultrasonographic abnormality is the lack of contact between the wing of the thyroid and the cricoid, yet there are other abnormalities too. Because of the variability of the abnormalities associated with dysplasias it is often impossible to accurately predict what will happen to the horse's throat under dynamic conditions and thus all dysplastic horses should undergo a dynamic endoscopy assessment before drawing conclusions on treatment. Even horses with apparent total immobility of an arytenoid may be able to perform successfully (**Fig. 4**).

Chondropathies impact performance because the deformation of the arytenoid cartilage impairs full abduction and depending on the degree of deformation obstructs a larger area of the glottis. Similar to dysplasias this also precipitates adjacent soft tissue structures to collapse into the airway during exercise and similar to dysplasias ultrasound is helpful in making the correct diagnosis.[29] More often the chondropathy may go unnoticed until the cartilage itself becomes large enough to impair a large part of the glottic opening or acutely becomes a chondritis with marked edema associated with the larynx and cause respiratory compromise even at rest. When there is marked inflammation and edema associated with a chondritis, the first line of defense should be minimizing oxygen demand (keeping the horse quiet in the stall) and treating aggressively with antimicrobials and anti-inflammatories. A tracheostomy that may seem necessary can often be avoided in most cases. Most horses resolve the acute edema within the first few days of treatment and then one can have a better assessment of the degree of permanent damage to the larynx (**Fig. 5**). In some patients the chondritis is rendered to a more chronic chondropathy and if there is minimal glottic

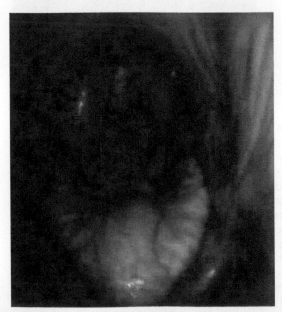

Fig. 4. Still frame from the exercising endoscopy of an event horse with right-sided laryngeal dysplasia that was competing successfully after only right-sided vocal cordectomy.

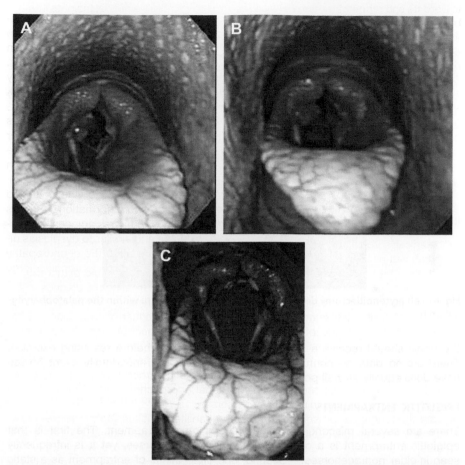

Fig. 5. (*A*) Acute arytenoid chondritis with a small glottis. (*B*) The same horse with an improved glottis after only 2 days of medical treatment. (*C*) The same horse 2 years after initial treatment with a static chondropathy. The horse had raced successfully despite the residual chondropathy.

impingement the horse can resume performance without further treatment. More commonly an arytenoidectomy is required to improve the horse's airway to allow for resumption of performance, but if the disease is bilateral the prognosis is much worse.

Although different forms of arytenoidectomies have been described,[12,30–32] the partial arytenoidectomy has been shown to provide the least postoperative obstruction.[30–33] A temporary tracheotomy is required to administer the inhalant anesthesia for a partial arytenoidectomy, because the surgery is performed through a laryngotomy. This author prefers to perform the arytenoidectomy through a dorsally based mucosal flap and use a primary closure.[13] Although this approach is more challenging the outcome is not dependent on the variability of second intention healing of the defect, and the results are favorable for returning to racing.[13] Postoperatively, a thin rim of mucosa should be seen just under the palatopharyngeal arch that should minimize any risk of aspiration and still provide an adequate glottis for performance (**Fig. 6**). If granulation tissue is present at a 1-month follow-up, it is transendoscopically removed with a laser on an outpatient basis. Once there is complete mucosal healing,

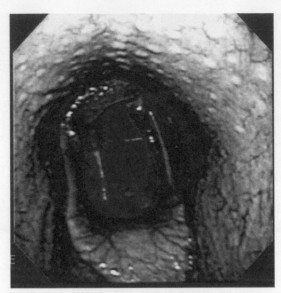

Fig. 6. Left arytenoidectomy demonstrating a thin rim of mucosa within the palatopharyngeal arch.

the horse should receive a second month with turnout before resuming exercise. There are no data on nonracehorses to draw from but anecdotally event horses have done equally as well postoperatively.

EPIGLOTTIC ENTRAPMENTS

There are several misconceptions about epiglottic entrapment. The first is that epiglottic entrapment is a disease of just young racehorses, yet it is infrequently seen in older nonracehorses.[34] Second, one often thinks of entrapment as a static condition because most frequently it is seen as such on a resting endoscopy, but it likely starts as an intermittent entrapment that then becomes persistent. Third, it is assumed that the epiglottic entrapment causes abnormal noise and/or exercise Intolerance, whereas a simple entrapment does neither. Finally, it is assumed that epiglottic entrapments are treated easily with axial division of the membrane and have an excellent prognosis, whereas in reality not all entrapments are the same and the prognosis is variable based on the pathology of the entrapping membrane and possibly the epiglottis itself.[35]

It is true that epiglottic entrapments are most commonly observed in racehorses, but are seen in nonracing performance horses and even older retired horses. Typically, the entrapment in racehorses is found on resting endoscopy performed for performance issues or abnormal respiratory noise. Interestingly, a simple entrapment alone does not cause significant respiratory compromise or abnormal noise,[36] but the entrapment can often precipitate or be associated with displacement of the soft palate that compromises performance and creates noise.[37] It is likely that a secondary displacement that causes significant respiratory obstruction and noise is what prompts the resting endoscopic examination. In the nonracehorses a more common complaint that prompts the endoscopic examination is coughing.[34]

Most entrapments are persistent at the time they are diagnosed. Infrequently they are seen dynamically associated with swallowing at rest or are diagnosed dynamically during exercise. If the horse is not experiencing exercise intolerance or abnormal respiratory noise (likely not displacing their palate during exercise) the entrapment does not need to be resolved immediately and the horse can continue to compete successfully for a short period of time. It is not advised to leave an entrapment for an extended period of time if the outline of the tip of the epiglottis is not well delineated or if the membranes are particularly thick because these conditions could lead to more permanent deformation of the epiglottis or subepiglottic membranes.

Local anti-inflammatory medication and rest may be beneficial for simple entrapments diagnosed early, but more often entrapments diagnosed during resting endoscopy are treated surgically. In one study, 4 out of 38 horses with epiglottic entrapment were treated with anti-inflammatory throat spray alone, with resolution of the entrapment without any further treatment in three out of four of these horses.[38] A variety of techniques have been described for the surgical treatment of epiglottic entrapment. Axial division of the entrapping membrane with slightly differing techniques is most commonly performed using a curved bistoury or laser.[39–43] Alternatively, resection of the entrapping membrane is performed via laryngotomy under general anesthesia,[41] but the results seem less favorable. Some entrapments cannot be resolved with axial division of the membrane and resection of tissue is sometimes necessary. This is performed under general anesthesia or with the horse standing via transendoscopic laser surgery. It is preferred to do it standing rather than under general anesthesia because the natural position of the tissues is better appreciated in the standing transnasal approach. Regardless, resection of tissues should be reserved for only those cases in which it is required because resection of tissue requires a longer postoperative time for healing and can lead to a decreased prognosis.[35]

INTERMITTENT DORSAL DISPLACEMENT OF THE SOFT PALATE

This is truly a dynamic abnormality that cannot be reliably diagnosed on a resting endoscopic examination. There may be strong suggestions of this abnormality based on the resting endoscopic examination and history of poor performance associated with an abnormal expiratory noise, yet an exercise examination is required to make a definitive diagnosis. Furthermore, a horse that displaces during some performance may not reliably displace during an exercising endoscopic examination. Head and neck position, the degree of stress, and speed and interaction with the rider or driver can have a major impact on whether or not a horse displaces their palate. Nonsurgical management by changing the way the horse is used, or medical treatment are successful in some horses.

Not all horses displace for the same reason.[37] This is likely part of the reason there is not one universal treatment of all horses. Most displace secondary to a relative position of the larynx to the pharynx that was reproduced experimentally.[44] There could be multiple structural abnormalities that precipitate dorsal displacement of the soft palate and the clinician should determine if any of these abnormalities are present before formulating a treatment plan. Both guttural pouches should be evaluated because disease of the pouches could impact neural structures that affect pharyngeal function.[45] Any subepiglottic abnormality can result in intermittent or even persistent palate displacement. The more common abnormalities may be cysts or thickened membranes associated with ulceration or previous surgery. These may not be evident on standard endoscopic evaluations and manipulation of the epiglottis under endoscopic observation may be necessary (**Fig. 7**). Previous laryngoplasty has also been shown to precipitate displacement of the palate during exercise.[46] This may be a response to a level of aspiration. Addressing these abnormalities (if possible) should be part of any plan of treatment.

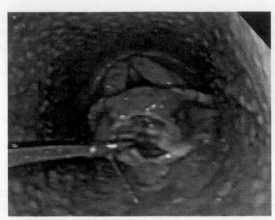

Fig. 7. Exposure of subepiglottic ulceration and thickened membranes by elevation of the epiglottis with long equine laryngeal forceps while the horse is sedated and the throat topically anesthetized.

The main surgical goal for treatment of displacement is to control the position of the larynx within the pharynx. A sternothyroid tenectomy is an easy procedure to perform with minimal recuperation time that decreases the caudal traction on the larynx during exercise. It seems to be successful in many horses. A more active approach is a tie-forward. This procedure restricts the position of the larynx to the hyoid apparatus and thus it is hoped maintains its position within the pharynx relative to the palate. Most horses have demonstrated an improvement in performance.[47]

OTHER ABNORMALITIES

Other abnormalities that are seen that could compromise performance horses are less common and require exercising examination to make a diagnosis. They include pharyngeal collapse, rostral billowing of the soft palate, medial deviation of the aryepiglottic folds, overriding corniculate processes, and epiglottic retroversion.[48–52] Not only do these abnormalities require exercising examination to make the diagnosis, but head and neck position is often critical to the presence or absence of these abnormalities.

These abnormalities are documented with increasing frequency as the spread of overground exercising endoscopy becomes more common. Yet, there should be some caution in attributing a performance problem to some or all of these abnormalities without critical evaluation. Despite the frequency of diagnosis there is limited experimental evidence about the degree of respiratory obstruction caused by some of these abnormalities and there is a range for each abnormality. If these abnormalities are seen endoscopically but do not cause abnormal respiratory noise the question should be raised about how much obstruction it can cause and how much is performance truly being affected.

The pathophysiology behind these abnormalities is still unclear and likely multifaceted. Neuromuscular strength, the physical geometry of an individual horse's airway, and the respiratory demand on the airway to maintain its integrity are the three main variables. There have been no proven methods to improve the neuromuscular strength that may resolve various forms of pharyngeal collapse, but there is some evidence that younger horses may resolve their condition over time.[48] Although the pathophysiology of aryepiglottic fold deviation is unknown, transendoscopic laser resection offers a treatment that has some proven success.[50] Epiglottic retroversion is likely a dysfunction of the hyoepiglotticus muscle or innervation and there is an unpublished surgical technique that has allowed two racehorses to return to racing successfully.

SUMMARY

There is no question upper airway dysfunction is performance limiting or even performance ruining. Fortunately, improved understanding and technology continues to enable clinicians to more accurately diagnose and effectively treat upper airway abnormalities. Yet the challenge continues to be more than just improved performance relative to the ailed performance, it is returning to completely normal function. Given the functional complexity of the upper respiratory tract, that goal remains more elusive.

REFERENCES

1. Hackett RP, Ducharme NG, Fubini SL, et al. The reliability of endoscopic examination in assessment of arytenoid cartilage movement in horses. Part I: subjective and objective laryngeal evaluation. Vet Surg 1991;20(3):174–9.
2. Perkins JD, Salz RO, Schumacher J, et al. Variability of resting endoscopic grading for assessment of recurrent laryngeal neuropathy in horses. Equine Vet J 2009;41(4):342–6.
3. Robinson NE. Consensus statements on equine recurrent laryngeal neuropathy: conclusions of the Havemeyer Workshop. Stratford Upon Avon. Equine Vet Educ 2004;16:333–6.
4. Parente E, Martin B. Correlation between standing endoscopic examinations and those made during high speed exercise in horses: 150 cases. Proc Ann Convention Am Assoc Equine Pract 1995;41:170–1.
5. Lane JG, Bladon B, Little DR, et al. Dynamic obstructions of the equine upper respiratory tract. Part 2: comparison of endoscopic findings at rest and during high speed treadmill exercise of 600 thoroughbred racehorses. Equine Vet J 2006;38:401–7.
6. Barakzai SZ, Dixon PM. Correlation of resting and exercising endoscopic findings for horses with dynamic laryngeal collapse and palatal dysfunction. Equine Vet J 2011;43:18–23.
7. Davison JA, Lumsden JM, Boston RC, et al. Overground endoscopy in 311 thoroughbred racehorses: findings and correlation to resting laryngeal function. Aust Vet J 2017;95(9):338–42.
8. Van Erck E. Dynamic respiratory videoendoscopy in ridden sport horses: effect of head flexion, riding and airway inflammation in 129 cases. Equine Vet J Suppl 2011;40:18–24.
9. Chalmers HJ, Yeager AE, Cheetham J, et al. Diagnostic sensitivity of subjective and quantitative laryngeal ultrasonography for recurrent laryngeal neuropathy in horses. Vet Radiol Ultrasound 2012;53(6):660–6.
10. Garrett KS, Woodie JB, Embertson RM. Association of treadmill upper airway endoscopic evaluation with results of ultrasonography and resting upper airway endoscopic evaluation. Equine Vet J 2011;43(3):365–71.
11. Taylor SE, Barakzai SZ, Dixon P. Ventriculocordectomy as the sole treatment for recurrent laryngeal neuropathy: long-term results from ninety-two horses. Vet Surg 2006;35(7):653–7.
12. Barnes AJ, Slone DE, Lynch TM. Performance after partial arytenoidectomy without mucosal closure in 27 thoroughbred racehorses. Vet Surg 2004;33:398–403.
13. Parente EJ, Tulleners EP, Southwood LL. Long-term study of partial arytenoidectomy with primary mucosal closure in 76 thoroughbred racehorses (1992-2006). Equine Vet J 2008;40:214–8.

14. Witte TH, Mohammed HO, Radcliffe CH, et al. Racing performance after combined prosthetic laryngoplasty and ipsilateral ventriculocordectomy or partial arytenoidectomy: 135 thoroughbred racehorses competing at less than 2400 m (1997-2007). Equine Vet J 2009;41:70–5.

15. Radcliffe CH, Woodie JB, Hackett RP, et al. A comparison of laryngoplasty and modified partial arytenoidectomy as treatments for laryngeal hemiplegia in exercising horses. Vet Surg 2006;35:643–52.

16. Rakesh V, Ducharme NG, Cheetham J, et al. Implications of different degrees of arytenoid cartilage abduction on equine upper airway characteristics. Equine Vet J 2008;40(7):629–35.

17. Hawkins JF, Tulleners EP, Ross MW, et al. Laryngoplasty with or without ventriculectomy for treatment of left laryngeal hemiplegia in 230 racehorses. Vet Surg 1997;26:484–91.

18. Davenport CL, Tulleners EP, Parente EJ. The effect of recurrent laryngeal neurectomy in conjunction with laryngoplasty and unilateral ventriculocordectomy in thoroughbred racehorses. Vet Surg 2001;30:417–21.

19. Kidd JA, Slone DE. Treatment of laryngeal hemiplegia in horses by prosthetic laryngoplasty, ventriculectomy, and vocal cordectomy. Vet Rec 2002;150:481–4.

20. Dixon RM, McGorum BC, Railton DI, et al. Long-term survey of laryngoplasty and ventriculocordectomy in an older, mixed-breed population of 200 horses. Part 1: maintenance of surgical arytenoid abduction and complications of surgery. Equine Vet J 2003;35(4):389–96.

21. Rossignol F, Vitte A, Boening J, et al. Laryngoplasty in standing horses. Vet Surg 2015;44(3):341–7.

22. Brown JA, Derksen FJ, Stick JA, et al. Effect of laryngoplasty on respiratory noise reduction in horses with laryngeal hemiplegia. Equine Vet J 2004;36(5):420–5.

23. Barakzai SZ, Boden LA, Dixon PM. Race performance after laryngoplasty and ventriculocordectomy in National Hunt racehorses. Vet Surg 2009;38(8):941–5.

24. Davidson EJ, Martin BB, Rieger RH, et al. Exercising videoendoscopic evaluation of 45 horses with respiratory noise and/or poor performance after laryngoplasty. Vet Surg 2010;39(8):942–8.

25. Parente EJ, Birks EK, Habecker P. A modified laryngoplasty approach promoting ankylosis of the cricoarytenoid joint. Vet Surg 2011;40(2):204–10.

26. Aceto H, Parente EJ. Using quarterly earnings to assess racing performance in 70 thoroughbreds after modified laryngoplasty for treatment of recurrent laryngeal neuropathy. Vet Surg 2012;41(6):689–95.

27. Leutton JL, Lumsden JM. Dynamic respiratory endoscopic findings pre- and post laryngoplasty in thoroughbred racehorses. Equine Vet J 2015;47(5):531–6.

28. Garrett KS, Woodie JB, Embertson RM, et al. Diagnosis of laryngeal dysplasia in five horses using magnetic resonance imaging and ultrasonography. Equine Vet J 2009;41(8):766–71.

29. Garrett KS, Embertson RM, Woodie JB, et al. Ultrasound features of arytenoid chondritis in thoroughbred horses. Equine Vet J 2013;45(5):598–603.

30. Belknap JK, Derksen FJ, Nickels FA, et al. Failure of subtotal arytenoidectomy to improve upper airway flow mechanics in exercising Standardbreds with induced laryngeal hemiplegia. Am J Vet Res 1990;51:1481–6.

31. Tulleners EP, Harrison IW, Mann P. Partial arytenoidectomy in the horse with and without mucosal closure. Vet Surg 1988;17:252–7.

32. Hay WP, Tulleners EP, Ducharme NG. Partial arytenoidectomy in the horse using an extra-laryngeal approach. Vet Surg 1993;22:50–6.

33. Lumsden JM, Derksen FJ, Stick JA, et al. Evaluation of partial arytenoidectomy as a treatment for equine laryngeal hemiplegia. Equine Vet J 1994;26:125–9.
34. Aitken MR, Parente EJ. Epiglottic abnormalities in mature nonracehorses: 23 cases (1990-2009). J Am Vet Med Assoc 2011;238(12):1634–8.
35. Keiffer PJ, Aceto H, Stefanovski D, et al. Using quarterly earnings to assess racing performance in 66 thoroughbreds after transendoscopic laser surgery for treatment of epiglottic entrapment. Vet Surg, in press.
36. Williams JW, Meagher DM, Pascoe JR, et al. Upper airway function during maximal exercise in horses with obstructive upper airway lesions. Effect of surgical treatment. Vet Surg 1990;19(2):142–7.
37. Parente EJ, Martin BB, Tulleners EP, et al. Dorsal displacement of the soft palate in 92 horses during high speed treadmill examination (1993–1998). Vet Surg 2002;31:507–12.
38. Greet TRC. Experiences in treatment of epiglottal entrapment using a hook knife per nasum. Equine Vet J 1995;27(2):122–6.
39. Tulleners EP. Transendoscopic contact neodymium:yttrium aluminum garnet laser correction of epiglottic entrapment in standing horses. J Am Vet Med Assoc 1990; 196(12):1971–80.
40. Ross MW, Gentile DG, Evans LH. Transoral axial division, under endoscopic guidance, for correction of epiglottic entrapment in horses. J Am Vet Med Assoc 1993; 203(3):416–20.
41. Lumsden JM, Stick JA, Caron JP, et al. Surgical treatment for epiglottic entrapment in horses: 51 cases (1981-1992). J Am Vet Med Assoc 1994;205(5):729–35.
42. Perkins JD, Hughes TK, Brain B. Endoscope-guided, transoral axial division of an entrapping epiglottic fold in fifteen standing horses. Vet Surg 2007;36(8):800–3.
43. Lacourt M, Marcoux M. Treatment of epiglottic entrapment by transnasal axial division in standing sedated horses using a shielded hook bistoury. Vet Surg 2011; 40(3):299–304.
44. Ducharme NG, Hackett RP, Woodie JB, et al. Investigations into the role of the thyrohyoid muscles in the pathogenesis of dorsal displacement of the soft palate in horses. Equine Vet J 2003;35(3):258–63.
45. Holcombe SJ, Derksen FJ, Stick JA, et al. Effect of bilateral blockade of the pharyngeal branch of the vagus nerve on soft palate function in horses. Am J Vet Res 1998;59(4):504–8.
46. Barnett TP, O'Leary JM, Dixon PM, et al. Characterisation of palatal dysfunction after laryngoplasty. Equine Vet J 2014;46(1):60–3.
47. Cheetham J, Pigott JH, Thorson LM, et al. Racing performance following the laryngeal tie-forward procedure: a case-controlled study. Equine Vet J 2008;40(5):501–7.
48. Boyle AG, Martin BB Jr, Davidson EJ, et al. Dynamic pharyngeal collapse in racehorses. Equine Vet J Suppl 2006;36:546–50.
49. Allen KJ, Lane JG, Woodford NS, et al. Severe collapse of the rostral soft palate as a source of abnormal respiratory noise in six ponies and horses. Equine Vet J 2007;39(6):562–6.
50. King DS, Tulleners E, Martin BB Jr, et al. Clinical experiences with axial deviation of the aryepiglottic folds in 52 racehorses. Vet Surg 2001;30:151–60.
51. Dart AJ, Dowling BA, Smith CL. Upper airway dysfunction associated with collapse of the apex of the corniculate process of the left arytenoid cartilage during exercise in 15 horses. Vet Surg 2005;34(6):543–7.
52. Parente EJ, Martin BB, Tulleners EP. Epiglottic retroversion as a cause of upper airway obstruction in two horses. Equine Vet J 1998;30(3):270–2.

Lower Airway Disease in the Athletic Horse

Melissa R. Mazan, DVM

KEYWORDS

- EIPH • IAD • Equine asthma • Respiratory • Exercise • Performance

KEY POINTS

- Exercise-induced pulmonary hemorrhage (EIPH) and inflammatory airway disease (IAD) are the two most important lower airway diseases of the athletic horse.
- EIPH may be considered, at least at the onset, as a problem of physiology rather than a disease, and IAD is a disease primarily of domestication.
- Both EIPH and IAD are widespread among the athletic horse population and account for an impressive number of horses that fail to perform to their potential.
- Because of the high demands for oxygen in the athletic horse, even minor insults to the oxygen-carrying capacity of the body can affect performance, so it is of critical importance to keep the lungs as healthy as possible.

EXERCISE-INDUCED PULMONARY HEMORRHAGE

Exercise-induced pulmonary hemorrhage (EIPH), or bleeding that comes from the horse's lungs during exercise, is certainly the most dramatic of the lower airway diseases that affect equine athletes and the one that causes most consternation in the lay population. It is commonly held by both veterinarians and the lay population that EIPH is a major cause of wastage for equine athletes, especially in the racing industry, and that, when severe, it can result in sudden death. Despite this accepted knowledge, in reality, the connection between performance and EIPH is still poorly understood and sudden death due to EIPH occurs in less than 0.029% of the racing population. There is, indeed, debate as to whether EIPH is even a disease or whether it is an inevitable outcome of the remarkable physiology that allows the horse to be an elite athlete.

Epidemiology: Who Gets It and What Are the Risk Factors?

Bleeding Childers, the grand progenitor of Eclipse, who is ubiquitous in the pedigree of almost all modern racehorses, was eponymously named because he bled so often.

Disclosure Statement: No conflicts or commercial affiliations to disclose.
Department of Clinical Sciences, Tufts University Cummings School of Veterinary Medicine, 200 Westboro Road, North Grafton, MA 01536, USA
E-mail address: melissa.mazan@tufts.edu

Vet Clin Equine 34 (2018) 443–460
https://doi.org/10.1016/j.cveq.2018.04.010
0749-0739/18/© 2018 Elsevier Inc. All rights reserved.

Although EIPH is well-recognized in the equine racing population, with the vast majority of racing Thoroughbreds and Standardbreds affected,[1] it has become increasingly clear that this is a disease that any horse that performs strenuous exercise at speed has. Populations of horses that perform bursts of work at speed are those that have most recently been identified as experiencing EIPH, including barrel horses whose runs generally last less than 20 seconds[2] and polo ponies that run for short bursts of speed during a 7-minute chukka.[3] Reported prevalences depend on the method used for diagnosis. For instance, if tracheobronchoscopy is used within 2 hours of racing, up to 75% of racehorses are found to be bleeders,[4] whereas with examination of cytology from bronchoalveolar lavage (BAL) to detect evidence of recent and more chronic hemorrhage from the lungs, the number approaches 100%.[5] One population of highly competitive horses that does not regularly experience EIPH, however, is the endurance horse even at high levels of competition.[6] The putative reasons for this will be more fully explored in the later discussion of pathogenesis.

The biggest risk factor for a horse developing EIPH is going at high speed or undergoing very intense exercise. This is most easily appreciated in Thoroughbred racehorses, where it has been found that more horses have evidence of pulmonary hemorrhage after racing than they do after breezing.[7] Horses jumping at speed, such as steeplechasers, are more likely to develop EIPH than horses that race on the flat.[8] Although older horses are commonly thought to be more susceptible to EIPH, it is years spent racing rather than age itself that is associated with EIPH. Other risk factors that have been identified include exercise when temperatures are less than 68F and wearing bar shoes.[9]

Pathogenesis: Why Do Horses Bleed from the Lungs?

The prevailing theory for the cause of EIPH posits that stress failure of pulmonary capillaries occurs because of very high transmural pressures or the pressure that develops across the wall of the pulmonary capillary. It is easiest to think of this as a push and a pull—the push comes from a very high pulmonary artery pressure at intense exercise, and the pull comes from a negative alveolar pressure at the same time as the horse breathes in. This, in turn, is mandated in order to accommodate the horse's phenomenal exercise capacity; in order to supply the amount of oxygen that the horse needs to perform at its extraordinary levels of Vo_{2max}, the heart rate must be high and pulmonary capillary pressures skyrocket from approximately 25 mm Hg to up to 90 mm Hg because high left ventricular filling pressures are necessary to maintain cardiac output in these conditions. Simultaneously, in order to accommodate the need for increased ventilation that is coupled to the horse's stride, the respiratory system is forced to exert tremendous negative pressures in the pleural space—up to −60 cm H_2O or approximately 45 mm Hg. These pressures summate to more than 120 mm Hg transmural pressure, making it easy to understand why pulmonary capillaries then rupture.[10] For perspective, in human athletes, 20 to 25 mm Hg threshold for pulmonary capillary pressures is associated with interstitial lung edema and altered ventilation/perfusion relationships, and maximum pulmonary arterial pressures (PAPs) of 40 to 50 mm Hg, which elite human athletes can achieve at maximal exercise, are considered to correspond to the extreme of tolerable right ventricular afterload.[11] These numbers seem positively puny with respect to the exercise physiology of the horse.

Anything, therefore, that either increases pulmonary artery pressures or decreases (creates a larger negative pressure) alveolar pressures will potentiate EIPH in the equine athlete. The most logical comorbidities that would contribute, therefore, would be dynamic upper airway obstructions, such as laryngeal hemiplegia or dorsal displacement of the soft palate. The tendency of steeplechasers to hold their breath over the jump, thus causing a greater negative pressure during great exertion, may help to explain their increased likelihood to bleed. Human athletes who hold their breath, such as sprint swimmers and divers, also have an increased likelihood to experience alveolar hemorrhage.[12]

Although clinicians commonly associate lower airway inflammation with EIPH, there is more clear evidence of EIPH as a cause of lower airway inflammation, rather than as a result.[13] It is important to remember that association between airway inflammation and EIPH, as has been seen in racehorses,[8] is not an evidence of causation. In a recent study looking at tracheal mucus accumulation (TMA) as a marker of lower airway inflammation in barrel horses and EIPH, the presence of both was high, but that of TMA was almost twice that of EIPH, thus there was no linear correlation between the two.[14] It is likely that EIPH has multifactorial causes, and it will be difficult to sort them out.

Heritability

It is difficult to detect heritability of a condition or a physiology when virtually all members of a cohort experience the problem to some degree. Two studies, done in countries where race-day treatment is not allowed, suggested a component of heritability.[15,16] Very recently, single nucleotide polymorphisms in CD39 and CD39L1, which are important in maintaining normal hemostasis and limiting inflammation, were shown to be highly prevalent in horses with pathologic evidence of EIPH on post-mortem examination,[17] which is suggestive of but does not prove a genetic basis for the disease.

Pathology: What Do We See?

When the lungs of a horse with chronic EIPH are seen on post-mortem examination, gross abnormalities, in the form of gun-metal discoloration, are easily seen on the dorsal border, but not on the cranioventral area of the lung. This area of the lung is usually obviously stiff as well. On microscopic examination, the abnormalities are seen to be due to accumulation of hemosiderin as well as pleural and septal fibrosis and angiogenesis.[18] It has been shown that the pulmonary veins in this region are extensively remodeled, termed veno-occlusive remodeling, which results in increased resistance and may contribute to mechanical stress failure.[19]

Effect on Performance

When assessing the literature, it is important to see where the study was done. Furosemide is an accepted race-day medication (within 4 hours of racing) in North America, but is generally not accepted internationally. So when you are looking at performance in North America, you are generally looking at medicated horses. It is also important to remember that races and other competitions are won and lost by hundredths of seconds, so it can be exceedingly difficult to sort out what is contributing to success or failure, and a large number of horses are necessary for a strong study. With this in mind, a very large study out of South Africa, looking at 1000 horses using trachea bronchoscopy, found that 68% had EIPH greater than grade 1, and horses with grade 0 were two times more likely to win.[20] In contrast, a study looking at 3794 racing Thoroughbreds in Australia (with, again, no use of furosemide or nasal strips) found that mild to moderate EIPH did not impair performance.[21] The latter study did show, however, that the highest grades of EIPH did significantly worse. Indeed, horses with grade 4 or higher EIPH were less likely to collect race earning and had lower race earnings overall, had slower overall speed in the last 600 m, and were more likely to be passed at the end of the race. In barrel racing horses, there appeared to be no real impact of EIPH on performance, but the numbers were smaller in that study.[14] EIPH of grade 1 to 3 does not shorten a horse's racing career, but horses with grade 4 or more have fewer race starts after diagnosis and fewer lifetime starts.[22,23]

A very large study showed that horses with low-grade EIPH, thus the population in which disease did not affect performance, tended to improve their position in the latter part of the race, whereas those with high-grade EIPH were significantly faster in the first part and more likely to deteriorate in the last half.[21] This may explain why performance in barrel racers, who usually run for fewer than 20 seconds, was unaffected. It raises the question, as well, as to whether race strategy determines development of EIPH. Crispe and colleagues[21] (2017) demonstrated that rapid acceleration triggers high PAP, which appears in turn to be highly connected to mechanical stress failure of the pulmonary capillaries, thus it may be that the strategy of a fast early pace actually causes alveolar hemorrhage in these horses. It certainly provides intriguing food for thought.

Clinical Signs

Overt epistaxis is really the only clinical sign that can be reported without use of more advanced techniques such as tracheobronchoscopy or BAL. Coughing is anecdotally thought to be a clinical sign, as is increased RR or poor respiratory recovery, but there is no real evidence for this.[1]

Treatment: What Do We Do About It?

Racehorses have been treated with furosemide since the 1970s, and since that time, a positive effect on race performance has been noted, to the extent that bettors like to spot horses that are running for the first time on furosemide. This diuretic is permitted on race day within 4 hours of racing in North America but generally not elsewhere.[24] Although there is certainly an effect of furosemide on red blood cell counts on BAL and reduced evidence of bleeding on tracheobronchoscopy,[24] and furosemide is noted to attenuate the increase in PAP,[25] the mechanism of effect is still not completely understood, and no treatment actually abolishes the alveolar hemorrhage that characterizes the condition. The effect is noted to be present when treatment is administered at 4 hours before racing, but not when it is administered 24 hours beforehand. On the other hand, there is no effect of treatment on performance in barrel racing horses.[2]

In a recently published ACVIM Consensus Statement, it was noted that despite frequent use in the racing population, the list of drugs or treatments that have no good evidence for efficacy include bronchodilators, aminocaproic acid, pentoxifylline, estrogens, corticosteroids, nonsteroidal antiinflammatory drugs, herbs, inhaled water vapor, carbazochrome, serum concentrates, endothelin 1-A antagonist, nedocromil, nitric oxide, sildenafil, and nasal strips, which is an impressively long list.

Exercise-Induced Pulmonary Hemorrhage: Summary

EIPH, at least in its early stages, is likely less a disease and more a consequence of the physiology that is mandated by the development of the horse as a superb athlete. The combination of the need for high left ventricular filling pressures in order to fulfill the demand for oxygen culminating in high pulmonary capillary pressures along with very large pleural and thus alveolar pressure swings results in mechanical stress and rupture of pulmonary capillaries. This explains the old adage that "if a horse doesn't bleed it isn't running fast enough." Indeed, alveolar hemorrhage with exercise is not limited to horses—it seems to be the province of elite athletes. Because horses endure repeated bouts of EIPH, it is likely that veno-occlusive remodeling renders the susceptible portion of the lung even more fragile, with the result that bleeding becomes more frequent and severe. Recent findings that horses with severe EIPH tend to run faster in the first part of the race and horses with milder EIPH tend to take over during the latter part of the race may give us a hint as to improved racing strategies or may merely reflect the inevitability, yet again, of physiology.

INFLAMMATORY AIRWAY DISEASE

Although EIPH is the most publicly recognized lower airway disease of sport horses, inflammatory airway disease (IAD) has a more pervasive and broad impact on the sport horse population. IAD, as a disease of domestication and exposure to particulate matter, affects all groups of horses, including those, such as endurance horses, that do not perform under conditions that produce high pulmonary artery pressures. IAD was recently categorized as being under the umbrella of equine asthma[26] and is described as an inflammatory but nonseptic disease of the equine respiratory system. The more severe form, recurrent airway obstruction, otherwise known as RAO or heaves, will not be discussed here.

Epidemiology and Etiology: Who Gets Inflammatory Airway Disease and What Causes It?

Many different causes likely contribute to the constellation of signs that we recognize as IAD. The most commonly invoked contributors remain high levels of particulates in the environment, viral disease, air pollution, genetic predisposition, and bacterial infection.

It has long been noted that racehorses with clinical signs of IAD often live in poorly ventilated stables, and organic dusts and molds are at least partly to blame.[27] Organic dust in the barn environment, including hay, manure, shavings, molds, fungi, animal dander, mites, and plant material, is very good at eliciting an inflammatory response, and ammonia, which can be extremely high even in well-managed stables, contributes to lung inflammation and damage. Endotoxin and particulates likely act in concert to exert the most profound inflammatory effect. This idea was given considerable support when previously unaffected horses were shown in multiple studies to develop BAL neutrophilia when introduced to a stable environment.[28,29] It is unsurprising that hay eating has been identified as a risk factor for increased tracheal mucus in pleasure horses.[30] Horses that are stabled near a trainer's office, near entrances to the stable, or where there are fans are all at increased risk for developing IAD.[28] The worst offender in increasing exposure to airborne particulates is the hay net, as it is directly in the horse's breathing zone.[31] Inorganic particulates are of less importance, but still contribute, with silicates from dusty arenas or oil fly ash from diesel machinery being used inside large barns.

Veterinarians and trainers have long suspected that respiratory viral disease can trigger IAD. Recent infection with a respiratory virus is the most common trigger for exacerbation of the similar disease, asthma, in humans, so it is logical to make the connection to IAD, and evidence is building to support this hypothesis. Both alphaherpesviruses (equine herpesvirus [EHV] 1 and EHV-4) and gammaherpesvirus (EHV-2) have been associated with more long-lasting airway inflammation.[32] A recent study in the author's laboratory has shown that horses with hyperresponsive airways have a correspondingly higher titer to equine rhinitis A virus.[33] The role of bacterial infection in IAD remains a point of contention. A strong relationship between inflammation of the lower respiratory tract and the presence of Streptococcal species has been noted.[34] A recent study shows that the lower respiratory tract microbiota differs between horses with IAD and those without.[35] It is debatable whether there is a causal relationship or whether poor clearance secondary to airway inflammation allows a transient population of bacteria to accumulate. There are multiple other possible contributors to the development of airway inflammation in horses, including cold air and pulmonary hemorrhage, but again, there are few data to either refute or support these etiologies.[36]

Clinical Signs

Clinical signs are often hard to detect in horses with IAD, indeed, by definition they do not have episodes of air hunger or respiratory embarrassment, and they tend to be younger horses expected to do athletic work. The most common owner-reported signs are coughing and failure to perform at an expected level. With sport horses such as dressage horses, a complaint might be that the horse has "lost its brilliance". This is a subjective but not unimportant statement that can be very difficult to parse out. If endoscopic examination is used, excessive airway mucus is often seen, ranging from multiple specks to streams of mucus.[37] Other clinical signs that may be noticed include prolonged respiratory recovery; respiratory embarrassment at exercise; worsening of signs during hot, humid weather; and inability to perform work during collection. Racehorses with IAD are typically described as fading during the last quarter of the race (personal observation). Horses with dorsal displacement of the soft palate (DDSP) have a higher prevalence of IAD than control horses. This brings into play a chicken-or-egg argument, as we cannot determine whether IAD is a risk factor for DDSP, or if DDSP is a risk factor for IAD.[38]

The extent to which IAD affects performance depends on the use of the horse and the expectations of the owner or trainer. Practitioners who work primarily with pleasure or show horses might report a low incidence of IAD in young horses, but will see more cases as horses age and the disease progresses. This is because these horses do not work sufficiently close to their Vo_{2max} to unmask subclinical IAD. Practitioners working with young horses working near or at Vo_{2max}, such as racehorses, will notice exercise intolerance far more frequently. Indeed, in a National Hunt racing population, excessive mucus was detected endoscopically in 68% of horses,[39] and IAD was one of the top two reasons cited for horses not running.[40] Cough, rather than overt exercise intolerance, is more commonly reported in sport horses other than racehorses.

Lung Function—Inflammatory Airway Disease

Although it is reasonable to deduce that physical airway obstruction due to mucus plugging, bronchoconstriction, or epithelial hyperplasia might cause abnormalities in respiratory resistance, these changes still are often too subtle to be measurable in the average horse with IAD. Physical airway obstruction due to mucus plugging or epithelial hyperplasia, for instance, and reversible bronchospasm will result in increases in respiratory resistance that cannot be measured at rest in horses with IAD. This low-grade obstruction may cause impaired gas exchange during exercise; however, horses with obvious evidence of airway inflammation do not necessarily have a history of exercise intolerance.[41] This may reflect the difficulty of diagnosing low-grade respiratory impairment and the trainer's failure to recognize poorer performance than nature intended, however, rather than the benign nature of the underlying disease.

Lung Function Challenge in the Horse with Inflammatory Airway Disease

Because subtle airway obstruction is difficult to detect with our current methods of lung function testing in IAD, we look for airway hyperresponsiveness when horses are exposed to nonspecific agents such as histamine aerosol. In our clinical laboratory, horses with a clinical history and signs compatible with IAD have significantly greater airway reactivity than controls, although some control horses, similar to some humans without asthma, display airway hyperresponsiveness as well. This phenomenon in people is associated with a greater risk of eventual development of asthma[42] and may be tied into the recent finding of signs of IAD being strong risk factors for eventual development of RAO.[43]

Cytologic Diagnosis of Airway Inflammation

The presence of airway inflammation at the cellular level is best diagnosed with BAL. Many practitioners continue to use the tracheal wash to assess inflammation in both diseases, even though with a little practice, a BAL is no harder to perform in the field than is a tracheal wash. Inflammation in the lower airway as seen with BAL does not correlate well with what is found on tracheal wash.[44] In all, the evidence points to the BAL as a superior method of assessing airway inflammation.

How, then, do we diagnose airway inflammation using the BAL? IAD is generally held to be consistent with mild neutrophilia (>5%), eosinophilia (>0.5%), mastocytosis (2%), or combinations of these in the BAL fluid.[45] The question of whether morphologic differences in BAL identify different IAD syndromes is not clear. In a study from the laboratory, horses with neutrophilic BAL tended to be older and have a cough, whereas horses with mastocytosis were more likely to have airway hyperresponsiveness when assessed with histamine bronchoprovocation.[46] A recent study showed that Thoroughbred racehorses were more likely to have mastocytosis-eosinophilia with increased amounts of mucus evident in the BAL cytology, whereas Standardbreds of the same age were more likely to have neutrophilic inflammation. Neither group was different with respect to exercising hypoxemia or any other physiologic variable such as exercising heart rate or blood lactate levels.[47] Other studies have also shown that horses with neutrophilic disease were more likely to have greater levels of hypoxemia when exercising.[5]

When evaluating BAL cytology for mast cells in particular, it is important to remember that fast Romanowsky stains such as Dif-quick are not suitable. In the laboratory, we routinely stain one slide with a fast Romanowsky stain and one with toluidine blue. This latter stain is easily done by using the first phase of Dif-quick fixative and then leaving the slide in toluidine blue solution for a minimum of 15 minutes. The granules of the mast cells will stain a variety of brilliant magenta colors and will thus be easily identifiable. It is also critical to count a sufficient number of cells, as small differences in mast cells and eosinophils can make or break a diagnosis of IAD. Recent evidence suggests that using 500× and evaluating five dense fields yields the most repeatable results.[48]

Endoscopy

Endoscopy is important in ruling out contributions from upper airway disease and is also the best method for assessing mucus accumulation in the trachea. Endoscopic evaluation of tracheal septum thickness and mucus accumulation are reasonably good distinguishing the horse with RAO from the horse with IAD.[49,50] Tracheal mucus has been associated with cough and is very common in stabled horses, with all horses in one study having abnormal findings despite having no clinical complaint.[51] It is important to keep in mind, however, that the horses in these studies were nonracing sport horses; the lower necessary Vo_{2max} accompanying their workload likely masked the subclinical disease that would have affected performance in a racehorse. Indeed, in other studies, poor performance in racehorses has been associated with increased tracheal mucus.[52]

Diagnostic Imaging

Radiographs do not correlate well with results of lung function testing or BAL in horses with IAD, and thus, again, are useful only in ruling out other diseases.[53] Ultrasound may show roughening of the pleura, but is unlikely to be of use in the diagnosis of heaves or IAD.

Treatment

The therapeutic goals for treating IAD include (1) immediate relief of the broncho-spasm that causes cough and bronchoconstriction that impairs; (2) reduction of lower airway inflammation, mucus production, and airway plugging, and (3) long-term pre-vention of worsening of IAD by control of lower airway inflammation and airway obstruction.

For treatment to be successful, the practitioner must develop a treatment strategy with recognizable and achievable goals in place that is approved by both the attending veterinarian and the owner or trainer. Owners should also recognize that this may be a chronic problem that may require management of some kind for the life of the horse. Clear expectations of what the outcome of successful treatment will be should also be set in place. It is entirely reasonable, for instance, to expect that a young racehorse would be able to return to racing after a short, targeted period of treatment. The owner of the older horse with heaves, however, must recognize that a much more modest return to light pleasure riding is a reasonable goal.

Environmental Remediation

The barn environment is replete with organic particulate matter, respirable endotoxin, molds, and volatile gases such as ammonia. The worst offenders appear to be hay and straw. Multiple studies have shown that significant improvements can be made by replacing dusty substrates and feed with less dusty substitutes.[54] For instance, pel-leted hay and wood shavings are often better than regular hay and straw bedding, but outdoor living, in most cases, is the best. What is not clear to many owners is that even small or transient contacts with hay can initiate severe signs and should be avoided.[55] In addition to changing to low dust feeds and beddings, the following recommendations to owners should be made:

- Feed hay from the ground, not from a hay net
- Soak hay well before feeding or use ensiled or baked hay products
- Wet any dusty grain (eg, pellets) before feeding
- Sprinkle aisle ways with water before sweeping
- Avoid storing hay overhead. If unavoidable, lay a tarp under the hay to avoid dust raining down on the horses
- Use a humectant or hygroscopic agent to reduce dust in the indoor and outdoor arenas
- Remove horses from the barn while cleaning stalls or moving hay
- Do not use blowers to clean aisles
- Remove cobwebs and other dust collectors routinely when horses are out of the barn

An overarching principle that can be derived from the OSHA Dust Control Handbook is that prevention is better than cure. In addition to the well-known presentation of summer pasture–associated recurrent airway obstruction in hot, humid southern states, it is important to remember that horses in New England can also have disease that presents primarily in the spring and summer and that seems to improve when horses are kept temporarily in clean, nondusty indoor environments.

It is of critical importance to take an in-depth history to try to document environmental triggers. For instance, particulates associated with feeding from a hay net versus feeding from the ground is one of the most important risk factors for the development of airway inflammation, so identifying a simple-to-fix risk factor could be of considerable help. A very thorough inspection and assessment of the horse's environment will be important for remediation. For instance, if the history suggests that the horse is consistently worse in the spring, whereas clinical signs are abated in the barn in the winter, it suggests that the worst culprits for this horse are the molds and pollens associated with moist warm weather, and the clinician may prescribe clean indoor living for the horse during that period. It is very useful for the owner or trainer to keep a diary for the affected horse, noting when exacerbations occur. Simple interventions, such as opening the barn doors or making sure to feed hay on the ground, can significantly decrease the number of particulates that a horse breathes. Endotoxin levels are lower at the breathing zone in horses at pasture than in stables, which may explain why outdoor living benefits many horses with lower airway inflammation.

A recent review of environmental factors in equine asthma shows that using haylage versus hay results in a 60% to 70% decrease in exposure to particulates and that even soaking hay results in a 50% decrease in exposure to particulates. Other things that help significantly are feeding a pelleted feed and late harvest or second cutting hay.[31] Similarly, nondusty shavings for bedding are better than straw and paper or pelleted bedding is better than shavings. Good ventilation in the barn is also important, and a trained barn architect can be very useful in this regard. Recently it has been shown that omega-3 fatty acids confer added protection to a low-dust environment.[56]

Drug Therapy

There is strong evidence for the efficacy of treatment of both bronchodilators and glucocorticoids in heaves, and we have a reasonably good idea of how and why they work in this disease. This knowledge has largely been extrapolated to the treatment of IAD. For both, the mainstay of treatment has become a combination of environmental remediation, corticosteroid therapy, and bronchodilators. We must acknowledge, however, that our understanding of these drugs in horses with IAD is much less complete.

Corticosteroid therapy

Corticosteroids remain the cornerstone of successful treatment of IAD, because it is important to counteract the inflammation that characterizes this disease. Bronchodilator drugs will help to relieve coughing due to acute bronchospasm, but only consistent antiinflammatory therapy, in conjunction with avoidance of environmental triggers, will break the vicious cycle of inflammation, airway hyperreactivity, and bronchoconstriction. Corticosteroids activate glucocorticoid receptors, thus putting into motion a profound inhibition of the arachidonic acid cascade and limiting production of leukotrienes and other inflammatory molecules. Response to steroids can vary considerably from horse to horse.

The choice of whether to use systemic drugs in combination with inhaled drugs or alone may depend on a number of factors, including severity of disease and finances, because aerosolized drugs and their delivery devices are quite expensive, as well as known and putative side effects. It is important to remember that corticosteroids can, among other things, adversely affect tissue growth and protein use, impair the barrier function of the intestinal mucosa, cause immune suppression, and suppress adrenal function, so they must be used with caution.

Systemic corticosteroids Multiple studies have demonstrated the positive effects of corticosteroid drugs on horses with heaves, but the evidence for their use in IAD, despite good clinical response anecdotally, is less robust. Prednisolone and dexamethasone are the corticosteroids used most frequently in the treatment of RAO and IAD. Triamcinolone acetonide has also been shown to relieve airway obstruction in heaves. Triamcinolone, however, is anecdotally more closely associated with the development of laminitis in horses than other corticosteroids and has been shown to cause profound and persistent hyperglycemia and hypertriglyceridemia (3–4 days) in horses after a single injection of triamcinolone, which may explain the anecdotal reports.[57] Thus its use is discouraged in the treatment of IAD.

Inhaled corticosteroids The use of inhaled corticosteroids has truly revolutionized the treatment of IAD. Whereas initial systemic tapered corticosteroid therapy is often necessary with all but very mild IAD, regular inhaled therapy is essential for long-term success in most cases. The most important factor that limits regular use of inhaled corticosteroids is cost, because drugs such as fluticasone and beclomethasone are very expensive. When assessing the effects of corticosteroids on horses with airway disease, the delivery device and drug formulation used should be noted because certain devices deliver more drug to the lower airways, and certain drug formulations, such as QVAR, a proprietary formulation of beclomethasone, have been shown to reach the lower airways more reliably, at least in humans. For this reason, it is very difficult to make comparisons of drugs across studies that used different delivery devices. Moreover, the FDA has phased out the use of chlorofluorocarbon (CFC) propellants in metered dose inhalers (MDIs) in accordance with the Montreal protocol in order to protect the ozone layer. Thus studies using CFC inhalers are not directly comparable to those using the currently available hydrofluoroalkane inhalers.

Aerosolized corticosteroids are stated to be preferred over systemic in order to decrease potential side effects. This is well-documented in humans, but although this is a rational approach in horses, there is little documentation to support it. It is important to point out for sport horses that may undergo testing that fluticasone propionate or its metabolites can be detected in blood for a minimum of 72 hours after being given by inhalation and urine for approximately 18 hours after inhalation.[58]

Fluticasone propionate is thought to be the most potent of the inhaled steroids, has the longest pulmonary residence time, and causes the least adrenal suppression. On the other hand, newer formulations of beclomethasone dipropionate that incorporate HPA as the propellant have more uniform particle size and are more uniformly mixed. A recent study found that both dexamethasone (0.05 mg/kg IM q 24 hours) and inhaled fluticasone (3000 ug q12 hours) were effective at decreasing airway hyperreactivity in horses with IAD, but neither had a significant effect on clinical signs or the number of inflammatory cells in the BAL fluid. Moreover, the treatments had no residual effect 3 weeks after discontinuation.[59]

In the author's clinic, both QVAR and Flovent are used and the deciding factor as to which one is used is often the cost. For reasons that are not well understood, some horses seem to do better on one drug versus the other, and the clinician must maintain a certain flexibility in choosing drugs. The author frequently treats with an initial course of parenteral corticosteroids, typically, a 4-week decreasing course of prednisolone, followed by inhaled corticosteroids.

Delivery devices Spacers that can be used with metered dose inhalers that are currently on the market for use in horses include the Aerohippus (Trudell, Ontario, Canada) and the EquineHaler (Equine HealthCare, Horsholm, Denmark). The choice as to which to use is largely determined by cost and which device will best suit the particular horse in question. Although a recent study showed a trend for there to be a larger decrease in pulmonary resistance after treatment with albuterol using the Aerohippus, there were no statistical differences between the two devices. Regardless of the type of mask/spacer device used, actual delivery of particles to the lower airways is poor in the horse, as indeed it is even in humans, and the least efficacious means of delivering aerosolized drugs is by nebulization. An alternative to the MDI is the jet nebulizer, such as the Flexineb (Flexineb, Inc, Union City TN). Unfortunately, strategies that we know improve lung deposition of aerosolized drugs in humans, such as slow deep breathing and breath holding, are not practical in the horse. However, keeping the horse calm and the respiratory rate low may help.

Bronchodilators

Bronchodilators, as with corticosteroids, can be administered both systemically and via aerosol; however, aerosolization is by far the preferred method. Both beta-2 agonists (B2-adrenergic receptors [ARs] [sympathomimetics]) and parasympatholytics are used in horses. Of the B2-ARs commonly used in equine medicine, albuterol, which is known as salbutamol everywhere but in the United States, is primarily administered by inhalation and clenbuterol is administered orally. For the parasympatholytic agents, ipratropium is administered by inhalation and atropine and N-butylscopolammonium (Buscopan) are administered parenterally.

Although N-butylscopolammonium bromide can be used for rapid relief of bronchospasm, its effect is only short lasting.[60] The only longer lasting systemically administered bronchodilator is clenbuterol, a B2-AR that was approved for use in horses in the United States in 1998 under the brand name Ventipulmin (Boehringer Ingelheim Vetmedica, Inc, St Joseph, MO, USA). Severe toxicities have occurred when improperly compounded clenbuterol was administered to horses. The safety and efficacy of chronic administration of clenbuterol is controversial. Chronic administration of clenbuterol at 2.4 µg/kg (5 days on, 2 days off, for 8 weeks) was reported to have a negative impact on aerobic performance in horses.[61] Tachyphylaxis also appears to be a problem with chronic administration of clenbuterol. For example, a recent study demonstrated that after 3 weeks of clenbuterol administration at 0.8 µg/kg bwt po, q12 hr increased airway reactivity was evident and the horses were refractory to the bronchodilatory effects of clenbuterol.[62]

Most horses appear to tolerate the lower doses of clenbuterol well, but with higher doses horses may have tremors, tachycardia, sweating, and an appearance of anxiousness, among other signs. Together, these findings suggest that the practice of administering clenbuterol to horses in order to enhance performance is probably misguided at best and harmful at worst. It is also important to recognize that the recommended duration of treatment is 30 days. Clenbuterol can be best used as a short-term bronchodilator in horses that cannot tolerate aerosolized devices. Clenbuterol is not appropriate and should not be used as a chronic therapy.

Inhaled bronchodilators Albuterol is commonly used to elicit bronchodilation in IAD. It is important to remember that the inflammatory condition will persist despite apparent improvement due to transient bronchodilation, and the disease will worsen if the other two legs of treatment—corticosteroid (anti-inflammatory) therapy and avoidance of environmental triggers—are not pursued. Regular use of B_2 agonists in the absence of antiinflammatory medication may mask symptoms that would otherwise indicate progressive worsening of the disease, in particular further airway obstruction with mucus. Albuterol is the most affordable of the short-acting B_2 agonists; however, levalbuterol, the R-enantiomer of albuterol, has recently become more affordable (trade name Xopenex). There is a possibility that albuterol may cause unexpected bronchoconstriction because of action of the L-enantiomer. Levalbuterol may prevent this, but paradoxic bronchoconstriction has occurred even with the use of levalbuterol. Although regular use of inhaled albuterol for 10 days does not result in tachyphylaxis, it may be that longer use would result in treatment failure.

The preponderance of evidence shows that short-acting B_2 agonists are not performance-enhancing in humans, and there is little evidence to indicate that they are performance-enhancing in horses,[63] with one study showing a small increase in aerobic performance in Thoroughbred horses in a treadmill study, whereas the other failed to show any effect of albuterol administration on aerobic performance in Standardbreds on a treadmill.[64] Nonetheless, all equine sporting events ban albuterol, and due care should be taken to stop drug administration before competition, noting that albuterol can be detected in urine for at least 48 hours after administration via metered dose inhaler. A recent study showed that budesonide is found in greater concentrations systemically when it is inhaled during exercise (an interesting concept), likely reflecting the depth of breathing, so this should be taken into account when determining withdrawal times.[65] Short-acting B_2 agonists can be useful in horses with a cough due to bronchoconstriction to improve the return to training. No more than 450 mg of albuterol by inhalation is necessary to bronchodilate most horses, irrespective of the delivery device chosen.

Although aerosolized B_2 agonists have a relatively low incidence of side effects, excessive use or sensitive individuals may experience systemic effects such as trembling, anxiety, and cardiac arrhythmias. The author has noted all these in individuals treated with 900 µg of albuterol, whereas other individuals show no signs of intolerance. Repeated use of the drug tends to decrease side effects as the body downregulates receptors.

Long-acting inhaled B_2-AR therapy We occasionally treat moderate IAD with long-acting B_2-AR therapy in addition to inhaled corticosteroids, with the initial impression of enhanced performance and quality of life. It cannot be emphasized enough, however, that regular use of long-acting B_2-ARs must be accompanied with regular use of inhaled corticosteroids. The most commonly used long-acting B_2-ARs are salmeterol and formoterol, whose basic mechanism of action is the familiar cAMP pathway. Their duration of action in horses is 6 to 8 hours.

Inhaled parasympatholytic therapy The most commonly used inhaled parasympatholytic drug is ipratropium, a quaternary ammonium derivative of atropine, which produces bronchodilation lasting approximately 6 hours, which is at least 2 hours longer than albuterol. Although adverse side effects, such as thickened mucus, tachycardia, and decreased ciliary beat frequency, are possible with parasympatholytics, no such side effects have been reported in horses up to a dose of 1200 µg. Ipratropium cannot be considered a rescue drug, unlike atropine, because it has much longer onset of action; however, the effect may last somewhat longer than atropine. It is unusual for ipratropium to be necessary in IAD.

Mast cell stabilizers These agents are chromones that block calcium channels preventing the release of histamine and tryptase, and the subsequent downstream cascade of prostaglandin and leukotriene formulation that eventually cause bronchoconstriction. Sodium cromoglycate can be efficacious in treating known mast cell–mediated IAD, but will not be of use for treating most of the horses with neutrophil-mediated disease. Their use, however, requires considerable owner compliance, because the maximum response to this drug occurs at 1 to 2 weeks after beginning treatment.

Evaluation of therapeutic outcome It is important to have a baseline assessment of the horse before initiating therapy. Ideally, this would include auscultation with and without a rebreathing bag, careful physical examination, observation during exercise, and baseline pulmonary function testing and measure of airway reactivity (IAD) followed by BAL. The goal of a thorough baseline assessment is to facilitate a treatment regimen tailored to the individual horse and to monitor response to therapy. Horses should then be evaluated one to 2 months after initiation of therapy to assess response and guide therapy for the upcoming months. If there is poor response to therapy, it is important to do some detective work to determine why treatment has been unsuccessful. For example, it is essential to check the client's technique for using the drug delivery device. Failure to modify the environment may, in some horses, negate any attempts at drug therapy. Some horses with chronic, severe pathology may be resistant to corticosteroids or may have irreversible changes in the lungs that prevent response to bronchodilators. Finally, lack of response to therapy may be because of underlying infectious disease and may indicate the need for further diagnostics and perhaps an entirely different approach or concomitant antibiotic use.

FURTHER THOUGHTS

Although these are soft data observations, generally speaking, horses with EIPH or IAD do not look "sick". They should have a good appetite, a bright eye and attitude; they are eager to work but do not perform at their highest ability or coughing interrupts their work. Horses that have a fever, are listless, lose weight, have a poor appetite, or develop a putrid or discolored nasal discharge do not have IAD or at least do not have IAD alone and should be worked up for infectious disease. It can be useful in these cases to perform a CBC with a fibrinogen or an serum amyloid A (SAA) assay, as the latter has been shown to be significantly lower in noninfectious than in infectious respiratory disease.[66]

That said, horses that present for IAD may be harboring subclinical viral respiratory disease or may have early-stage equine multinodular pulmonary fibrosis associated with equine herpesvirus 5. The former may be a trigger for more chronic airway hyperreactivity and cough[33] or will resolve as the disease runs its course, and the latter will inexorably progress to life-threatening disease. It is equally important to remember that all horses that cough do not necessarily have IAD—coughing can be caused by dorsal displacement of the soft palate, epiglottic entrapment, rhinitis, and foreign bodies among other things. When the usual treatment does not ameliorate the condition, it is necessary to take a step back and extend the diagnostic approach in order to figure out what the problem actually is.

SUMMARY

Lower airway disease in the form of IAD and EIPH is pervasive in the athletic horse population, and because both can initially present as subtle impediments to athletic performance, they are often missed or discounted. Because the lower airways form the critical and last barrier to the passage of oxygen to the blood, any diminution in their function results in exercise impairment. An understanding of the physiology of the equine athlete's respiratory and cardiac system is critical to the diagnosis and management of EIPH and an understanding of the inadequacies in the way that we house horses is equally critical to the diagnosis and treatment of IAD. There is no single effective treatment for either condition, and both are best approached with changes in management along with judicious use of pharmacologic therapies.

REFERENCES

1. Hinchcliff KW, Couetil LL, Knight PK, et al. Exercise induced pulmonary hemorrhage in horses: American College of Veterinary Internal Medicine consensus statement. J Vet Intern Med 2015;29(3):743–58.

2. Gold JR, Knowles DP, Coffey T, et al. Exercise-induced pulmonary hemorrhage in barrel racing horses in the Pacific Northwest region of the United States. J Vet Intern Med 2018;32(2):839–45.

3. da Silva KM, Otaka JNP, Goncalves CAP, et al. Association between exercise-induced pulmonary hemorrhage and inflammatory airway disease in polo ponies. J Equine Sci 2017;28(2):55–9.

4. Hinchcliff KW, Morley PS, Guthrie AJ. Efficacy of furosemide for prevention of exercise-induced pulmonary hemorrhage in Thoroughbred racehorses. J Am Vet Med Assoc 2009;235(1):76–82.

5. McKane SA, Rose RJ, Evans DL. Comparison of bronchoalveolar lavage findings and measurements of gas exchange during exercise in horses with poor racing performance. N Z Vet J 1995;43(5):179–82.

6. Fraipont A, Van Erck E, Ramery E, et al. Subclinical diseases underlying poor performance in endurance horses: diagnostic methods and predictive tests. Vet Rec 2011;169(6):154.

7. Raphel CF, Soma LR. Exercise-induced pulmonary hemorrhage in Thoroughbreds after racing and breezing. Am J Vet Res 1982;43(7):1123–7.

8. Newton JR, Rogers K, Marlin DJ, et al. Risk factors for epistaxis on British racecourses: evidence for locomotory impact-induced trauma contributing to the aetiology of exercise-induced pulmonary haemorrhage. Equine Vet J 2005;37(5): 402–11.

9. Crispe EJ, Lester GD, Robertson ID, et al. Bar shoes and ambient temperature are risk factors for exercise-induced pulmonary haemorrhage in Thoroughbred racehorses. Equine Vet J 2016;48(4):438–41.

10. West JB, Mathieu-Costello O, Jones JH, et al. Stress failure of pulmonary capillaries in racehorses with exercise-induced pulmonary hemorrhage. J Appl Physiol (1985) 1993;75(3):1097–109.

11. Naeije R, Chesler N. Pulmonary circulation at exercise. Compr Physiol 2012;2(1): 711–41.

12. Cross TJ, Breskovic T, Sabapathy S, et al. Respiratory muscle pressure development during breath holding in apnea divers. Med Sci Sports Exerc 2013;45(1): 93–101.

13. McKane SA, Slocombe RF. Experimental mild pulmonary inflammation promotes the development of exercise-induced pulmonary haemorrhage. Equine Vet J Suppl 2010;(38):235–9.
14. Leguillette R, Steinmann M, Bond SL, et al. Tracheobronchoscopic assessment of exercise-induced pulmonary hemorrhage and airway inflammation in barrel racing horses. J Vet Intern Med 2016;30(4):1327–32.
15. Weideman H, Schoeman SJ, Jordaan GF, et al. Epistaxis related to exercise-induced pulmonary haemorrhage in south African thoroughbreds. J S Afr Vet Assoc 2003;74(4):127–31.
16. Velie BD, Raadsma HW, Wade CM, et al. Heritability of epistaxis in the Australian thoroughbred racehorse population. Vet J 2014;202(2):274–8.
17. Boudreaux MK, Koehler J, Habecker PL, et al. Evaluation of the genes encoding CD39/NTPDase-1 and CD39L1/NTPDase-2 in horses with and without abnormal hemorrhage and in horses with pathologic evidence of exercise-induced pulmonary hemorrhage. Vet Clin Pathol 2015;44(4):617–25.
18. O'Callaghan MW, Pascoe JR, O'Brien TR, et al. Exercise-induced pulmonary haemorrhage in the horse: results of a detailed clinical, post mortem and imaging study. VI. Radiological/pathological correlations. Equine Vet J 1987;19(5):419–22.
19. Williams KJ, Robinson NE, Defeijter-Rupp H, et al. Distribution of venous remodeling in exercise-induced pulmonary hemorrhage of horses follows reported blood flow distribution in the equine lung. J Appl Physiol (1985) 2013;114(7): 869–78.
20. Morley PS, Bromberek JL, Saulez MN, et al. Exercise-induced pulmonary haemorrhage impairs racing performance in thoroughbred racehorses. Equine Vet J 2015;47(3):358–65.
21. Crispe EJ, Lester GD, Secombe CJ, et al. The association between exercise-induced pulmonary haemorrhage and race-day performance in thoroughbred racehorses. Equine Vet J 2017;49(5):584–9.
22. Sullivan S, Hinchcliff K. Update on exercise-induced pulmonary hemorrhage. Vet Clin North Am Equine Pract 2015;31(1):187–98.
23. Manohar M, Hutchens E, Coney E. Frusemide attenuates the exercise-induced rise in pulmonary capillary blood pressure in horses. Equine Vet J 1994;26(1): 51–4.
24. Knych HK, Vale A, Wilson WD, et al. Pharmacokinetics of furosemide administered 4 and 24 hours prior to high-speed exercise in horses. J Vet Pharmacol Ther 2018;41(2):224–9.
25. Goetz TE, Manohar M, Magid JH. Repeated administration of frusemide does not offer an advantage over single dosing in attenuating exercise-induced pulmonary hypertension in thoroughbred horses. Equine Vet J Suppl 1999;(30):539–45.
26. Couetil LL, Cardwell JM, Gerber V, et al. Inflammatory airway disease of horses–revised consensus statement. J Vet Intern Med 2016;30(2):503–15.
27. Sweeney CR, Humber KA, Roby KA. Cytologic findings of trachoobronchial aspirates from 66 thoroughbred racehorses. Am J Vet Res 1992;53(7):1172–5.
28. Millerick-May ML, Karmaus W, Derksen FJ, et al. Airborne particulates (PM10) and tracheal mucus: a case-control study at an American Thoroughbred racetrack. Equine Vet J 2015;47(4):410–4.
29. Tremblay GM, Ferland C, Lapointe JM, et al. Effect of stabling on bronchoalveolar cells obtained from normal and COPD horses. Equine Vet J 1993;25(3):194–7.
30. Robinson NE, Karmaus W, Holcombe SJ, et al. Airway inflammation in Michigan pleasure horses: prevalence and risk factors. Equine Vet J 2006;38(4):293–9.

31. Ivester KM, Couetil LL, Moore GE, et al. Environmental exposures and airway inflammation in young thoroughbred horses. J Vet Intern Med 2014;28(3):918–24.

32. Fortier G, Richard E, Hue E, et al. Long-lasting airway inflammation associated with equid herpesvirus-2 in experimentally challenged horses. Vet J 2013; 197(2):492–5.

33. Houtsma A, Bedenice D, Pusterla N, et al. Association between inflammatory airway disease of horses and exposure to respiratory viruses: a case control study. Multidiscip Respir Med 2015;10:33.

34. Cardwell JM, Smith KC, Wood JL, et al. Infectious risk factors and clinical indicators for tracheal mucus in British National Hunt racehorses. Equine Vet J 2014; 46(2):150–5.

35. Bond SL, Timsit E, Workentine M, et al. Upper and lower respiratory tract microbiota in horses: bacterial communities associated with health and mild asthma (inflammatory airway disease) and effects of dexamethasone. BMC Microbiol 2017;17(1):184.

36. Davis MS, Williams CC, Meinkoth JH, et al. Influx of neutrophils and persistence of cytokine expression in airways of horses after performing exercise while breathing cold air. Am J Vet Res 2007;68(2):185–9.

37. Koch C, Straub R, Ramseyer A, et al. Endoscopic scoring of the tracheal septum in horses and its clinical relevance for the evaluation of lower airway health in horses. Equine Vet J 2007;39(2):107–12.

38. Courouce-Malblanc A, Deniau V, Rossignol F, et al. Physiological measurements and prevalence of lower airway diseases in Trotters with dorsal displacement of the soft palate. Equine Vet J Suppl 2010;(38):246–55.

39. Allen KJ, Tremaine WH, Franklin SH. Prevalence of inflammatory airway disease in national hunt horses referred for investigation of poor athletic performance. Equine Vet J Suppl 2006;36:529–34.

40. Wilsher S, Allen WR, Wood JL. Factors associated with failure of thoroughbred horses to train and race. Equine Vet J 2006;38(2):113–8.

41. Couetil LL, Denicola DB. Blood gas, plasma lactate and bronchoalveolar lavage cytology analyses in racehorses with respiratory disease. Equine Vet J Suppl 1999;(30):77–82.

42. Boulet LP, Turcotte H, Prince P, et al. Benefits of low-dose inhaled fluticasone on airway response and inflammation in mild asthma. Respir Med 2009;103(10): 1554–63.

43. Gerber V, Tessier C, Marti E. Genetics of upper and lower airway diseases in the horse. Equine Vet J 2015;47(4):390–7.

44. Malikides N, Hughes KJ, Hodgson DR, et al. Comparison of tracheal aspirates and bronchoalveolar lavage in racehorses. 2. Evaluation of the diagnostic significance of neutrophil percentage. Aust Vet J 2003;81(11):685–7.

45. Couetil LL, Hoffman AM, Hodgson J, et al. Inflammatory airway disease of horses. J Vet Intern Med 2007;21(2):356–61.

46. Bedenice D, Mazan MR, Hoffman AM. Association between cough and cytology of bronchoalveolar lavage fluid and pulmonary function in horses diagnosed with inflammatory airway disease. J Vet Intern Med 2008;22(4):1022–8.

47. Nolen-Walston RD, Harris M, Agnew ME, et al. Clinical and diagnostic features of inflammatory airway disease subtypes in horses examined because of poor performance: 98 cases (2004-2010). J Am Vet Med Assoc 2013;242(8): 1138–45.

48. Fernandez NJ, Hecker KG, Gilroy CV, et al. Reliability of 400-cell and 5-field leukocyte differential counts for equine bronchoalveolar lavage fluid. Vet Clin Pathol 2013;42(1):92–8.
49. Wysocka B, Klucinski W. Usefulness of the assessment of discharge accumulation in the lower airways and tracheal septum thickening in the differential diagnosis of recurrent airway obstruction (RAO) and inflammatory airway disease (IAD) in the horse. Pol J Vet Sci 2014;17(2):247–53.
50. Holcombe SJ, Jackson C, Gerber V, et al. Stabling is associated with airway inflammation in young Arabian horses. Equine Vet J 2001;33(3):244–9.
51. Christley RM, Hodgson DR, Rose RJ, et al. Coughing in thoroughbred racehorses: risk factors and tracheal endoscopic and cytological findings. Vet Rec 2001;148(4):99–104.
52. Durando MM, Martin BB, Davidson EJ, et al. Correlations between exercising arterial blood gas values, tracheal wash findings and upper respiratory tract abnormalities in horses presented for poor performance. Equine Vet J Suppl 2006;(36):523–8.
53. Mazan MR, Vin R, Hoffman AM. Radiographic scoring lacks predictive value in inflammatory airway disease. Equine Vet J 2005;37(6):541–5.
54. Kirschvink N, Di Silvestro F, Sbai I, et al. The use of cardboard bedding material as part of an environmental control regime for heaves-affected horses: in vitro assessment of airborne dust and aeroallergen concentration and in vivo effects on lung function. Vet J 2002;163(3):319–25.
55. Fairbairn SM, Lees P, Page CP, et al. Duration of antigen-induced hyperresponsiveness in horses with allergic respiratory disease and possible links with early airway obstruction. J Vet Pharmacol Ther 1993;16(4):469–76.
56. Nogradi N, Couetil LL, Messick J, et al. Omega-3 fatty acid supplementation provides an additional benefit to a low-dust diet in the management of horses with chronic lower airway inflammatory disease. J Vet Intern Med 2015;29(1):299–306.
57. French K, Pollitt CC, Pass MA. Pharmacokinetics and metabolic effects of triamcinolone acetonide and their possible relationships to glucocorticoid-induced laminitis in horses. J Vet Pharmacol Ther 2000;23(5):287–92.
58. Gray BP, Biddle S, Pearce CM, et al. Detection of fluticasone propionate in horse plasma and urine following inhaled administration. Drug Test Anal 2013;5(5):306–14.
59. Leguillette R, Tohver T, Bond SL, et al. Effect of dexamethasone and fluticasone on airway hyperresponsiveness in horses with inflammatory airway disease. J Vet Intern Med 2017;31(4):1193–201.
60. Couetil L, Hammer J, Miskovic Feutz M, et al. Effects of N-butylscopolammonium bromide on lung function in horses with recurrent airway obstruction. J Vet Intern Med 2012;26(6):1433–8.
61. Sleeper MM, Kearns CF, McKeever KH. Chronic clenbuterol administration negatively alters cardiac function. Mod Sci Sports Exerc 2002;34(4):643–50.
62. Read JR, Boston RC, Abraham G, et al. Effect of prolonged administration of clenbuterol on airway reactivity and sweating in horses with inflammatory airway disease. Am J Vet Res 2012;73(1):140–5.
63. Bailey J, Colahan P, Kubilis P, et al. Effect of inhaled beta 2 adrenoceptor agonist, albuterol sulphate, on performance of horses. Equine Vet J Suppl 1999;(30):575–80.
64. Mazan MR, Hoffman AM. Effects of aerosolized albuterol on physiologic responses to exercise in standardbreds. Am J Vet Res 2001;62(11):1812–7.

65. Barton AK, Heinemann H, Schenk I, et al. Influence of respiratory tract disease and mode of inhalation on detectability of budesonide in equine urine and plasma. Am J Vet Res 2017;78(2):244–50.

66. Viner M, Mazan M, Bedenice D, et al. Comparison of serum amyloid A in horses with infectious and noninfectious inflammatory respiratory disease. J Equine Vet Sci 2017;49.

Printed and bound by CPI Group (UK) Ltd, Croydon, CR0 4YY

03/10/2024

01040391-0008